Hospital
Cost Containment

Hospital
Cost Containment
Selected Notes for Future Policy

EDITED BY MICHAEL ZUBKOFF,
IRA E. RASKIN, AND RUTH S. HANFT

Published for the Milbank Memorial Fund by
PRODIST
New York   1978

Published with the cooperation of
the National Center for Health Services Research
Department of Health, Education, and Welfare

Published for the
Milbank Memorial Fund
by
PRODIST
a division of
Neale Watson Academic Publications, Inc.
156 Fifth Avenue, New York, N.Y. 10010

Library of Congress Cataloging in Publication Data
Main entry under title:

Hospital cost containment.

Includes bibliographies and index.
1. Hospitals—Cost control.   2. Hospitals—United
States—Cost control.   I. Zubkoff, Michael.
II. Raskin, Ira E.   III. Hanft, Ruth S., 1929–
IV. Milbank Memorial Fund.   V. National Center for
Health Services Research.
RE971.3.H618   338.4′3   77-13041
ISBN 0-88202-068-4

Contents

Federal, State, and Local Experiences

Methodological Issues in Cost-Containment Procedures

Future Outlooks

Acknowledgments

Appreciation is expressed to David Willis of the Milbank Memorial Fund and Gerald Rosenthal of the National Center for Health Services Research for their support in the manuscript preparation and distribution of this volume.

We wish to thank the authors for their cooperation and patience during the process of readying this volume for publication. A personal note of thanks to Rose Migas, Patricia Berndt, Dona Heller, and Rosemary Richter, who were extremely helpful in preparing the essays for publication.

The outstanding editorial assistance of Betsy Pitha, as well as her preparation of the index, warrants special recognition and our deep personal appreciation.

MICHAEL ZUBKOFF
IRA E. RASKIN
RUTH S. HANFT

Contributors

Katharine G. Bauer
Lecturer
Department of Preventive Medicine
Harvard Medical School
Principal Associate
Center for Community Health
    and Medical Care
Harvard School of Public Health
Boston, Massachusetts

Ralph E. Berry, Jr.
Professor of Economics
Harvard School of Public Health
Boston, Massachusetts

Thomas W. Bice
Associate Director
Institute for Health Care Studies
    of United Hospital Fund
New York

James F. Blumstein
Professor of Law
Vanderbilt University
Nashville, Tennessee

William O. Cleverley
Associate Professor
Graduate Program in Hospital and
    Health Services Administration
College of Medicine
Ohio State University
Columbus, Ohio

Harold Cohen
Executive Director
Maryland Health Services
    Cost Review Commission
Baltimore, Maryland

David R. Drake
Director, Office of Program
    and Policy Development
American Hospital Association
Chicago, Illinois

William L. Dunn
Analyst for Hospital Reimbursement
Congressional Budget Office
Washington, D.C.

Joseph Eichenholz
Director, Health Economics Office for
    Deputy Assistant Secretary for
    Health Policy, Research and Statistics
U.S. Department of Health, Education,
    and Welfare

Paul B. Ginsburg
Associate Professor
Policy Sciences and Community
    Health Sciences
Duke University
Durham, North Carolina

Ruth S. Hanft
Deputy Assistant Secretary for
    Health Policy, Research and Statistics
U.S. Department of Health, Education,
    and Welfare

Fred J. Hellinger
Office of Policy, Planning
    and Research
Health Care Financing Administration
U.S. Department of Health, Education,
    and Welfare

Mary Lee Ingbar
Professor of Family and
    Community Medicine
University of Massachusetts
    Medical School
Worcester, Massachusetts
Principal Research Associate
    in Social and Preventive Medicine
Harvard University School of Medicine
Boston, Massachusetts

Judith R. Lave
Associate Professor of Economics
    and Urban Affairs

School of Urban and Public Affairs
Carnegie-Mellon University
Pittsburgh, Pennsylvania

Lester B. Lave
Professor and Head, Department of
    Economics
Graduate School of Industrial
    Administration
Carnegie-Mellon University
Pittsburgh, Pennsylvania

Bonnie Lefkowitz
formerly, Analyst for Resource Control,
    Congressional Budget Office
presently, Special Assistant to
    Deputy Assistant Secretary for Planning
    and Evaluation/Health
U.S. Department of Health, Education,
    and Welfare

Irving Leveson
Senior Professional Staff
Hudson Institute
Croton-on-Hudson, New York

Joseph Lipscomb
Assistant Professor
Institute of Policy Sciences and
    Public Affairs
Duke University
Durham, North Carolina

John Alexander McMahon
President
American Hospital Association
Chicago, Illinois

Ira E. Raskin
Associate Director for
    Policy Development
Bureau of Health Planning and
    Resources Development
Health Resources Administration
U.S. Department of Health, Education,
    and Welfare

Michael A. Redisch, Economist
U.S. General Accounting Office
Washington, D.C.

Gerald Rosenthal
Director, National Center for
    Health Services Research
Hyattsville, Maryland

David Salkever
Associate Professor
    School of Hygiene and Public Health
Department of Health Services
    Administration
The Johns Hopkins University
Baltimore, Maryland

Stuart O. Schweitzer
Division of Health Service and
    Hospital Administration
School of Public Health
University of California,
Los Angeles, California

Judith L. Wagner
Senior Research Associate
The Urban Institute
Washington, D.C.

Michael Zubkoff
Professor and Chairman
    Department of Community Medicine
Dartmouth Medical School
Professor of Health Economics
Amos Tuck School of Business
    Administration
Dartmouth College
Hanover, New Hampshire

William Zubkoff
Associate Director for
    Special Projects
South Shore Hospital and
    Medical Center
Miami Beach, Florida

Introduction

RUTH S. HANFT, IRA E. RASKIN, AND MICHAEL ZUBKOFF

The federal government has begun a new phase in its attempts during the last several years to contain rapidly escalating hospital costs. The latest effort may be a forerunner of future control mechanisms under national health insurance. Its success or failure may determine how quickly the nation moves toward national health insurance and the approach to it.

The papers in this book outline several of the steps taken to date to control hospital costs. The federal government's latest effort goes far beyond all previous efforts by placing controls on the total revenues per admission from all payers except for a major exception: wages of nonsupervisory personnel can be passed through. Heretofore, except for the brief Economic Stabilization Program, which affected all industries, rate regulation of hospitals has been confined to one or two payers. All of these partial rate regulation efforts have left the hospitals with the capability of shifting costs and charges to other third parties, largely the commercial insurers and self-pay patients who pay on a charge basis. In addition, the Administration, for the first time, has sought to place a cap on total capital expenditures. (See Dunn and Lefkowitz.)[1]

The final shape of cost-containment legislation is not clear. The pluralistic nature of the health and the hospital industry and the plethora of competing interests are such that the final version of the Carter Administration's proposal, if enacted into law, will reflect many compromises.

[1]All references are to papers in this book.

1

Pluralism and Problems of Size

The health care industry is the third largest in the nation, employing over 4 million people and consuming 8.6 percent of the Gross National Product. The largest sector of this industry is the hospital sector, which accounts for more than 40 percent of tot l health care expenditures. Hospital costs have been rising at approximately 14 to 15 percent per year during the last several years, more than twice as fast as the remainder of the economy. Although part of the increase can be attributed to rises in wages, in fuel and food prices, and in utilization, a large part can be attributed to the increased intensity of services; that is, advances in technology and changes in the product. In other industries, increased investment in technology usually results in labor and price saving; in the health industry the situation is reversed. Increased investment in health technology often carries with it greater labor intensity and requirements for more highly skilled labor. For each dollar invested in health care, an additional fifty cents per year is the consequence in operating costs.

The hospital industry is composed of more than 7,000 institutions that meet multiple needs. Hospitals vary widely in size, services offered, age and modernity of plant and equipment, mission (that is, service, education, and research), ownership, and unionization. There are acute general hospitals, chronic care hospitals, specialized hospitals, and psychiatric hospitals. Hospitals are owned and operated by state governments, counties, municipalities, universities, religious groups, corporations, and groups of physicians or private investors. They range in size from less than twenty-five to more than 1,000 beds and have occupancy rates ranging from 50 percent or less to full, even overfull, capacity. The scope of services varies from simple medical and surgical procedures to complete outpatient and emergency services, secondary care in all fields, and sophisticated tertiary care, such as neonatal intensive care, open-heart surgery, and so on. Some hospitals provide no educational programs; others provide a wide variety of them, training technicians, nurses, social workers, medical students, residents, dental surgeons, financing the programs by and large from patient care dollars. Some hospitals are great centers for biomedical research.

Some hospitals are the largest employers in an area, and a change in scope of services, number of employees, or wages affects the economy of the area. In fact, one of the greatest barriers to efforts to make these institutions more efficient—closing unneeded beds and reducing nursing and other staff—is the threat to the economy of the area. Indeed, cost-containment efforts have come at a time when unemployment is high and efforts are being made in all other parts of the economy to increase capital investment and to reduce unemployment, the reverse of the prescriptions proposed for the hospital industry. This volume does not contain a discussion of the employment-economy issues.

Compounding the complexity and diversity of the hospital field are the influences of the different decision makers: the administrators, the physicians, unions, trustees, third parties, and the consumers of care. Each plays a greater or lesser role in the decisions of the institutions, and the pluralistic nature of the decision making leaves no focus for final public accountability. The administrator finds himself caught between the hospital physicians' needs, desires, and pressures and those of the community (Zubkoff). The administrator believes he has little control over the decisions, yet he is responsible for the financial viability of the institution. The physicians often drive up the costs of the institution through their demands for new patient services, the most current equipment, and more ancillary personnel, and through their decisions on admissions and lengths of stay. A physician's training motivates him to do the utmost for the individual patient without much thought for the consequences of his actions in terms of cost and efficient use of services. The fee-for-service method of payment to the physician encourages the philosophy of when in doubt, do more (Redisch). Since without the cooperation of the physician the institution cannot function, the administrator is under the incentive to accede to the demands of the physician (Zubkoff). The consumer, who bears directly little of the cost of the hospital stay, wants the best in care and wants it to be as accessible as possible (Ingbar). Trustees, not explicitly discussed in this book, are motivated primarily by two factors, economic viability and prestige of the institution. In regard to viability, as long as the patient care revenues meet the expenditures, there is little incentive to impose restraints.

More than 90 percent of hospital costs in the country are paid for by third parties: the commercial insurance companies, government, and the Blue Cross associations. The commercials' primary incentive is to compete for group coverage and maintain their share of the market, yet under the antitrust laws they are constrained from combining to negotiate rates. Their bargaining position on rates with the hospitals is weak, since they hold the smallest share of the market and are a diverse, uncoordinated group of companies. Started by the hospitals, Blue Cross had overlapping boards of directors with hospitals until the late 1960s. Consequently, until then the focus was largely on the financial viability and stability of the hospitals. Both the Blues and the commercials were able to pass through all cost increases by way of increased premiums to their subscribers, and until recently the government did so by way of taxes. Government finances hospital in two ways, as a third-party payer and through deficit appropriations to government-owned institutions. Government is now the largest payer with the greatest potential clout. With a few exceptions, Medicare and Medicaid pay on a retroactive reasonable cost basis; in effect, theirs is a pass-through of costs met by increased general revenues and payroll tax expenditures.

With such a multiplicity of interests and interest groups who then should be responsible for accountability and cost control?

The federal and state governments have the strongest economic bargaining positions, paying for 53 percent of all hospital costs. Until the recent federal move, the lead in cost containment has come from the states in controlling Medicaid programs and development of rate regulation commissions. Faced with constraints on revenues, due to the combination of recession and inflation, rapidly escalating hospital costs, and the consequent rapidly escalating Medicaid expenditures, the states have cut Medicaid benefits and sought waivers from the federal government to establish maximum rates of hospital payment for their Medicaid beneficiaries. In many states, Medicaid payments exceed public assistance payments.

State efforts at rate regulation have been beset by lawsuits, lack of information on case mix, and to some extent crudeness of classification and exception systems (Cohen, Bauer, Hellinger). A major weakness has been the limited capability of the states to impose their rating systems on other third parties: Medicaid, the Blues in some states, and the commercials, allowing the hospitals to pass costs to self-pay patients, commercial charge payers, and to some extent Blue Cross. A further major weakness is the state of the art of prospective rate setting (Bauer, Hellinger).

Except for the ESP controls, the federal government until now has proceeded more conservatively than the states. The 1972 amendments to the Social Security Act allowed the government to classify hospitals and set maximum per diems, and permitted prospective reimbursement experiments (Bauer, Hellinger). The prospective reimbursement experiments have been slow in starting, few and far between, and not operational long enough for their impact to be tested fully.

Attempting to control hospital operating costs without controlling capital investment is futile, since capital borrowing, amortization, interest, and depreciation are translated into per diem costs, and, more important, influence manpower and the use and volume of services. Through the early comprehensive health planning structure, and now the Health Systems Agencies and certificate-of-need requirements imposed on the states, the federal government has attempted to gain some control over capital expansion. The results to date have been mixed (Salkever and Bice). The planning problems highlight the mixed motives of the physicians, hospital administrators, and consumers and the lack of an accountability focus (Redisch, Zubkoff, Ingbar, McMahon and Drake). Regrettably, we did not include a chapter on the sources of capital financing for hospitals and the economic tension generated when the general economy is sluggish and efforts are made to boost construction, encourage other capital investment, and expand employment. The conflict in the private insurance industry, seeking on the one hand to invest reserves and on the other to control hospital costs, is a fascinating example of the pluralism that retards cost containment. The same can be said of federal public works and economic investment policies conflicting with other federal efforts to contain hospital cost inflation.

Professional standards review is another effort to affect costs by monitoring the appropriate use of hospital services. But since the mechanism is that of peer review—one physician vis-à-vis another—the conflict of quality versus cost is immediately established, and with the emphasis on the maximizing of care, the net result may be increased rather than decreased services (Redisch, Blumstein).

The Public Policy Decision Makers: Federalism, Pluralism, and Fragmentation

Controlling hospital costs and the impact of the controls will depend on accommodation among competing interests: not only competition between the private and public sectors, and between the state and the federal governments but also among various federal objectives. The political decision-making apparatus can be characterized by federalism, pluralism, and fragmentation. At the federal level the committees of Congress that make decisions impacting on hospital costs are multiple and have conflicting interests. The Senate Finance Committee and the House Ways and Means Committee have direct input to the Medicare and Medicaid programs. Yet decisions made by the Senate Human Resources Committee and the House Commerce Committee on the size and the nature of the physician manpower pool, on investment in research resulting in new technologies, on the strength of the Health Systems Agencies, can act as countervailing influences on any direct cost-containment efforts and vice versa.

At the administrative level the success or failure of cost control efforts depends on multiple branches of the bureaucracy. If the Department of Housing and Urban Development is liberal in ensuring loans for hospital construction and in subsidizing interest, it will provide an incentive for continued capital expansion. If the Office of Management and Budget underfunds the Health Systems Agencies, even over the objections of DHEW, it will impede the agencies' ability to make rational local planning decisions because they will not be able to obtain staff and objective technical information. If the tax laws allow write-offs for construction loans that are tax-exempt, HSAs will have difficulties withstanding local pressures.

Within DHEW, professional standards review activities stressing quality and underutilization of services can adversely affect cost-containment activities. If the National Institutes of Health increase their investment in midlevel technology, with corresponding increase in capital and manpower, the ability to withhold the new developments for cost considerations will be limited. How does a society withhold potential life-saving and life-enhancing procedures even when the cost benefit is marginal? Although the ethical issues are not explicitly discussed in this volume, they will assume increasing importance.

Competition will inevitably exist between the federal government and the states. In large measure states have put in place rate regulation and certificate-of-need mechanisms as a response to their increasing Medicaid burden. The states pay for half of the Medicaid expenditures and some include those left out of third-party payments but uneligible for Medicaid. If federal cost-containment efforts are less restrictive than the state regulatory devices, the states will not gladly step aside for the federal substitute. What then will influence the costs—fifty different state systems or one national system? If New York, for example, decides to cut its support of teaching hospitals or residency programs, will this impact on the total manpower pool? Who sets national policy, the federal government or the states?

Hospitals must be interested in their own financial viability. Any regulatory action that will affect the ability of an individual hospital to control its own destiny or decisions, its cash flow and reserves, will be resisted. Which institution, for example, should get the burn unit for the community—the county hospital, the university hospital, the Methodist, Catholic, or Jewish hospital? Is there a need for five burn units?

Reimbursement controls are antithetical to the objective of maximizing revenues and reserves. Although the hospitals themselves have been proponents of prospective reimbursement (Drake and McMahon), prospective reimbursement means different things to different groups: individual budget review; classification; ceilings on per diem and ancillaries; ceilings on revenues. Hospital associations have not been reluctant to bring suit against the federal government and the states on prospective methods and rate regulation. Suits have been brought against the Medicare classification system under Section 223, the New York State rate system, the New Jersey rate system, the Maryland system, and it can be predicted that the American Hospital Association and the Federation of American Hospitals will seek to modify, to their perceived benefit, the new federal proposals. Certificate-of-need suits have been brought against many states by individual hospitals and hospital associations.

The resistance to PSROs by the American Medical Association and state medical societies need not be redescribed here. If cost containment or planning begins to affect the independence of physicians' decision making, it follows that there will be organized resistance on the part of the AMA and state medical societies throughout the land and understandably so.

Hospitals are rapidly unionizing. Cost-containment efforts will necessarily influence the number of jobs, layoffs, and wage and fringe-benefit advances. It can be anticipated that unions may combine with hospitals, if their interests are similar, to resist regulatory activities that affect jobs and pocketbooks. The greatest resistance to the closing of New York City Hospital Corporation hospitals has come from the unions affected. How organized labor will rationalize the impact on individual unions and resource constraints with its demands for a tightly controlled national health insurance plan remains to be seen. A wage pass-through was negotiated on the federal cost-containment proposal in the hope of winning labor support.

Private third-party payers at the moment have been supporting cost-containment efforts related to hospital care. But if these efforts extend to control over the third parties' way of doing business, their premiums and retentions, they too can be expected to join in resisting regulation.

And what of the consumer? Since he pays indirectly often only a small portion of the costs of his coverage if he is covered by his employer, what is his motivation to support capital or cost containment? The primary objective of the consumer is to have the best health services available when needed. What incentive, then, is there for the consumer to vote nay on adding a new service for the local hospital? If he does not feel the financial effect, why should he question the decisions of the physician to hospitalize him, order tests and medication, extend his length of stay? To the physician the hospital is an adjunct to his patient care capabilities. He does not pay for the decisions he makes within the institution.

In the decision-making process, therefore, there are competing interests, fragmented decision points that affect costs, incentives to resist cost controls at every level—all in all, a climate inimical to success.

Responsibility and Authority for Containing Hospital Costs and the Dynamics of the Economics of Hospitals

The first part of this volume provides an overview of perspectives on containing costs of health care in general and the hospital specifically.

In "Controlling the Cost of Health Care," Gerald Rosenthal describes the linkage between controlling health care costs and achieving the goals of public health policies. Many of the factors that have led to rising medical care costs stem from public health policy. But we have now reached the stage where trade-offs need to be made. Rosenthal points out that cost-containment strategies are not neutral with respect to these trade-offs and discusses the research findings highlighting those factors that affect cost-containment strategies. The research findings are organized into three categories.

The first category, supply incentives and disincentives, describes research findings addressed to hospital investment controls, incentives, and supply of ambulatory services. Next, Rosenthal outlines provider behavior incentives and disincentives, including changes in treatment patterns, effects of insurance, changes in physician productivity, physician reimbursement, and cost controls. Incentives and disincentives are equally important with respect to consumer behavior. Findings discussed are the role of insurance in the demand for services, and financing mechanisms.

In summary, Rosenthal asserts that the push and pull of conflicting incentives in the health industry lead to the expectation of future
inflation and sees the need for empirical analysis of the macroeconomic consequences of national health insurance.

Stuart Schweitzer presents a review of alternatives. He itemizes
the reasons for intervention: the government's role in delivering and
financing care; the feeling that expenditures are not getting value for
the dollars spent; inefficiencies and inflation fostered by government
financing systems; the threat to other social programs of the health
care cost inflation; and the nature of the health market where the
provider exerts a considerable influence on demand. Next, a series
of policy alternatives is presented. The issue of cost-sharing is raised
with the recognition that hospital care is the least price sensitive. The
fundamental question, he believes, is not one of reduction but of
"deflection" in care. A second alternative is to provide incentives for
more efficient, lower-cost care, using fees as signals to stimulate
production of selected services over other services, and noting the
relationship between fee-for-service and high resource use.
Schweitzer expands his discussion by reference to health care
systems of other countries.

Utilization review is seen as providing a potential for cost
containment, acting directly on the process of care rather than on
reimbursement. Schweitzer points out the unfortunate inadequacy
of analytical models in defining appropriate care. Utilization review,
however, does carry with it the fear of falsely accusing peers for
poor practice, and consequently its efficacy is somewhat doubtful.

The concept of planning or limiting inputs is based on the
underlying assumption that supply creates its own demand. However, there is the problem of withstanding the formidable professional and political pressures to expand and "improve quality." The
author concludes that a combination of cost-containment programs
acting in concert needs to be applied; a lone approach will not
succeed.

McMahon and Drake review the organized hospital view of cost
problems and cost-containment efforts and end up by advocating
the American Hospital Association's plan for national health insurance introduced by Congressman Al Ullman, Chairman of the Ways

and Means Committee. They claim that inflation is beyond the control of the individual hospital and is related to the organization of the entire health industry. Factors influencing inflation are well reviewed, with an explanation of the change from demand-pull to cost-push inflation. Nonlabor input factors such as malpractice, fuel prices, sophisticated technology, and extent of third-party coverage are cited, as are such factors as physician determination of demand—all valid concerns. The solutions, according to the authors, are greater organization and rationalization of the system with the hospital as the keystone or focus of the system: mission oriented hospitals. McMahon and Drake call for implementation of the Hospital Association's national health insurance plan—a mandated employer approach with the hospital as the center of the service system and essentially the controlling organization for all services. In effect, the latter half of the paper is an advocacy argument. Equal time probably should have been given to other proponents of national health insurance. McMahon and Drake do not indicate how hospitals, as the center of the new health universe, will exert control on costs at the expense of institutional objectives. Nor does their proposal indicate how consumer financial interests can be used to contain costs.

In her discussion of the consumer's perspective, Mary Lee Ingbar generally equates the consumer with the payer. She raises the important issue of who the consumer is and what the consumer's roles are as regulator and planner. The murkiest area in planning and certificate of need is definition of the consumer. In the health planning regulations, consumers are restricted to those with no financial interest in the health industry, thus excluding spouses of health professionals, health service researchers, and members of boards of trustees of hospitals even though they do not derive their livelihoods from the health industry per se. The consumer is not just one individual and consumers' interests will necessarily vary with their immediate perspectives of health care. If a consumer is ill and needs care, the more accessible that care is, the better. The last thing the consumer will question when he or a close family member is ill is the need for services and their costs. The consumer rarely directly negotiates for his health insurance benefits and often does not understand the scope of coverage, its restrictions and exclusions. He lacks information on alternative sources and sites of care, qualifications of providers, and price information. Yet he is expected, without strong staff assistance, to sit on Health Systems Agencies and determine the need for hospital beds, CAT scanners, or specific types of health manpower. He can only be overwhelmed in the decision-making process by the sophistication and backup resources of the provider. The consumer as representative of his local community is motivated to provide the best health services for that community, often with little knowledge of alternatives, the total costs, in terms of both capital and operating costs, of his decisions, and national trade-offs.

As the book was being completed in July 1977, the Congressional Budget Office issued "An Analysis of the Administration's Cost-Containment Proposal," which is now being "marked" up and modified by a series of congressional committees. William Dunn and Bonnie Lefkowitz in their introduction point out that hospitals have been singled out because the cost per patient day is increasing at double the rate of overall inflation. If nothing were done to stem this, hospital care expenditures would increase from $61 billion in 1978 to $104 billion by 1982.

"Excessive increases in the amount paid for hospital care are thought to be caused by operating inefficiencies, unnecessary growth in the intensity of services . . . and duplicative facilities." Capital expenditures are also part of the problem.

Title I of the Administration's bill seeks a ceiling on total inpatient revenues in nonfederal short-term hospitals with some adjustments for admissions increases, wage pass-throughs, and exceptions. Increases are expected to be limited to 10.6 percent in 1978 and 8.9 percent in 1981, as contrasted with today's 15 percent. The ceilings apply to all revenues and all payers. The Congressional Budget Office believes the proposal would achieve major savings, reduce growth in services, and be simple to administer.

Disadvantages of the proposal are that there are few incentives for efficiency; adverse selection and dumping of patients can occur; individualized treatment of hospitals is difficult. There is a possibility that hospitals can circumvent some of the pressure by alternating a high wage increase one year with no subsequent increase and in the second year apply the full revenue growth allowance for nonlabor purposes.

Alternatives are suggested including classification of hospitals; altering the exceptions process; altering or eliminating the wage pass through. Senator Herman Talmadge has also offered a control bill. It is possible to combine the bills.

Title II of the Administration's bill places a limit on capital expenditures of $2.5 billion allocated among the states based on population. A standard of four beds per 1,000 population and 80 percent occupancy is set, and no certificate of need can be issued if the standard is exceeded.

Five problems are discussed. Necessary improvements could be retarded because of the arbitrary limit. There is excess capacity at present. The proposal would not reduce the excess. There is no control of out of hospital procedures and there could be shifts. Small investments would not be controlled. It should be noted that the Administration has recently issued guidelines to reduce excess hospital capacity.

In the second part of the book the effects of different factors on costs are considered. Michael Redisch's "Physician Involvement in Hospital Decision Making" points out that the central feature of the hospital system is the relationship between the hospital and physician. With unconstrained cost reimbursement methods, the administrator has little incentive to resist physician demands for personnel, equipment, or use of ancillary services. The physician might be reluctant, however, to utilize the entire volume of inputs when he must bear the full costs or increase his managerial responsibility.

Redisch argues that the greatest cause of increase in aggregate costs of hospitalization is admission, because of physicians' uncertainty over the need for service and value of alternative therapies. This argument is the logical extension of recent conclusions by Rinehart and Ginsburg regarding the negative influence of the increased supply of physicians on costs. If it is the physicians who make the decisions on admission, diagnostic, and treatment patterns, and consequently length of stay and ancillary services, controls that exclude these decisions are at best short-range.

Redisch does not believe that certificate of need, rate review, or prospective reimbursement gives the administrator sufficient added rationale for confronting physicians' decisions and demand, and he believes that decisions will be based on the power of physicians' groups rather than on social efficacy. We believe the argument to be somewhat overstated. If prospective rates are set tightly enough and include ancillary services by diagnosis, they may bring enough financial pressure to act as a countervailing force. Redisch thinks that PSROs and utilization review might be more effective but cites the high cost of case-by-case review and concludes that PSRO might be a more efficacious quality-control than cost-control mechanism. Case-by-case review is not necessarily the only approach—sampling approaches might be more cost effective.

In his final sections, Redisch deals with the cost-containment aspects of physicians' training, fee-for-service payments, and office-based versus hospital-based physicians. Some incentive proposals are offered but not fully developed, including capitation for primary care with pool distribution of savings to the doctor. Also suggested is a plan for disbursements to physicians when hospital costs are below projections; but how such a plan could be administered is not clear. Redisch's conclusion—that there is no one magic solution to cost problems—is very much to the point.

In the paper on the role of the administrator, William Zubkoff, a hospital administrator, begins, discusses, and ends on the note that the administrator has no control. Zubkoff asks what the definition of cost containment is to a hospital administrator: slowing of research, better management of services, limiting nonessential ancillary services, lessening care and services, slowing down of personnel pay.

He asserts that no consumer desires to purchase cheaper medical care. This is a questionable statement for two reasons. First, the consumer pays little at the time of service and is never offered price comparisons. Second, the administrator has no incentive to provide cheaper care since he equates savings in costs with a reduction in quality of services (by itself a questionable assumption).

Zubkoff gives a laundry list of factors over which he says the administrator has minimal or no control; the lack of control over some of these factors can be questioned. He does indicate that the administrator can, however, introduce some efficiencies particularly in manpower. He points out that economies of scale in the hospital sector are not entirely clear and that there may be a lower optimal size than is generally believed. Efficiencies could probably be obtained through redistribution of patients according to hospital capabilities; that is, through regionalization. The overemphasis on the medical center model, that "bigger is better," should certainly be reduced. A section is devoted to cost quality and size; the author correctly emphasizes that "quality is not merely technical quality."

An interesting part of the paper concerns "planning the wrong way." Zubkoff correctly cites the government's initial push for and support of more beds, and claims the same ill-planned expansion is now happening in emergency care. A number of current regulatory devices are criticized with some justification. For example, some inspection and accrediting programs and agencies impose a multitude of staffing and procedural standards. In fact, from this author's perspective, some attention should be devoted to the cost effects of multiple accrediting, inspection bodies, their requirements, the actual impact on outcomes versus the costs.

In the section "Pursuit of the costly impractical," the author points out the problem of terminating impractical nonproductive programs (often government-sponsored or required). Utilization review is used as the example. The expectation of cost-containment measures is limited from the hospital administrator's point of view. He claims that increased costs per patient day may be inherent in health care. However, he does believe that direct controls are needed over duplicative services, incentives are needed for referral and regionalization, and most important, changes in public values of medical care delivery are needed. Finally, he raises an important issue, not addressed adequately in this volume: who should benefit from the money saved, provider, consumer, or third-party payer?

In the past several years the influence of technology on hospital costs has been recognized. Judith Wagner and Michael Zubkoff discuss why technology has been singled out as a leading factor in cost inflation. They highlight the paucity of impact that many health services have on health outcomes and the disappointing record of controlling capital investment. They differentiate between problems in the way the health care system allocates resources and problems of technical change itself. Quality perceptions of patients and hospital decision makers influence behavior related to technology, with three factors considered critical: structural changes in medical education emphasizing tertiary care; failure of the reimbursement mechanisms to constrain investment; and patient demands. The importance of these factors leads to recommendations for over-hauling of the reimbursement systems: a federal agency to reevaluate medical practices and report the results to physicians and patients; a change in medical education to prepare clinicians to take account of efficacy, effectiveness, and efficiency issues.

The authors then discuss the distinctions between changes that enhance quality and those that lower cost, and the dichotomy between those who think there is too much technology and those who think more is better.

Dialogues on the role of technology and health care costs have rarely raised the point that the economic impact is mixed and not always of a cost-generating nature. In a review of the literature, Wagner and Zubkoff point out that the basic problem is the misallocation of resources rather than the impact of technology. They conclude that there are major gaps in what we know about technology and its dissemination; that increasing federal attention needs to be paid to efficacy; and that the major policy problem is the trade-off between costs and effectiveness and the rationing process.

Cost Containment and Regulatory Efforts

Part three of the volume explores experiences with hospital cost control mechanisms, including planning and rate regulation. Paul Ginsburg begins by reviewing the impact of the Economic Stabilization Program (ESP). He points out that a major retrenchment in inflation in the health industry occurred just before the program was initiated. In terms of what happened during the control period several important findings are presented. Input use accelerated very rapidly. Wages followed expenditures but there was little difference in wage trends in the period preceding the controls.

Ginsburg differs with the Wage-Price Control Council analysis, because the council focused on prices rather than cost. He believes that revenue per unit of output should be the measure of success and indicates that the regulations were not designed to influence service intensity. (The current Administration proposal for cost control recognizes the importance of this factor and attempts controls on the rate of growth of revenues per admission.) Further criticisms include the problem of ambiguities in the ESP regulations: hospitals were given no incentives when their increases were below 6 percent. (This is also a problem with the current cost control proposal.) Gains in efficiency could not be used to increase profit margins and the hospitals feared that current costs would be used as the basis of future prices, removing the incentive to hold costs. The regulations also introduced incentives to alter case mix toward less complex cases. The author concludes that ESP was effective in reducing rates of increase in hospital wages but not costs. Input intensity did not decline.

In "Hospital Rate Setting—This Way to Salvation?" Katharine Bauer punctures the balloon of easy answers. She begins by pointing out what rate setting is *not* doing; it does not target on the physician, the key decision maker; there is no systematic case-mix control; there is no medical audit. The rationale for rate setting is reviewed and the following assumptions of proponents of rate setting are discussed: rising costs are associated with inefficiencies; inefficiencies can be controlled; visible rate determination can provide the motivation to control costs; rate setters will have skills and resources to accomplish the task; there can be an exactness to the rates.

Bauer points out that none of the above is based on empirical evidence, but she is kind enough not to say it is all wishful thinking. Each of the proponents of rate setting has different expectations ranging from curbing unit costs to total expenditures. The paper thoroughly reviews current rate setting conducted by Blue Cross plans, and state rate-setting authorities. Bauer discusses the nature of the different rate-setting bodies as well as the advantages and disadvantages of private versus public rate review. She reviews the objectives and processes of rate setting, their problems, and the crude state of the art. An important section of the paper is devoted to risks and incentives in rate setting, deliberate and unintentional. The great weakness in rate setting, which should be recognized and given great attention, is that in no rate-setting scheme to date has there been any incentive for cost consciousness on the part of the physician, a theme that runs through many of the papers.

Bauer herself concludes that rate setting is not the way to salvation. "Rate setting per se is a highly complicated tinkering operation, plugging up leaks in one small section of a rudderless ship, cracking at the seams."

Fred Hellinger explores experiences with prospective rate-setting experiments and demonstrations and produces a mixed review; yet prospective rate setting is still at an early stage. He reviews the legislation authorizing Medicare and Medicaid to develop demonstrations and experiments in prospective reimbursement and indicates that natural experiments were taking place even before this authorization. The chapter evaluates four prospective reimbursement plans: Western Pennsylvania, Rhode Island, New Jersey, and New York Blue Cross. The major limitation of the paper is that the detailed findings go only until 1974. Since then prospective reimbursement methodology has progressed and shows more promising results.

Harold Cohen is a pioneer in the field of hospital rate regulation and has headed the Maryland Health Services Cost Review Commission for several years. His paper reviews the experience of this commission. The task of the commission is threefold: (1) public disclosure of the financial condition of a hospital and development of a uniform accounting and reporting system (without the latter it is not possible to make valid comparisons among hospitals); (2) rate review of institutional costs related to services offered and aggregate rates (rates are to be set equitably among all purchasers or classes of purchasers); (3) trustee disclosure.

Cohen reviews in detail the process the commission uses for review. Highlights of the Maryland system include a new method of treating depreciation—a replacement cost concept. Money for expansion is not provided. The Maryland commission also has challenged contracts for hospital-based physicians and has succeeded in reducing some of the large percentage arrangements for pathology and radiology services. Also, except for a few types of services, the Maryland method attempts to reduce cross-subsidization within the hospital. Each patient care area is expected to be self-supporting. The overall aim of hospital review is to achieve a break-even budget.

Cohen discusses the important relationship between capital planning and rate setting. Unfortunately, Maryland's comprehensive health planning effort has lagged behind that of other states. He concludes that it is too early to assess the public utility model but notes that Maryland rates have increased slightly less than 7 percent overall and 10 percent per inpatient day, substantially below national figures.

In the mid 1960s, the concept of capital control began with the Partnership for Health Act and the formation of areawide and statewide health planning agencies. These agencies relied on voluntary compliance and were beset with problems of underfinancing, understaffing, and lack of adequate planning guidelines and tools. An attempt was made to strengthen planning through the Health Planning and Resources Development Act of 1974, which was designed to establish certificate-of-need authority in each of the states. In their paper, David Salkever and Thomas Bice review planning and certificate-of-need experiences up to 1974 and come to some important conclusions.

There are two types of possible controls over capital expenditure: direct and indirect. Direct controls are certificate of need or other legal means to prohibit capital projects. Indirect controls are economic sanctions, usually refusal to reimburse for capital expansion as permitted by Section 1122 of the Social Security Act. Currently both forms of control are in operation; the indirect controls will probably be replaced as certificate of need spreads.

Salkever and Bice outline the various theories regarding certificate of need. First, there is the capture theory—the capture of the control mechanism by those to be controlled and the danger that new entrants to the market will be excluded. Next, Roger Noll's political economic theory postulates that regulation may fail to serve the public interest because of the inability to identify just what is the public interest and the compulsion to avoid conflict. The third theory is that of perverse provider response, a preemptive response; favored providers will increase their expansion and switch to less regulated investment options.

In examining the literature and the effect of certification of need, the authors found that there was no appreciable effect on total investment, but rather a shift in investment that exacerbated inflation. In fact, there has been an increase in plant assets per bed. However, they also found that inpatient utilization had been reduced. Unfortunately it is impossible to compare what occurred with what would have occurred without certificate of need. In addition, the combination of technical ability and cost consciousness required to enhance the certificate-of-need review process may itself be a function of time.

Salkever's and Bice's conclusions may be valid where certificate of need is the only control but perhaps not where there are complementary controls. Capital planning, while a critical variable, must be combined with rate regulation, control of utilization by both provider and consumer, and control of physician manpower supply to be an effective cost-containment strategy.

Professional Standards Review Organizations are still fairly new. The legislation was part of the Social Security Amendments of 1972 but only recently have PSROs actually come into being. Although PSRO activities are officially limited to Medicare and Medicaid, they could be universally used if proved successful. James Blumstein reviews the charter of PSROs, the local and state bodies, and the National Council. He discusses the sanctions and incentives and the interrelationships with other regulatory mechanisms.

The PSRO legislation seemed to require that nationally approved norms be used by local PSROs. Now, DHEW has modified the legislation to accede to the profession's demand for greater local autonomy and fewer national norms. Blumstein points out the potential conflicts between cost-containment objectives and so-called waste control. The statutes call for consideration of economic factors in developing norms. But reliance on professionally developed norms might tend to impose on health care the best available practice rather than cost containment. PSROs have no options to reallocate resources. Therefore "micro" rather than "macro" quality is promoted. The consumer in one region receives no reward or incentive for forgoing very expensive medical services—a disincentive to economize, when consumers in other areas are receiving the services. In the long run PSROs "might well become potent and virtually unopposed political instruments for increasing rather than containing costs."

Technical Problems

Part four of this book deals with the methodological issues that can make the difference between the success and failure of specific cost-containment proposals. Most of the papers preceding this part dealt with the conceptual framework or historical developments. But without knowledge of how to implement cost containment, all concepts remain theoretical.

William Cleverley discusses a critical issue: without uniform cost accounting how can rational controls be attempted? Two factors are essential for cost control: normative measures of what costs should be, and measures of actual costs. Cost-accounting systems that are comparable are essential to cost-containment programs. Four methods of establishing normative costs have been used: formulas applied to past actual cost data for a specific hospital; similar formulas for groups of hospitals; submitted individual budgets; and industrial engineering cost analysis.

Cleverley next discusses the costing process, describing the alternatives for each of the factors in the process and evaluating those alternatives. In conclusion, he recommends the type of cost information that a hospital cost-containment agency should receive. All hospital cost-accounting systems should use general price level, adjusted historical costs as the basis for valuing resources. All hospital cost reports should present measures of direct departmental cost for direct and indirect departments. Hospital cost-accounting standards should be established by the federal government. Annual certified public accountant audits should be required of all hospital cost reports.

Joseph Lipscomb, Ira E. Raskin, and Joseph Eichenholz discuss the use of marginal cost estimates in cost-containment policy. Their paper focuses on the concept of the marginal cost of hospital services and the role designed for the use of marginal cost in Phase IV of the Economic Stabilization Program.

Phase II controls are considered an oversimplification of hospital cost and revenue functions. A volume index was used, which results in disincentives for control of total costs. In layman's language this means that whatever the volume of service, the cost of care was considered equal for each admission. Thus, there was no encouragement to control volume; indeed incentives were created to expand it and thus lead to additional cost.

Phase IV was intended to minimize the undesirable incentives of Phase II. Changes were made in the regulations, including the use of admissions as a measure of hospital volume; separate controls were put on inpatient and outpatient services; add-on cost adjustments were permitted for complex patient mix and enlarged capital outlay. A more flexible assumption was introduced for the differences between fixed and variable costs. The regulations directly incorporated the assumption that marginal costs (costs attributable to increased volume) were on the average 40 percent of average hospital costs. This was modified by variations in minimum and maximum constraints on cost increases per admission and varied by hospital size.

The authors review various methodological issues, such as:

- Hospitals are multiproduct (also joint product) firms. Case mix varies and using any single variable to represent output implies a homogeneity that does not exist. Indices of case mix need to be developed.
- The manner in which a hospital combines inputs relates to the objectives of the hospital. Linkages of the institutional characteristics and objectives are necessary.
- The failure to account for changes in services can lead to biased estimates.

The authors conclude that future cost control policies should reflect the fact that a significant portion of hospital cost does not vary in the short term with volume. This has been recognized in the Administration's proposed cost control program, where there are financial disincentives for increased volume. Clearly the experience under the four phases of ESP has contributed to recent efforts to design cost containment.

Judith Lave and Lester Lave have made major contributions to the understanding of the behavior of hospitals. They continue to do so in their paper on "Hospital Cost Function Analysis: Implications for Cost Controls." Using a variety of techniques, the authors have tested their hypotheses against ten years of data from over 1,000 hospitals, thus making a major contribution to the dialogue on how to control hospital costs.

Lave and Lave begin with a brief general description of the evolution of the ESP regulations. Their purpose is to estimate hospital cost functions and to answer critical questions necessary to the implementation of cost containment. These questions include: what is the cost of an additional patient or patient day; what are the effects of other factors on costs; what similarity is there in cost functions by geography and by size of hospital; what is the extent of pure cost increases?

After presenting their theory of the hospital cost function, outlining the problems associated with estimating cost functions, and describing the methodology of their econometric analysis, the Laves arrive at certain specific conclusions:

- There is a stable hospital cost structure and marginal costs can be estimated while controlling for various hospital characteristics.

- There is evidence of economies of scale, but not in the largest hospitals. Teaching hospitals add cost, but rates of inflation are similar to those of nonteaching hospitals. The cost structure is constant across regions, but not across size of institution.

- The Economic Stabilization Program did not stop inflation but did slow it. However, a slowdown in hospital inflation began before 1970. In the postcontrol period the rate of inflation has accelerated.

• All cost control schemes are not equivalent. Freezing costs per patient day is inequitable. Phase IV was considered a step toward equity and feasibility, but it ignored factors such as outpatient services and geography.

The final section of the volume contains two articles, one on research needs and one on policy choices. Ralph Berry places research requirements in the context of what the questions really are. The first and overriding question is what do we really want to contain: price increases, total expenditures, percent of GNP, size of the government budget for health, rate of increase in per capita expenditures, or (what is not mentioned) none of the above?

Another basic question is what is the right rate of output of hospital services? Berry believes the policy intent of cost containment is based on either of two implicit assumptions: whatever the right rate of output, it is less than the actual output; or, the actual rate is acceptable but the only tolerated increases should be generated by real productivity increases. We believe that the first is the public policy makers' assumption; the current rate of output is producing too much of one product and the wrong product, although no one seems to be able to define the product that is to be produced. It is described as utilization, quality, per capita expenditures evenly distributed, but the basic output is undefined, especially in the context of the total national economic output.

In calling for more research, Berry points out the need for a better understanding of the market for hospital service; more information about supply responses; and refinement of measures of demand elasticity. Little has been done to account for product difference or the quality and complexity of hospital services in demand function analysis. The role of physicians in demand for services and their influence on hospital costs—a theme constant in this book—needs research. Perhaps the most interesting part of the paper is in the last section. Berry comments that the exuberance of cost containment reflects the growing dissatisfaction with the performance of the hospital sector—the sector is not producing at the right rate and the extreme market imperfections preclude acceptable performance without external intervention.

What form should this intervention take? Should the hospital industry as now structured be replaced, regulated, or repaired? Berry claims the volume is skewed toward regulation, and points out that the choice of whether to regulate, replace, or repair the health market depends on what is known and what needs to be known to affect desired outcome. We feel that political and social objectives enter into the choice and would rephrase the whole question to read that the choice depends on the political-economic views of the policy maker and even the researcher. It is not a value-free question. Data are important in deciding among alternatives and in refining them, *but*, regrettably, data can be designed and selected to bias toward certain alternatives. There are no value-free data in this field or in most others in social science. One often starts with a value system and manipulates, albeit subconsciously, the research questions, the data findings and conclusions accordingly.

Irving Leveson's paper on policy coordination and the choice of policy mix summarizes the basic strategies for containing costs; presents a public choice model and elements of effective cost containment; and ends with a list of actions that should be taken next.

He states that efforts to contain hospital costs are of two types: those that provide a basic resource constraint and allow hospitals to decide the details; and those that exert controls over certain aspects of hospital operations. Some present strategies for containing costs are evaluated as follows:

Almost all commentators agree that the basic hospital insurance structure, first-dollar coverage, places no constraint on either consumer or provider demand. Leveson discusses increasing co-insurance and admits the difficulty of overcoming consumer resistance.

Capital control is currently the focus of much cost-containment effort and he summarizes some of the problems with this approach. In the area of manpower he reiterates the need to limit supply. He points out some of the problems regarding hospital rate regulation discussed in earlier papers, and he examines proposals to place a cap on total expenditures and the difficulties of distributing the dollars among the hospitals while controlling for quality.

The competitive alternatives to regulation, rarely discussed in this volume, are acknowledged by Leveson, as he examines the potential role of HMOs (and other forms of competitive organizations) and points out that they are particularly vulnerable to regulation and can be blocked by limitations on new entrants and services. Utilization review is seen as too spotty; PSROs he feels are too new.

Leveson presents his view of an effective cost-containment policy containing the following elements: a definite resource constraint broadly imposed; optional ways of producing output; careful details of implementation; incentives and policy interaction. In regard to the importance of policy interaction, he cites as examples length of stay reimbursement and the connection between Health Systems Agencies and the reimbursement process. He concludes with a list of actions that can immediately be carried out:

- Change in reimbursement criteria from reasonable cost to efficient production of services
- Definition of need under certificate-of-need legislation at a target level
- Uniform accounting
- Incremental cost reimbursement for changes in length of stay
- Coupling of Medicare and Medicaid reimbursement rates
- Experiments with case-mix reimbursement systems
- Efficacy testing of technology

Economic, Political, and Ethical Choices

The Administration's recent cost-containment proposal for hospitals is a classic example of the difficulties of imposing cost constraints on hospitals or the health industry. It contains many of the suggestions presented in this volume—a ceiling on capital expenditures; a cap on hospital revenues per admission with admission and length of stay controls; coverage of all third parties—and is a major effort toward rational cost containment, yet it has serious limitations. There is a wage pass-through for all nonsupervisory employees, including nurses and technicians. No controls are placed on outpatient services. It can be predicted that hospitals will manipulate preadmission testing and length of stay, outpatient surgery, and a number of activities such as payment of physicians, because their motivation is that to be successful means to maximize revenue. Capital funds within a total will have to be distributed by HSAs, many of which are not yet functioning and none of which has faced a total dollar constraint. The potential for fierce local political battles as to who gets the capital will be strong, as well as the potential for locking out all new entrants, particularly innovative delivery systems. No constraints are placed on the supply of manpower, nor are economic penalties or incentives offered to physicians, who largely control hospital demand. Finally, the states' role in rate regulation is limited and it is questionable as to whether some existing state rate regulation agencies will qualify under the bill.

To date Congress has had mixed reactions about the proposal, and many modifications are proposed. Undoubtedly, if anything like it is enacted, it will be only after a long series of compromises with the states, hospitals, physicians, and third-party payers. Until the federal government controls the vast bulk of expenditures for health, either directly or through requirements imposed on the private sector, or until the consumer and employer are equally concerned about national health expenditures, general economic and political forces militate against strong cost containment.

Perhaps a different perspective toward health care and its importance to the public and economy can solve the dilemma. The health care industry and the hospital industry could be viewed as a consumer good; a growth industry and a source of employment for a large part of the working population. With all the dialogue recently on the marginal value of new health care development, on health status, and on life expectancy, perhaps the consumer does not view health care only as a *curing* industry but also values the absence of disability, pain, and discomfort and the *caring* aspect of medical care. First-dollar insurance coverage has evolved over the years as the result of consumer choice, not merely because of the tax benefits. Consumers through choice in both the private and the public sectors have deemed health care a worthy consumer good, have forgone other fringe benefits, and have chosen health care. Even as costs have inflated, private health insurance benefits have continued to expand into new areas: drugs, dental care, mental health.

So we might ask is there a right amount of GNP we should be spending on health and health-related matters—8 percent, 10 percent, 12 percent? And what of the larger economic consequences? The vast proportion of health and hospital industry employment is in semiskilled jobs. Wages in the industry were depressed until 1967, and a large number of hospital workers in urban areas earned wages so low that they received supplementary public assistance payments or housing subsidies. The wage picture has changed dramatically with the imposition of minimum wages and unionization, and wages largely have caught up.

The industry, furthermore, is one of the largest employers of women and minority workers, unfortunately not yet in the more senior positions, but even this is beginning to change. What then are the macroeconomic consequences of strong restraints that may result in cutbacks in employment, increased unemployment, increased public assistance loads, other social welfare consequences? How do we balance out concerns with the inflationary trends and the economic and social consequences of stringent controls? What are the trade-offs?

We pose these questions as important issues that have not surfaced in the cost-containment dialogues to date and submit that until there is either a national health insurance program or a serious consumer movement to constrain costs, all the current efforts will operate only at the margin and at cross-purposes with general economic objectives. This is not to say that the problems are to be ignored, but that the chances of success are limited, unless there is a groundswell of consumer concern and a dramatic change in the public view of the value of health care services.

There is little doubt that to create efficiency in the delivery of health services major changes are needed across the spectrum of the organization of services, the supply and use of manpower, and financing. First the public must consciously define in the political and the social arenas what services it values, the quantity and quality of these services, and how much of its income it is willing to forgo to achieve its goals. The inflation in health care is worldwide, not merely a phenomenon of the United States. It is equally severe in nations like Sweden with tightly controlled supply and financing systems. The problem is a reflection of rising incomes and standards of living, rising consumer expectations, and technological advances, that appear to reduce disability and provide relief from discomfort, even though they may not actually prolong life.

If conscious political and social choices are made, the regulatory devices that we have put in place in the last few years are forerunners of devices to control expenditures under national health insurance. Capital control is conceded by all to be necessary to control total supply, regulate demand, and affect costs. However, capital control has not yet been imposed on manpower and without controlling the behavior of manpower, there will continue to be leakages in the system. The techniques of placing strong controls on capital are not yet well developed and the success of certificate of need without a total resource constraint is not yet known.

On the manpower side, particularly physician manpower, supply continues to escalate with a number of new medical schools on the drawing boards. In addition, the number of midlevel practitioners in primary care is also growing and by 1990 the pool of both will create real cost problems unless utilization and income controls are imposed. The alternative is to begin to reduce the production of manpower, a difficult task.

While rate regulation of hospitals can be an important tool in future cost containment, without similar regulation of long-term or outpatient care, there are bound to be problems in these other sectors as hospital cost containment tightens. Little attention, except for the extending of PSROs to outpatient services, has been given to rate or cost controls in the nonhospital sector.

Finally, the issues of technology are only just being addressed. Everyone is talking about requiring efficacy testing before the proliferation of high-cost technology. Unfortunately, there are several serious issues in control of technology. It often takes many years to test fully a new machine, procedure, or practice. It is even harder to measure the cost-benefit and cost-effectiveness consequences over time. How then do you withhold a technology once developed if there are indications that it can save lives, extend life, reduce disability and pain? Who will make what are essentially ethical choices and, assuming the technology is introduced, who then will determine who benefits? These same concerns pertain to the PSRO cost-quality tensions.

The issues of hospital cost containment go far beyond the issues of the rate of inflation, techniques of control, and the success of control mechanisms. They extend to issues of consumer social and political choices, whether and what type of national health insurance we will develop, the impact on employment in a diverse industry, and ultimately the underlying social and ethical choices of a nation.

An
Overview
of Perspectives

Controlling the Cost

of Health Care*

GERALD ROSENTHAL

The rising costs of medical care have come, increasingly, to command attention in public discussions of health care. It is not surprising, therefore, that the goal of constraining and moderating the rise
in health care expenditures comes more and more to be articulated
as the central objective of public health care policy. It is important
to remember that such an emphasis for public policy is a recent
phenomenon.

Traditionally, public health care policy has focused on control
and eradication of communicable disease, expanding access to
medical care services, enhancing the ability of medical science to
respond to illness, assuring a more equitable distribution of services
to the poor, improving and assuring the quality of care, and
encouraging the rapid application of new technological capabilities
in the control and treatment of illness. Each of these objectives has
been pursued by means of public policies and strategies characterized in the main by the use of incentives and stimuli rather than
coercion and prohibition.

The coexistence within the American medical care system of a

*This paper was recently disseminated as the first Policy Research Series Report of
the National Center for Health Services Research. Its relatively quick but extensive
synthesis of the literature has received a rather enthusiastic public response. The
National Center would like to extend its appreciation to Ira E. Raskin and Pam
Farley, who helped to make this paper possible.

wide variety of providers, organizational forms, and financing sources has traditionally been viewed as a positive attribute which contributes to the rapid diffusion of new technology, enhancement of the quality of care, and the capacity of the system to adapt to change. Strategies to achieve public health care objectives were designed, typically, to be consistent with a diverse and decentralized system of care provision. The use of fiscal stimuli through grants-in-aid, the commitment in major financing programs to retrospective reimbursement of costs on a fee-for-service basis, and the reliance on peer review for quality assurance all reflect a preference for achievement of public objectives through strategies that offer positive rewards to providers for compliance rather than impose costs for failure to comply. Such strategies are inherently expansive and minimize the need for deliberate allocative choices by increasing the flow of resources into the health care system.

In many ways, then, the current emphasis on cost containment is a reflection of the success of past policy coupled with a growing awareness of the limitations of simple expansion of resources for achieving health care goals. As the opportunity costs associated with rapidly rising health care expenditures begin to impinge on the achievement of other public objectives, there is created a need for reassessing policies with an eye toward moderating the incentives for expanded expenditures while protecting the central public commitment to the achievement of positive health goals. *Rather than being the central goal of health care policy, cost containment has become the context within which the basic, positive goals of public health care policy must be pursued.*

This distinction is critical. Many of the incentives for rising medical care expenditures are the result of public policy. Cost-containment strategies that are designed to modify these incentives will limit the achievement of other health objectives. Such a circumstance is not necessarily undesirable. We are moving from pursuing health goals "at any price" to a realization that limited resources require deliberate choices. The goal of "the best for everyone" provides no guidance for making trade-offs among alternative uses of resources when that goal cannot be immediately achieved. The reality of resource constraints makes trade-offs inevitable, and the choices which will be exercised in the system will reflect the options available and the incentives and disincentives faced by the decision maker.

As a matter of public policy, we may not wish to regard all trade-offs as equally acceptable. Some health care policy objectives might be more important than others. Is "equity of access" more or less important than "quality of care"? Should we commit to a minimum adequate "floor" of care below which no trade-offs could be made? *No cost-containment strategy is neutral with respect to these issues.* Therefore, no cost-containment strategy should be initiated without assessing how incentives and disincentives currently influencing behavior in the health care system will respond to its imposition. Conversely, expectations of the positive impact of particular instruments of cost containment must reflect the influence of incentives and disincentives that may offset that impact. It is hoped that this paper provides a framework for such an assessment. It arrays selected research findings that highlight the large number of factors which affect attempts to constrain cost increases in the health sector. The findings are not meant to be exhaustive or free of the usual panoply of caveat and counterargument. They have been drawn, however, from the work of recognized experts in the field and tend to reflect the prevailing climate of analytical opinion.

Supply Incentives and Disincentives

Hospital Investment Controls

Certificate of need is designed to give government some control over investment in the health sector. To date the approach has been used primarily to limit hospital construction.

- Analysis of the impact of early certificate-of-need programs suggests that this approach has not substantially affected total investment in the hospital sector. Although there has been some reduction in the use of capital to increase bed capacity, investment in new and costly equipment and services has increased. This redirection of investment capital has reduced the utilization of inpatient services by reducing the availability of hospital beds. The net effect, however, has been an increase in the cost of each day of care that is provided (Salkever and Bice, 1977).

- Existing hospitals are protected to some degree from new competition by the tight restrictions on bed expansion that result from certificate-of-need programs. As a result, hospitals are able to raise the price of services without experiencing a decline in utilization. By increasing the price of services for all patients, hospitals are able to acquire the capital needed to finance sophisticated new services of sometimes limited applicability (Salkever and Bice, 1977).
- A further problem with certificate-of-need programs derives from a failure to define in many instances what constitutes an appropriate supply of services. The agencies that administer these programs have no review standards and little information on the use of and need for facilities, equipment, and services. Typically the investment plans of one institution are reviewed without information on or regard for the plans of other institutions in the area. Lacking useful concepts and operational measures of need as well as a knowledge of potential investment opportunities, certificate-of-need agencies are unable to select a set of proposals which, when taken together, will produce an optimal pattern of investment (Salkever and Bice, 1977).

Hospital Investment Incentives

Federal programs to support and encourage hospital investment have had mixed results.

- Federal financial assistance for construction of health care facilities under the Hill-Burton program succeeded in equalizing the relative availability of hospital facilities among the states. Further, by changing the pattern of distribution of hospital beds, federal intervention also influenced changes in the national distribution of physicians (Lave and Lave, 1974).
- Since 1970 the federal programs to assist health facility con-

struction efforts have emphasized guaranteed loans and reduced interest rates. This approach has introduced various distortions in the market for hospital investment capital. Should a hospital default on a guaranteed loan, the government is obligated to pay the interest and mortgage. Because there is little indication that the government intends to assume control of the hospital in such situations, there is no obvious threat to hospital management in the event of default. The potential consequences are clear. Management has no immediate incentive to make wise investment decisions. Similarly, since they are also protected from loss, private capital lenders have little incentive to analyze the financial feasibility and risks of a proposed investment (Lave and Lave, 1974).

- However, in the absence of government guarantees, the acquisition of private capital for hospital investment becomes extremely difficult. The present level of cash flow is inadequate to finance facility development directly or to cover the growing costs of debt. Moreover, the possibility that government financing programs will place upper limits on reimbursement; that periodic reviews for appropriateness by Health Systems Agencies will eliminate some reimbursable services; that the rising costs of malpractice and self-insuring programs will increase the financial risks of institutions; that third-party reimbursements will not be sufficient to meet replacement costs of equipment and facilities; and that the precarious financial state of local government will make local support problematic should compound the problems currently facing hospitals that are forced to rely upon private capital markets. The immediate consequence of these uncertainties and risks is the rising cost of debt (Raskin, 1976).

The Supply of Ambulatory Services

Federal support for medical education and new programs to alter the distribution of physicians geographically and by specialty are likely to have somewhat of a favorable effect on physician fee inflation.

- With respect to general practitioners and surgeons, an increase in the physician-population ratio of an area seems to temper fee increases. Whether the same effect can be expected in the case of internists, specialists in obstetrics and gynecology, or pediatricians is not yet clear (Sloan, 1976; Sloan and Steinwald, 1974).
- Even with significant increases in the number of medical school graduates and a shift toward general practice, the supply of ambulatory services is not likely to be able to increase enough in the short run to meet the anticipated demand for such services under a comprehensive national health insurance program. Offering providers more money will produce neither an effective nor an equitable solution to the immediate problem. Rationing through a variety of non-price mechanisms will take place. These will include longer waits for appointments, longer waiting room delays, a reduction in the time spent with each patient, fewer return visits, and an increased reliance on telephone consultations. The degree to which each of these mechanisms will be called into play is unknown (Newhouse and Phelps, 1974a, b).

Provider Behavior—Incentives and Disincentives

Changes in Treatment Patterns

Overall, it appears that changing treatment practices will not have the effect of reducing health care costs. Expenditures for new services and equipment outweigh the savings from reductions in hospital utilization.

- It appears that hospitals compete with each other in the adoption of technical innovations. Those in competitive environments, where there are large numbers of hospitals relative to the population, tend to adopt new technologies earlier and to acquire more expensive equipment than other hospitals (Rapoport, 1976).

- Empirical evidence for selected illnesses shows that the only significant trends toward lower costs are the reduction in length of hospital stays and the increased tendency to treat patients in an ambulatory setting. Every other change in the treatment of these selected illnesses—the use of tests, the level of training of the physician, the nature of the medical or surgical therapy—tends to increase costs. For example, changes from 1964 to 1971 in caring for otitis media in children, appendicitis, maternity care, cancer of the breast, forearm fractures in children, pneumonia, duodenal ulcer, and myocardial infarction were, *in general*, cost-raising. That is to say, costs rose more than they would have if only the price of inputs had changed. The total cost of treatment for myocardial infarction rose 126 percent during 1964–1971, with an increase in input prices of 70 percent and a net increase in inputs of 33 percent (Scitovsky and McCall, 1977).

- Although some preliminary research suggests the substitutability of outpatient for inpatient care in the Medicare program and elsewhere (Russell, 1973; Davis and Russell, 1972; Huang, 1975), the strength of the evidence is limited by the methodological problems of these studies. The Canadians did not experience cost saving in the substitution of extended-care facilities for hospital care. What was saved in lower acute care stays per episode was lost in longer extended-care stays (Evans, 1976a; Feldstein, 1971). Furthermore, Canadian evidence (Evans, 1976a, b) supports the paradox that ambulatory medical care insurance increases hospital utilization by promoting the detection of medical problems (Lewis and Keairnes, 1970) and that the provision of outpatient benefits does not lower hospitalization rates (Newhouse and Phelps, 1974a; Freiburg and Scutchfield, 1976). However, because these studies were not able to measure the efficacy of treatment or changes in health outcome, what appears to be no cost saving may be an improvement in health status for the same expenditure on health services.

- There is considerable empirical evidence to suggest that the Health Maintenance Organization (HMO) tends to reduce hospital utilization and generate a *net* savings in total per capita health care costs. Major questions, however, remain unanswered with respect to differences between HMO and fee-for-service arrangements in terms of the quality of care received, accessibility and continuity of care, patient satisfaction, and economic viability. We still do not know to what extent differences in the characteristics of patients who are enrolled in HMOs account for the results of evaluation studies (Mechanic, 1976; Reidel et al., 1975; Gaus, Cooper, and Hirschman, 1976; Ellwood and Schlenker, 1973).

● Capitation payment in HMOs may not be the significant factor that alone produces major changes in hospital utilization; that an HMO is an organized, multispecialty group-practice arrangement largely with salaried physicians may be more significant (Gaus, Cooper, and Hirschman, 1976).

The Effects of Insurance

Physicians will tend to recommend and patients will tend to use any service covered by insurance that promises some benefit. Increased insurance coverage, as a result, is associated with increased demand for services. As service demands become heavier and the patient's ability to pay is no longer of concern, providers are likely to respond by raising their prices.

● Physician fees will increase by 0.19 to 0.30 percent for every 1.0 percent increase in the proportion of the population having major medical insurance. Even with coinsurance and deductibles, a national health insurance program that extended this type of coverage to the entire population would stimulate an increase in demand large enough to cause a significant increase in physician fees (Sloan and Steinwald, 1974).

● Increases in major medical insurance coverage are associated with greater increases in the average total bill for physicians' visits than in the size of professional fees. This suggests that more services (laboratory tests, for example) are provided per visit, or that physicians elect to itemize charges for services that were previously included as part of the professional fee (Sloan and Steinwald, 1974).

- Increases in Medicare Supplemental Insurance Benefits have also been associated with increases in the average total bill for a physician visit. A 1.0 percent increase in benefits per capita has been accompanied by a 0.60 to 0.75 percent increase in the average cost of a visit (Sloan and Steinwald, 1974).
- Existing patterns of insurance coverage, where more people are insured more extensively against the cost of hospital care, may partly explain the large increases in expenditures for hospital care. The general willingness to pay more for hospital care and the increased threat of malpractice suits have led to the offering of a more technologically sophisticated, and more expensive, hospital product. Another source of historical increases in hospital costs has been the rise in hospital wages. Since hospitals are reimbursed by insurance companies and other third-party payers for whatever costs they incur, they have had little reason to resist or alter these trends.

Changes in Physician Productivity and Workload

The productivity of physicians and the number of hours they choose to work can seriously affect the price of physician services. To the extent that fees increase in response to demand pressures, efforts on the part of physicians to treat more patients will help to combat inflation. On the other hand, when fees increase it is possible for doctors to work fewer hours, carry a smaller patient load, and yet maintain or gradually increase their income. This type of response exacerbates an already inflationary situation.

- Substantial gains in physician productivity appear to be possible through the increased use of ancillary personnel. Potential productivity increases are greatest in areas having relative shortages of physicians; physicians are more likely to utilize ancillaries, the heavier the demands on their time. Primary care practices appear to have the greatest potential for increasing productivity through the use of allied health personnel (Hadley, 1974).
- Physicians tend not to hire as many ancillaries as is technically warranted. The factors which deter the full utilization of allied personnel include the possibility of quality deterioration,

patient resistance, weakening of the patient-doctor relationship, and malpractice suits; the costs of on-the-job training;
space limitations and problems of office design; the added
managerial burden on the physician; and licensure policies
that restrict the potential range of ancillary tasks (Human
Resources Research Center, 1972).

- The evidence is varied regarding the responsiveness of physician work effort to a rise in prices. One study shows that the
level of physician effort (hours per week per year) does not
appear to be sensitive to *short-run* changes in earnings. (However, changes in earnings may over time affect the choice of
medicine as a specialty, the choice of specialties within
medicine, and the choice of practice locations.) While there
will be fee inflation under national health insurance, physician
workloads will not change enough to either exacerbate or
dampen the upward trend in prices (Sloan, 1975).

- Another study has, however, suggested that at some targeted
level of physician income, the quantity of services provided
by physicians may decline as prices increase (Feldstein, 1971).

- In response to the introduction of a compulsory, universal
health services insurance program in Quebec, Canadian physicians reduced the length of their work-week by an average of
8.5 hours, increased vacation time and days off, reduced
patient contacts, and hired more ancillary personnel. Average
waiting time to appointment increased from 6.0 to 11.0 days,
and waiting time in physicians' offices also increased. All of
these factors suggest that the number and mix of procedures
per visit may have changed quite substantially in response to
the increased demand pressure (Enterline et al., 1975).

- On balance, employed physicians devote less time to professional activities. Whether or not these work patterns reflect a
systematic response to financial incentives cannot, however,
be determined with available data. The possibility remains
that physicians with a preference for shorter work-weeks opt
for employed practice and that this segment would not be
responsive to financial incentives if they were offered. But

there is reason to think that government efforts to promote large-scale institutional practices in which the physician is an employee (rather than self-employed) may well lead to a decline in the average time that each physician works (Sloan, 1975).

- Salaried practice can be very unattractive in terms of increasing physician effort. The incentive to work long hours is reduced as the number of physicians in the group increases. Unless such measures as unequal income sharing and centralized decision making by a board of directors or a business manager are instituted, physician workloads may be expected to fall to a minimum "acceptable" level (Sloan, 1974).

Physician Reimbursement

Physician reimbursement policies are critical to the design of any cost-controlled national health insurance program.

- The usual-customary-reasonable method of reimbursement tends to reinforce inflationary trends in physician fees. In effect, such reimbursement plans are more generous than fixed fee schedules and have a greater inflationary effect (Sloan and Steinwald, 1975).
- Nearly all Western European countries using fee schedules to reimburse physicians under national health insurance have sooner or later adopted the fee schedule as the *maximum* allowable charge to the patient, primarily to control health care costs through physicians' fees (Glaser, 1976).
- Establishing maximum allowable charges also helps to assure equitable access to care. Under Medicare in the United States, where they have a choice, physicians will accept assignments (agreeing to limit *total* charges to the charges reimbursed by the carrier) only as long as the payments are consistent with the general level of reimbursement (Gornick, 1976).
- If a maximum allowable fee schedule is to be instituted with national health insurance, a method must be devised for allowing increases in such schedules. On the other hand, if no

counterdvailing power confronts the medical profession, fees will continue to rise faster than overall consumer prices. Negotiation between providers and consumers (or third-party payers) is essential (Glaser, 1976).

- Certain types of physicians are more likely to participate in Blue Shield service benefit programs. By inference they are also more likely to participate in other service benefit programs, such as Medicaid, which are an important source of care for many low-income persons. Foreign medical school graduates are more likely to participate; board-certified and/or medical school–affiliated physicians are less likely to do so. Holding physician characteristics constant, the extent of participation increases as the fee schedule does. These results indicate that trade-offs between costs, quality, and access must be faced in the design of a national health insurance plan (Sloan and Steinwald, forthcoming).

Hospital Reimbursement

- Traditionally, hospitals have been reimbursed retrospectively on the basis of whatever costs they incurred. Experiments involving *prospective reimbursement* for hospitals (amounts or rates of payment are established in advance and paid regardless of the costs actually incurred) have not had a demonstrably significant effect on hospital costs. Any definitive interpretation of these experiments with regard to the magnitude and potential of cost savings is impossible. Much additional work is required to delineate the multiple objectives and the interaction of decision makers in the hospital sector. These factors may in fact counteract the cost-saving incentives introduced by prospective reimbursement (Gaus and Hellinger, 1976; Hellinger, this book).
- In New Jersey, the method of prospective rate setting for hospitals encouraged cost *increases*. Because the prospective rate was established on the basis of the previous year's actual costs, the program tended to reinforce existing inflationary trends (Worthington, 1976).

Hospital Cost Controls

The results of research on the effectiveness of programs designed to control the inflation of hospital costs and prices have not been encouraging.

- While the Economic Stabilization Program (ESP) administered by the Cost of Living Council (COLC) was very effective in reducing wage increases for hospital employees, this was not the case for overall hospital costs. Reasons for ESP's minimal impact on costs include perverse disincentives and incentives under Phase II (Lipscomb, Raskin, and Eichenholz, this book), ambiguity of the regulations, and the expectation that the controls would be short-lived and, therefore, would not necessitate cost-saving managerial changes (Ginsburg, this book).
- Hospital cost inflation did slow appreciably during the period of COLC regulation. However, it is not clear to what extent this can be attributed to COLC, since the decline in the hospital inflation rate started in 1970 *before* COLC was established (Lave and Lave, this book).
- Per diem charge data (available as part of the Consumer Price Index) may have limited relevance in assessing the impact of the Economic Stabilization Program. Under a system of cost-based or retrospective reimbursement, few hospital patients actually pay these charges (Lave and Lave; Ginsburg, this book).

Consumer Behavior—Incentives and Disincentives

Insurance and the Demand for Health Services

Consumers are more likely to use health services for which they have insurance coverage. To expand insurance coverage is therefore likely to encourage a great increase in demand. Deductibles and co-insurance will tend to reduce the inflationary effect of insurance by deterring utilization. Such cost-sharing devices place consumers in a position where they must decide whether or not their need for health care warrants the additional, direct payment that is required. These devices also reduce the expense of public insurance programs, since they shift part of the cost to those who use the services. However, it is necessary to weigh the desirable effects of cost-sharing against its effect of deterring the use of services that are really needed, particularly by those with low incomes.

- As catastrophic coverage has become more common, the anticipated effect of a national catastrophic insurance program on the demand for services has been reduced. Coverage of persons with large medical expenses increased sharply between 1963 and 1970. Over 75 percent of "catastrophic expense" (that is, expenditures of $5,000 or more as recorded in the CHAS-NORC survey) was covered by insurance in 1970 as compared with 50 percent in 1963 (Phelps and Newhouse, 1974).

- Under rather restrictive assumptions (a population similar to that using the FEHBA high-option plan), the provision of catastrophic health insurance on a national basis, with unlimited ceiling and very high deductible, would not lead to a substantial increase in demand for medical care. Annual expenses of $3,000 or more were relatively infrequent in the group of federal employees studied; increasing the annual deductible from $50 to $3,000 would have reduced the number of claimants in an insurance program by 97 percent. Claims would have fallen by two-thirds as a result of increasing the annual deductible to $1,000 (Arthur D. Little, Inc.).

- A *comprehensive* national health insurance program should not lead to large price increases or trigger rationing mechanisms in the hospital sector. Insurance coverage for hospitals is already quite extensive, and hospitals are operating at historically low capacity levels. A full coverage insurance plan would lead to a 5 to 15 percent increase in demand for hospital care (Phelps and Newhouse, 1974).

- By contrast, national health insurance will have a dramatic impact on the demand for ambulatory services (Phelps and Newhouse, 1974; Newhouse and Phelps, 1974a; Scitovsky and

Snyder, 1972; Sloan and Steinwald, 1975). A full coverage health insurance plan would add at least 75 percent to the existing demands for physician services outside of the hospital. A plan with 25 percent co-insurance would add at least 30 percent to the existing demand for physician services outside of hospitals (Phelps and Newhouse, 1974; Newhouse and Phelps, 1974a; Scitovsky and Snyder, 1972).

- An AMA physician survey revealed that 65 percent of surgical specialists' billing was covered by insurance, as compared with 45 percent of medical specialists' billings and even less of general practitioners' and pediatricians' billing. This further supports the contention that comprehensive national health insurance will have a much more dramatic effect on the demand for office visits relative to hospital visits (Sloan and Steinwald, 1975).

- Insurance plans with a deductible are not likely to cause a major increase in the demand for ambulatory care, if the deductible is greater than the amount that most individuals spend on medical care (approximately $150 per year). Because the individual does not expect to exceed the deductible, he acts as if he were uninsured when contemplating the use of routine, lower priced services (Newhouse and Phelps, 1974a).

- It is difficult to determine to what extent the lower utilization rates observed with cost-sharing insurance plans are actually due to cost-sharing. Much of the difference may be due to self-selection, whereby those who are healthier choose less costly, lower coverage plans (Kaplan and Lave, 1971).

- Even allowing for their poorer health, Medicaid recipients received 30 to 40 percent more Medicare services in 1969 than did low-income patients who did not receive public assistance in meeting the patient's share of the cost of Medicare supplemental benefits. This implies that the co-insurance rate and deductible imposed under the program deterred low-income families from using Medicare services (Davis, 1975).

- Factors other than cost-sharing may help to dampen increases in demand associated with expanded insurance coverage. As money becomes less of a consideration, time becomes a more significant factor in the decision to seek health care. Expected increases in office waiting time will to some extent offset the tendency to demand more services when care is "free." Furthermore, it appears that waiting time is more likely to affect the service demands of higher income groups. Unless they have better protection against such losses in earnings, higher income (higher paid) workers lose more money when they are kept waiting in doctors' offices. Hence, if waiting time increases as expected, increases in utilization under national health insurance are likely to be relatively greater among low-income groups (Phelps and Newhouse, 1974).

- Furthermore, there is empirical evidence to suggest that structured patient education can contribute to the reduction of health care costs by speeding recovery in certain types of cases, decreasing emergency room utilization and inpatient readmissions, promoting self-care, and encouraging more informed decisions regarding the use and selection of acute care services (Fogarty, 1976).

Financing Public Health Care Programs

Carefully designed financing mechanisms are critical to the efficiency and equity of public health care programs. Associated with every tax are incentives and disincentives that alter the real costs and benefits of the program being financed.

- The federal government has for a long time encouraged its citizens to purchase health insurance by offering a personal income tax deduction for health insurance premiums. These deductions substantially reduce the price paid by consumers for health insurance; the subsidy averages 18 percent of total premiums. Higher income families in higher tax brackets receive the biggest subsidies, since their deductions are other-wise subject to progressive tax rates. Furthermore, the tax subsidy is *greater* than the difference between total premiums and total benefits (this difference is the total fee charged by insurance companies for their services). In effect, the government bears all of the expense associated with private insurance *and* offsets part of the cost of services as well. If the personal income tax deduction for health insurance premiums had been eliminated and if employer premium contributions had been treated as taxpayer's income, federal revenues would have been $6.4 billion higher in 1975. Taking into consideration the cost of excess insurance and the need for other taxes to regain the revenue lost from the subsidy, it is estimated that the total loss resulting from the 1970 subsidy of $4 billion was approximately $8 billion (Feldstein and Friedman, 1974).

- Even if administratively possible, a national health insurance program requiring copayments and deductibles that are proportional to income would impose a heavy burden on middle-class families. Under such a policy a substantial part of the revenue necessary to pay for taking care of the poor is exacted from families who use a great deal of care themselves. High-income families fare best under a system of high deductibles and copayments that are fixed without regard to income. Because they tend to have low utilization rates, their out-of-pocket expenditures do not increase greatly, and yet the reduction in program expenditures that results from cost-sharing means a reduction in tax burden (Wilensky and Holahan, 1972).

- Requiring employers to provide health insurance coverage will not be without significant budgetary effects. A substantial increase in employer health insurance premium contributions has the effect of increasing wage costs and will result in transitory increases in the unemployment rate. Tax revenues will decline as the taxable income of employees is reduced. Because mandated coverage hides the real cost of health insurance to the consumer, it is likely to inflate the demand for health insurance benefits by unions and employees (Mitchell and Phelps, 1976; Hornbrook and Coffey, 1976).

- Employers and state governments, who currently contribute to the cost of health insurance, will gain from a federal takeover of insurance financing. The magnitude of this windfall has been estimated at $20 billion for employers in 1975 and $6.3 billion for the states. Any reduction in such contributions should be phased out gradually to allow time for the adjustment in wages and revenue structure that will avoid such windfall gains (Davis, 1975).

- Three major roles have been proposed for state governments under national health insurance: regulation of the private health insurance industry; establishment of standards of participation and methods and levels of reimbursement for providers; and administration and subsidization of health insurance coverage for low-income families. Combining these roles may introduce counteracting incentives: the setting of higher physician fees to attract more physicians to a state must be balanced against the resultant higher program costs for health care to low-income populations. Moreover, those states most in need of physicians are the most unable to sustain higher program costs. Physician reimbursement policy should be determined at a federal level in order to prevent competition among the states for scarce doctors (Davis, 1975).

- Under the Medicaid program, state governments already share the financial burden of providing health care for the poor. In the face of tight budgets, many states have been tightening eligibility criteria and reducing Medicaid benefits (Taft, 1976). Yet, approximately 9.5 million persons below the poverty level, or 39 percent of the poor, are not covered by Medicaid (Davis, 1975). Since Medicaid is tied to welfare eligibility, families that do not meet welfare criteria are also ineligible for Medicaid. Thus, in many states, the working poor, families without dependent children, and poor families with an unemployed father living at home are ineligible for Medicaid. The problem of coverage gaps is exacerbated because public assistance income eligibility limits are not automatically adjusted to reflect rising prices and money incomes (Davis, 1975).

Summary

The push and pull of private and public incentives and disincentives in the health sector inevitably lead one to expect that inflation will continue and that health care will claim an increasing share of the country's resources. As some long-term observers of the scene have noted:

> Our apparent successes—in developing new technologies and training people better to use more of them—are part of our problem. . . . If we equate more with better in medical care we have to pay the price. . . . No one simple solution is in sight, not even one as difficult ethically and politically as limiting the number of expensive procedures. We are, rather, being nickeled and dimed to death, except that the nickels and dimes are five, ten and twenty dollar bills.
>
> To the extent that high quality care costs more, our national ability to provide it to those who cannot pay is lessened. Existing measures to achieve equity, such as the Medicare program, slowly erode away. As economic conditions and governmental commitments put increasing pressure on governmental budgets, new attempts to achieve equity are too expensive and must be shelved [Lee and Butler, in Scitovsky and McCall, 1977].

The degree to which this may be a legitimate societal concern is magnified by the anticipated onset of national health insurance. The potential for NHI as an engine of inflation merits not only further empirical analysis but a much better sense of viable policy measures prior to enactment. It is crucial that some a priori sense of its macroeconomic impact be considered. Unlike the mid-1960s, with the introduction of Medicare and Medicaid, the present is actively engaged in assessing cost-containment protocol and at least the need to instill a cost consciousness in all components of the health sector.

The urgency and activity of this cost concern were evidenced in recent congressional testimony prepared by the National Center for Health Services Research, in which the inflationary potential of NHI was highlighted:

> A national health insurance plan, with deductibles and co-insurance, will still have an inflationary impact on the health services system. This will be particularly evident in the case of

ambulatory care. Inflation will evolve not only from a sharp increase in demand for physician services but a supplier's response in which physicians tend to trade off increased revenue for greater leisure time and institutions invest in costly equipment and facilities at the institutional level. Regulatory mechanisms (in the past) have not been successful in curbing this inflation [Rosenthal, 1976].

The research findings described earlier are supportive of this outlook. Yet, we still are not certain as to what buttons to press or what *coordinated* initiatives to set in motion to contain costs and still secure an equitable and efficacious health care delivery system.

A cost-conscious mental set is new in the health sector. Its maturation will require hard evaluations of the different configurations of manpower, facilities, and services that will make the most effective use of limited resources. Its orchestration will necessitate a synthesis of the impact and interaction of various cost-containment strategies for informed decision making, and a realistic assessment of the behavioral and political underpinnings of the system as it responds to such strategies.

References

Davis, K.
   1975   National Health Insurance: Benefits, Costs and Consequences. Washington, D.C.: The Brookings Institution.
Davis, K., and L.B. Russell
   1972   "The substitution of hospital outpatient care for inpatient care." Review of Economics and Statistics 54 (May): 109–120.
Ellwood, P.M., and R.E. Schlenker
   1973   Medical Inflation: Causes and Policy Options for Control. Minneapolis: InterStudy.
°Enterline, P.E., et al.
   1975   "Physicians' working hours and patients seen before and after national health insurance: 'Free' medical care and medical practice." Medical Care 13 (February): 95–103.

°Supported by National Center for Health Services Research.

Evans, R.G.
  1976a   "Beyond the medical market place: Expenditure, utilization and
           pricing of insured health care in Canada." In R. Rosett, ed., The
           Role of Health Insurance in the Health Services Sector. New
           York: National Bureau of Economic Research.
  1976b   "Health costs and expenditures in Canada." in T.W. Hu, ed.,
           International Health Costs and Expenditures. Fogarty Interna-
           tional Center, DHEW Publication No. (NIH) 76-1067.
°Feldstein, M.
  1971   "An econometric model of the Medicare system." Quarterly
           Journal of Economics 85 (February): 1–20.
°Feldstein, M., and B. Friedman
  1974   "Tax subsidies, the rational demand for insurance and the health
           care crisis." Discussion Paper No. 382. Cambridge, Mass.: Har-
           vard Institute of Economic Research.
Feldstein, M., et al.
  1972   "Distributional aspects of national health insurance benefits and
           finance." National Tax Journal 25 (December): 497–510.
Fogarty International Center and the American College of Preventive
Medicine
  1976   Preventive Medicine USA. Task Force Report. New York:
           Prodist.
Freiburg, L., Jr., and D.F. Scutchfield
  1976   "Insurance and the demand for hospital care: An examination of
           the moral hazard." Inquiry 13 (March): 54–60.
Gaus, C.R., B.S. Cooper, and C.G. Hirschman
  1976   "Contrasts in HMO and fee-for-service performance." Social
           Security Bulletin 39 (May): 3–14.
Gaus, C.R., and F.J. Hellinger
  1976   "Results of hospital prospective reimbursement in the United
           States." Paper presented to the International Conference on
           Policies for the Containment of Health Care Costs and Expendi-
           tures. Fogarty International Center, DHEW, June.
Glaser, W.A.
  1976   "Controlling costs through methods of paying doctors: Experi-
           ences from abroad." Prepared for the International Conference
           on Policies for the Containment of Health Care Costs and
           Expenditures. Fogarty International Center, DHEW, June.

°Supported by National Center for Health Services Research.

Gornick, M.
   1976   "Ten years of Medicare: Impact on the covered population."
           Social Security Bulletin 39 (July): 3-21.
°Hadley, J.
   1974   "Research on health manpower productivity: A general over-
           view." In J. Rafferty, ed., Health Manpower and Productivity.
           Lexington, Mass.: D.C. Heath & Co.
°Hornbrook, M.C., and R.M. Coffey
   1976   "National health insurance: Recent evidence on policy issues."
           Staff paper prepared for National Center for Health Services
           Research, October.
°Huang, Lien-Fu
   1975   "An analysis of the effects of demand and supply factors on the
           utilization of health services in short-stay hospitals." Final Re-
           port, Contract No. HRA 106-74-190, NCHSR, September.
Human Resources Research Center
   1972   "Utilization of ancillary personnel by physicians in private
           practice." Working Paper, Human Resources Research Center,
           University of Southern California, March.
Kaplan, R.S., and L.B. Lave
   1971   "Patient incentives and hospital insurance." Health Services
           Research 6 (Winter): 288-300.
°Lave, J.R., and L.B. Lave
   1974   The Hospital Construction Act. American Enterprise Institute,
           Evaluative Study 16.
Lewis, C.E., and H.W. Keairnes
   1970   "Controlling costs of medical care by expanding insurance
           average: Study of paradox." The New England Journal of
           Medicine 282 (June): 1405-1412.
°Little, A.D., Inc.
   n.d.   "Financing of catastrophically expensive health care." Final
           Report, Contract No. HSM 110-71-197, NCHSR.
Mechanic, D.
   1976   Growth of Bureaucratic Medicine. Lexington, Mass.: Lexington
           Books, D.C. Heath & Co.
°Mitchell, B.M., and C.E. Phelps
   1976   "National health insurance: Some costs and effects of mandated
           employee coverage." Journal of Political Economy 84 (June):
           533-571.

°Supported by National Center for Health Services Research.

*National Center for Health Services Research
  1976   The Program in Health Services Research. DHEW Publication No. (HRA) 76-3136.

*Newhouse, J.P., and C.E. Phelps
  1974a   On Having Your Cake and Eating It Too: An Analysis of Estimated Effects of Insurance on Demand for Medical Care. Santa Monica: The RAND Corporation, R-1149-NC, April.
  1974b   "Price and income elasticities for medical care services." In M. Perlman, ed., The Economics of Health and Medical Care. London: Macmillan & Co.

*Phelps, C.E., and J.P. Newhouse
  1974   "Coinsurance, the price of time, and the demand for medical services." Review of Economics and Statistics 56 (August): 334–342.

*Rapoport, J.
  1976   "Diffusion of technological innovation in hospitals: A case study of nuclear medicine." Final Report, Grant No. HS 01238, NCHSR, September.

*Raskin, I.E.
  1976   "Financial structure and viability of health care institutions." BHPRD Issue/Transition Summary, November.

*Reidel, D.C., et al.
  1975   Federal Employees Health Benefits Program. DHEW Publication No. (HRA) 75-3125.

*Rosenthal, G.
  1976   Statement before Congress of the United States, Senate, Subcommittee on Public Health and Environment, Committee on Interstate and Foreign Commerce, February 10.

Russell, L.B.
  1973   "The impact of the extended care facility benefit on hospital use and reimbursement under Medicare." Journal of Human Resources 8 (Winter): 57–72.

*Salkever, D.S., and T.W. Bice
  1977   Impact of State Certificate-of-need Laws on Health Care Costs and Utilization. Research Digest Series, NCHSR, DHEW Publication No. (HRA) 77-3163.

*Scitovsky, A.A., and N. McCall
  1977   Changes in the Cost of Treatment of Selected Illnesses

*Supported by National Center for Health Services Research.

1951-1964-1971. Research Digest Series, NCHSR, DHEW Publication No. (HRA) 77-3161.

Scitovsky, A.A., and N.M. Snyder

1972 "Effect of coinsurance on use of physician services." Social Security Bulletin 35 (June): 3-19.

°1975 Medical Care Use by a Group of Fully Insured Aged. Research Digest Series, NCHSR, DHEW Publication No. (HRA) 75-3129.

°Sloan, F.A.

1974 "Effects of incentives on physician performance." In J. Rafferty, ed., Health Manpower and Productivity. Lexington, Mass.: D.C. Heath & Co.

1975 "Physician supply behavior in the short run." Industrial and Labor Relations Review 28 (July): 549-569.

1976 "Physician fee inflation: Evidence from the late 1960's." In R. Rosett, ed., The Role of Health Insurance in the Health Services Sector. New York: National Bureau of Economic Research.

°Sloan, F.A., and B. Steinwald

1974 "Determinants of physicians' fees." Journal of Business 47 (October): 443-451.

1975 "The role of health insurance in the physicians' services market." Inquiry 12 (December): 275-299.

forth- "Physician participation in health insurance plans." Journal
coming of Human Resources, 1978.

Taft, J.

1976 "States put scalpel to Medicaid in budget-cutting operation." National Journal 8 (May 1): 581-586.

Wilensky, G., and J. Holahan

1972 National Health Insurance: Costs and Distributional Effects. Washington, D.C.: The Urban Institute.

Worthington, P.

1976 "Prospective reimbursement of hospitals to promote efficiency: New Jersey." Inquiry 13 (September): 302-308.

Zubkoff, M., ed.

1976 Health: A Victim or Cause of Inflation? New York: Prodist for Milbank Memorial Fund.

°Supported by National Center for Health Services Research.

Health Care

Cost-Containment Programs:

An International Perspective

STUART O. SCHWEITZER

Current American health policy is focusing upon a number of objectives. Some deal with problems of access to care, both financial and geographic, while others attempt to improve the quality of care being delivered. Common to these efforts and the underlying force behind a number of recent and proposed policies is the perceived need to contain the rapid increase in health care costs and expenditures. Thus, certificate of need, comprehensive health planning, improved Medicaid data systems, and admission and length-of-stay certification are all programs with a strong cost-containment intent. This paper will describe some recent experience in the United States and other selected countries in designing and implementing cost-containment programs.

The Justification of a Cost-Constraint Strategy

Before considering specific cost-containment activities, however, one must subject the cost-containment strategy to some scrutiny and skeptical questioning. Why should a society attempt to intervene in the health care budget in the first place? After all, health care is surely a "good," valued positively, as opposed to harmful or immoral activities like drinking, smoking, or prostitution. Why should we be concerned with prices and expenditures in the health industry when we choose not to have so active a concern with other life-sustaining sectors, including food, clothing, and shelter? The answers to these questions are really the same. One is simply that society has chosen to assume an increasing role in both the financing and delivery of health care services for several segments of the population. One may criticize this decision, perhaps, but obviously it has been made. The government's role in the United States in delivering and financing health care has grown dramatically, so that in 1976 over 42 percent of national health expenditures came from public sources. The rate of increase of this public share has been two and one-half times as great as the rate of growth of the private component (Gibson and Mueller, 1977). The government share of per capita personal health expenditures was over $109 in 1974. This commitment to finance such a large portion of both total and personal health care has created the drive to economize in these expenditures.

A second answer emanates from the widespread feeling that health expenditures (both public and private) are not buying full value for the dollar expended. Furthermore, it is now apparent that much of the economic inefficiency and inflationary pressures existing in the market as a whole has been fostered by the very nature of the government financing systems, especially the Hill-Burton program, Medicare, and Medicaid. The spillover from the public portion of the programs to the private sector has undoubtedly been enormous, though as yet unquantified. It may be that with an understanding of how inflationary forces have been generated will come an understanding of how to dampen these pressures and gain control over recent price behavior.

A third justification for government intervention in the health sector is based upon the prevalent pattern in most countries of incorporating health sector expenditures, along with other social welfare programs such as income assistance for the indigent and the elderly, into a social welfare budget. An effort to increase economic efficiency of the health sector would be a socially useful goal in its own right, but within a political context it is even more important. The social budgets in many Western countries recently have been increasing rapidly, bringing political demands for constraint and, perhaps, reallocation of resources (see Fulcher, forthcoming). To some, the health component is the only one amenable to reduction through improved efficiency, since the Social Security (pension) and public assistance (income supplementation) programs are generally held sacrosanct. Recent developments in the United States, however, challenge that view; welfare and Social Security programs are both in jeopardy of being cut back because the *health* component of the social budget is seen as increasing at an uncontrollable rate. Regardless of which item in this sector's budget is seen as a dependent variable and which items are seen as exogenous and fixed, the necessity to allocate a stringent budget among alternative social goals defines a substantial shadow price for cost containment in the health sector.

A more fundamental justification than these, however, must be given for the imposition of regulation and intervention in the health care marketplace. This justification is based upon underlying characteristics of this market which are thought to preclude performance approximating that of a competitive market. Perhaps the most basic characteristic is the degree to which demand for health service is determined by the providers themselves, especially physicians. Consumer ignorance, reduced bargaining power of patients at time of decision to purchase care, and a pervasive acceptance of a "mystique" of medical care and those who deliver it (Illich, 1976) all conspire to deprive consumers of the sovereignty presumed to exist in other markets. The role of third-party payers in advocating patients' economic interests is an interesting topic, and one which deserves additional consideration. Legal and institutional aspects of this problem have been studied by Goldberg and Greenberg (1977). An "interventionist" third-party payer would act through the mechanisms illustrated in Fig. 1, leaving unanswered the questions whether the government or the private sector can better assume this role and if the latter, whether the insurer should be a single entity or a group of several.

What is evident is that the market for health care is highly

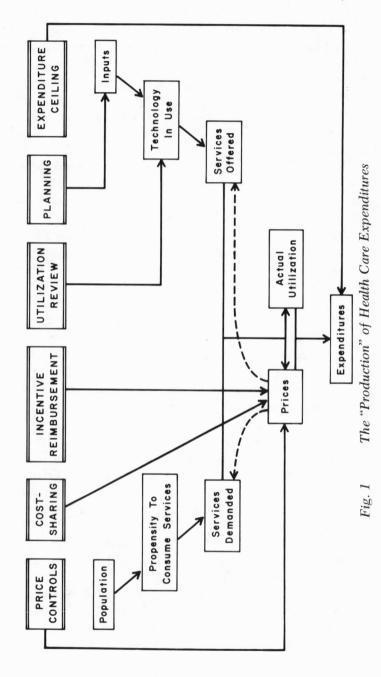

Fig. 1   The "Production" of Health Care Expenditures

noncompetitive at present and this has led to inefficiency, often combined with danger to consumers, especially in the areas of unnecessary surgery and irrational prescribing of medicines.

Health Care Expenditures and Their Control

The array of health care cost-containment programs can best be understood by presenting them within the context of a model of health care expenditures such as Fig. 1.

Expenditures are produced jointly by consumers and providers, as in any market, though unique characteristics of the medical marketplace give providers an unusual degree of control over the demand side of the market as well as over their own supply side (Fuchs, 1974). Aside from this extension of authority of the producer, the health care market is little different from other markets, though institutional arrangements such as nonprofit hospitals, professional associations, and third-party payers create a different environment for control mechanisms.

The process by which health care prices and expenditures are generated is fairly straightforward. Cost containment can theoretically result from intervention anywhere along the process or at the end. Cost-containment measures are classified into four "process" types and two "outcome-oriented" approaches.

Policy Alternatives

Cost-sharing

Of the four "process" policies only one, cost-sharing, seeks to ration services through a traditional demand-side variable: net price. Cost-sharing imposes direct payment of one sort or another on consumers so as to discourage needless utilization. The literature is already extensive on demand elasticities (both price and income) for various health services, and one hopes to learn more about the impact of cost-sharing on utilization patterns with the conclusion of the RAND health insurance experiment. Both price and income elasticities have been found to be low within a country (Newhouse, forthcoming); when one differentiates between sectors, however, the elasticities show considerable variation, with that for hospital care (constituting 42 percent of all health services expenditures) being least price- or income-sensitive. Not only does economic efficiency determine the impact of cost-sharing for health care, but also equity affects it: the burden of cost-sharing falls uniquely upon one class of consumers, those who seek medical care. If one attempts to redress the burden by exempting certain groups from the cost-sharing requirement, such as the elderly, the young, pregnant women, and the chronically ill, the tax base falls to perhaps half of the population.

The overriding problems in evaluating the impact of a cost-sharing method of rationing health care, however, are not by how much demand for health care is reduced, or which population groups pay the tax and which do not. More fundamental is the question of which care is "deflected" and which is not. Aggregate health care consumption is not the real target of cost-sharing, because health care consumed covers a wide range of medical necessity. Conceptually one would want the demand rationing system to deflect only nonessential services, while "necessary" care would be demanded as before. Attempts to discriminate among consumers are predictably difficult; the usual ones create exemptions for some of those groups referred to previously—the young, the elderly, the pregnant, and the chronically ill (Forsyth, 1975). The French, for example, have exempted twenty-five drugs from prescription copayment requirements (Rosch and Sandier, forthcoming). If criteria were established whereby medical services could be judged as either necessary or unnecessary, based, for example, on current diagnosis and medical history, one could be sanguine about measures to restrict demand through the market mechanism.

Provider Reimbursement

The other cost-containment policy directed at maintaining the market mechanism, as opposed to replacing it, is use of alternative methods to reimburse providers so as to give incentives for more efficient, lower cost forms of care. That the present structure of third-party financing encourages use of high-cost hospital care, when ambulatory care would be equally satisfactory, is a well-known failing of the American system. Some third-party payers are attempting to stimulate use of alternative treatment modes such as outpatient surgery or day hospital care, but all too often opposition to these innovations emanates from the very institutions housing the new programs, the voluntary hospitals. The reason for this, of course, is that the hospitals are not at risk for the total cost of hospital care. They are typically reimbursed at full cost for care delivered, leaving as a loss the fixed costs associated with unfilled beds. Savings from use of innovative admission substitutes therefore do not accrue to the hospital, but to the third-party payer (or, rarely, to the patient). Thus the new service is perceived as a threat to the hospital, and the obvious economies to the system as a whole become of secondary import.

Payment to U.S. physicians has generally followed the fee-for-service approach, though the salary mode, in existence in HMOs for over forty years, is growing and claims jurisdiction over substantial portions of the population in some regions. The reimbursement system has never been employed in any significant manner as a device to allocate physician services either geographically or among services. The closest attempts have been efforts to attract physicians to underserved areas. These efforts have not been noted for their success, however, as the magnitude of the "inducement" has always been small, relative to lifetime earnings potentials perceived by new physicians. Physicians have set their own fees by tradition, and so the vector of relative prices for medical services has been beyond the control of any force other than the providers themselves.

In order to reduce expenditures, state Medicaid authorities have attempted to set fee schedules that are more restrictive, based usually upon the distribution of existing fees and taking a fraction (for example, 80 percent) of some fixed percentile (for example, the 60th) of this distribution. The voluntary nature of Medicaid participation has had the effect of limiting the supply of providers available to the indigent. For many physicians, acceptance of

Medicaid patients has led to a practice style that produces a high-volume, less personal sort of care. This reaction has been a natural response to a reduced fee system, where maintenance of a target income is a more powerful component within a physician's objective function than is quality of care. But again, these fee schedules have never been used as "signals" to stimulate production of selected services at the expense of others; the formula has been applied rigidly to all services.

An alternative physician payment system has been employed in Denmark for the purpose of incorporating price "signals" as incentives to primary care physicians. This novel arrangement is a hybrid of customary capitation payment, typical in Europe, and fee-for-service payment, prevalent in the United States. Denmark is one country of many in Europe where primary care physicians, paid by capitation, are not allowed to practice within a hospital, and hospital-based physicians are not allowed to supply primary care. Any time a barrier is drawn between primary and secondary care physicians, one must ask whether one sector in the system (for example, the primary care physician) is performing its share of patient care adequately, or is passing on more difficult, time-consuming cases to the referral hospital sector. The economic incentive, of course, creates this potential spillover, since physicians are paid a fixed salary regardless of work performed. The Danes feared this phenomenon was occurring, thus raising costs of hospital care unnecessarily, so a compromise between the original capitation payment system and fee-for-service reimbursement method was struck. Capitation fees were reduced and primary care physicians were to be reimbursed for specific services rendered in addition to the capitation.[1] This reintroduction of the price system accomplished two things. In an aggregate sense, there is the impression that supply of office-based services was increased to an appropriate level. Second, the government created for itself a policy instrument to encourage delivery of certain services. When the rate of pediatric inoculations fell, for instance, fees for injections were raised to encourage this service. The program was apparently successful.

[1] Office-based physicians in Copenhagen now receive half of their income from capitation and half from fee-for-service reimbursement.

The Dutch use a mixed strategy of capitation and fee-for-service reimbursement, but in a manner exactly opposite to that of the United States, where primary care physicians are paid by fee-for-service while certain hospital-based specialists are paid by salary. In the Netherlands primary care physicians are paid by capitation and hospital-based specialists by fee-for-service (Fulcher, 1973). One would predict an overstimulation of hospital-based service, though the impact of this system on access to primary care and the referral rate to secondary care have not been studied thoroughly. Though the admission rate to Dutch hospitals (921 per 10,000 population) is very low, the average length of stay for patients who are admitted is extraordinarily long.[2] Detailed analysis of the impact of pricing and reimbursement methods on resource use, including case-mix variations that appear across many countries, has not been done; but the suggestion at least exists that there is a relationship between the fee-for-service payment system and high rates of resource use, whether in an ambulatory or inpatient setting.

Reference was made above to the problem of potentially high referral rates of patients from primary care physicians (often paid a fixed or capitation-based salary) to the hospital sector. We saw that the economic incentive to "dispose" of particularly difficult or time-consuming cases in this way exists, to the detriment of the health system in general. The division of labor between office-based and hospital-based physicians is the necessary condition for this problem, and the payment or reimbursement method for primary care physicians provides the incentive.[3] Countering the tendency toward excessive hospital referral is the "second opinion" chart review, which is inherent in the separated office/hospital model. A patient

[2]The 921 admissions per 10,000 population is exceeded by six countries in the Maxwell study (the comparable figure for the United States is 1,446 in 1969) and is less for only two. See Maxwell (1975), p. 27. The average length of stay was 17.9 days in 1969, which was among the highest noted in the study (p. 28). The comparable figure for the United States was 9.3 days.

[3]It has been argued that even in the United States, where office-based physicians continue to care for their hospitalized patients, availability of hospital capital stock and manpower encourage use of hospital services rather than a physician's own office. This would be particularly true during hours that the office is not normally open and staffed.

referred to a hospital specialist will automatically be examined and have his case reviewed, either before or after hospital admission, merely as a necessary requirement for hospital treatment. Whether this case "audit" accomplishes its subsidiary purpose of screening hospital admissions for necessity is a useful question to ask, especially in light of concern in the United States over admission certification, second surgical opinion, and so forth.

The experience in Great Britain seems to be that the referral process works well, with no serious problems of overuse or underuse of hospital care. The Danes, on the other hand, have observed a tendency toward excessive admissions, and hospital specialists show great reluctance to countermand a request by a primary care physician by refusing to admit a referral patient. Apparently a sense of courtesy leads to many short stays for "observation," though the admitting specialist feels that the admission was not needed. Of course, one would expect that a return to fee-for-service payment would lower the tendency to overhospitalize. In Israel there is widespread concern that many primary care physicians lack either the skill or the capital to provide comprehensive ambulatory care, so hospital referral is seen as a necessary complement to primary care. To reduce costs of the high rate of referral, however, hospitals have built outpatient departments that serve as secondary referral points. These departments are able to offer outpatient care of a more comprehensive nature than is available from many clinicians but without necessarily incurring the costs of a hospital admission.

Utilization Review

The discussion of reimbursement methods and their impact upon rates of resource use has emphasized the role of utilization review as either an integral aspect of a delivery system or a program that offers some control over rates of hospital use. Utilization review has a strong potential for cost containment, though its principal objective is often thought of as assuring quality of care. The cost implications could be either positive or negative, depending upon the distribution pattern of costs of care presently being offered and the position of the "norm" or "standard" determined by the review process relative to that distribution.

Utilization review acts *directly* upon the process of care rather than through the market mechanism. The philosophy of utilization review is that more rational patterns of medical practice and resource use can be induced through either formal or informal comparison between norms set by a peer review mechanism and existing practice. There is nothing new in peer review, of course, in spite of some of the dialogue concerning Professional Standards Review Organizations. Hospitals have had peer review committees for many years, and the hospital accreditation panel, the Joint Commission on Hospital Accreditation, requires these committees to conduct retrospective inquiry into some surgical procedures. Other review committees often exist to conduct in-house chart audit, but their effectiveness has been brought into question (Smith and Kaluzny, 1975: 226-227). The controversial aspects of the PSRO program are its attempts to stimulate objective criteria by which medical process can be evaluated and the threat that this review or assessment will be external to the hospital (and ultimately to the individual physician). Attempts to institute effective utilization review programs have so far looked at hospital admissions and length of stay (see Gertman and Eagle, and Platt, forthcoming). Since hospital expenditures constitute roughly two-thirds of total expenditures on personal health care, such a focus is not unreasonable.

A utilization review program confronts the basic problem of decision making under conditions of uncertainty: a decision must be made to classify a case as one of acceptable or unacceptable quality based upon a decision rule. In actuality, of course, the case may or may not be acceptable. In normal analysis of this type, a stochastic process creates a distribution of observations emanating from either a "good" or a "bad" production process. In health care, random variation among providers is compounded by variation among patients, so that acceptable care rendered one type of patient may not be acceptable at all for another. Thus, a three-day hospital stay may be good medical practice for a young patient with minor surgery, but the recuperative process for an elderly patient may warrant a much longer stay.

The number of variables determining the "appropriate" length of stay is extensive and includes patient demographic characteristics, medical history, family or home care setting, attendant medical conditions, and access to outpatient care. Only a sophisticated length-of-stay algorithm would be able to take into consideration all of these factors. One can safely say that just as existing utilization review procedures are simplistic, future ones will undoubtedly be so, as well. With that realization, what should be our expectations of how these guidelines are to be applied?

Given the weak prescriptive power of the length-of-stay guideline that forms the basic decision rule, and the political constraints requiring that physicians criticize one another only under the most serious circumstances, the decision rule is likely to be interpreted very loosely so as to minimize the probability of a "false positive" error. The false positive definition assumes a "good" standard of care being practiced, and an outlying observation (an unusually long length of stay), outside the decision rule, leads to an "out of control" judgment applied to the standard of care. Nothing could be less palatable for a medical review body than to falsely accuse one of its members of poor standards of care; so the decision rule, or level of acceptance, will be very liberal allowing, for example, twice the average length of stay, rather than having to call clinicians continually "on the carpet" and having them merely explain the circumstances, which were not included in the original hospital admission and length-of-stay protocol or certification.

What one sees, therefore, is that existing and incipient utilization review programs must labor under two handicaps: an inadequate analytical model defining "appropriate" care and a fear of falsely accusing physicians of poor practice. Given these preconditions, one can realistically expect that the programs will "flag" only the most egregious errors in practice and, hence, will have little impact upon costs of care delivered. In other terms, one can predict that a utilization review system is unlikely to impose constraints upon providers that are actually binding. Where constraints are not binding, their effect, of course, will not be significant. It may be that there will be an initial "Hawthorne" effect as physicians realize that their work is being reviewed by a panel of their peers.

While standards might tighten up somewhat, it will not be long before it becomes evident that the "tiger" is, in actuality, "toothless," and its bite is not likely to impact upon any but the fringe of physicians. Where utilization review has been instituted, this prediction has generally been accurate, including experience in the United States, Belgium, and the Netherlands. In Canada and in some sites in the United States, another utilization review mechanism has been undertaken. This is the construction of utilization profiles, which have the effect of conveying information to practitioners about their own practice patterns and those of their peers without necessarily conveying explicitly any pejorative significance to discrepancies that appear. These profiles have been used in connection with drug prescriptions and aspects of hospital use, especially within prepaid practice settings. There appears to be evidence that dissemination of these profiles has made physicians more aware of their use of resources and actually has seemed to reduce utilization, at least along the dimensions described by the profiles (see Hatcher, forthcoming; and Maronde et al., 1972). This could be viewed as a hopeful sign, as the distribution of these profiles is really only the transmission of technical knowledge among producers which, ideally, will serve to bring all producers onto the same, more efficient production possibility curve. If this can be accomplished without the inherent problems of a rigid application of algorithms, it shows that a market-like process of diffusion of technology can be simulated.

Health Care Planning

A more fundamental sort of alteration in the producer side of the market to contain costs avoids the pitfalls of attempting to change patterns of care by direct process intervention. Instead, by limiting facilities and other inputs, it is argued that the existing available inputs will be rationed among those in most need of treatment, and wasteful use of resources will be "squeezed" out of the system.

Underlying this supply control model is the assumption that supply creates its own demand and hence, use. In many countries, surplus hospital beds exist, together with increasing numbers of physicians. This combination of excess resources is viewed as explosive for health care utilization and expenditures. It is interesting that an outward shift in the supply schedule for physicians is viewed as explosive, but also as not likely to cause downward pressure upon prices (fees), which would be the predicted result of a competitive market. Rather, the demand schedule, fixed in the competitive model, is thought to be pushed outward too, creating a level of expenditures greater than would have been the case in a competitive setting. Quantity shifts out and price does not fall, so that expenditures rise. The rationing of facilities and providers is a major component of the cost-containment strategy of several countries, including Sweden, Denmark, and the United Kingdom. Carrying out these restraining policies is, of course, much more difficult than legislating them, though some success is apparent. The number of hospital beds in the United Kingdom is lower than it is for most European countries (95 per 10,000 population), but the figure is even lower for the United States, which had only 81 beds per 10,000 people in 1969 (Maxwell, 1975).[4] More important than looking at levels of hospital bed availability is to consider the role of the health planning effort in *altering* the level of the bed supply in recent years. When one compares 1959 rates of bed availability with those of a decade later, one finds far greater variation in the earlier period than in the latter, as several countries have apparently attempted to ration the access to hospital beds. For 10 selected countries, the mean number of beds per 10,000 fell from 112 to 99, a decline of 12 percent (Maxwell, 1975).

When one looks at hospital-related capital equipment, one finds the physicians demanding ever-increasing amounts of sophisticated equipment with which to produce their services, and hospitals facing political motivations to emulate the most sophisticated unit in the area. There is no present study that can document a rationing of capital equipment parallel to that having taken place for beds. The diffusion of technology, leading to excess capacity, has been best documented in the case of open-heart surgical units, which have proliferated well beyond an economically efficient or medically desirable extent.

In 1972 the Intersociety Commission for Heart Disease Re-

[4]The countries included in the Maxwell study are Sweden, Ireland, West Germany, U.S.S.R., Italy, France, the Netherlands, England, the United States, and Portugal.

sources recommended that "the workload for open-heart operations must be sufficient to allow physicians and surgeons the opportunity to maintain their clinical skill and research interests." This commission recommended that institutions perform at least four to six operations per week to maintain this standard. Yet in 1969 it was stated that "less than 4 percent of the hospitals performing open-heart procedures come close to this minimum standard. In fact, more than 70 percent average fewer than one such procedure per week, and more than 20 percent average fewer than ten per year" (Smith and Kaluzny, 1975).

Gaining control over the supply of health providers has been a formidable task in nearly every country. Though systems differ, the professional and political pressures appear to be ubiquitous. For many countries, health planning with the objective of containing costs remains an unfulfilled objective. The frustrations of administering the Comprehensive Health Planning Act were felt in other settings as well, and the initial legislative and judicial battles over the new Health Planning and Resources Development Act, P.L. 93-641, does not bode well for the ability of the Health Systems Agencies to become established and credible organizations.

Expenditures and Price Ceilings

Two additional strategies for cost containment have been adopted in various settings, perhaps in desperation. One is an effort to put a ceiling on aggregate health expenditures. The process is applicable, of course, only to that portion of the health sector under control of the budget authority. Thus, while the British can talk meaningfully of efforts to decrease and redistribute the global health budget (Pole, 1974), the jurisdiction for the American effort is limited to a much smaller public component of the health budget. In 1976 the combined expenditures for health from federal, state, and local sources amounted to just over 42 percent of total health expenditures (Gibson and Mueller, 1977). Whether this expenditure "cap" effort can be instituted through the long legislative process of both the Medicare and Medicaid programs, and through the state-oriented decentralization of the latter, is still open to question. But the temptation to approach cost containment this way is clear and understandable.

The other "frontal" attack on inflation is the institution of price controls directly limiting rates of increase of fees but leaving uncontrolled the quantity (and, of course, quality) of expenditure. The four basic tools discussed earlier for cost containment represent attempts either to reinstitute competitive market behavior in a situation where it has been missing or, short of that, to impose regulation that will achieve a "second-best solution" in which competitive market-like results can be induced in an inherently noncompetitive market. If we had an adequate understanding of the process by which health care is consumed and expenditures generated, there is little doubt that appropriate control mechanisms could be designed which would affect the "process" so as to effect desired changes in the "outcome." The evidence appears mixed that cost-sharing, incentive payments, utilization review, or planning are successful in actually moderating either prices or expenditures for health care. Much the same can be said concerning the impact of the expenditure ceiling or price control approaches as well. Though these two approaches are, in a sense, "guaranteed" to work (if one administers the programs strictly, they will succeed by definition), they have impacts that feed back into the delivery process in subtle ways.

One might argue that one of the difficulties in evaluating any of the cost-containment programs is that success is too narrowly defined, and indirect impacts upon the system are not recognized. The "side effects" may be so serious that, whereas the program objective (expenditure containment) is achieved, other objectives of the health system (access to care or quality maintenance) that are formally excluded from the policy initiative may be jeopardized. Our lack of a thorough understanding of the health system, its incentives, interconnections, and process for generating expenditures, thus threatens not only the "process-oriented" control programs but the "outcome-oriented" ones as well.

Conclusion

These subtle relationships may well dictate the sort of policy mix that would be appropriate for the United States to follow. And the need for some sort of cost-containment strategy will grow enormously as the system eventually encompasses national health insurance. Experience both abroad and within the United States indicates that application of a single program to regulate or control the health industry often suffers because the system is too easily manipulated to meet that regulatory effort while remaining essentially on the same course as before. To effect significant change, a system of programs will have to be employed that will not only consider the avowed objective of price or expenditure containment but will include as well other indicators of health system performance that are at least implicitly recognized. One must not fall into the trap of measuring success of a regulatory program tautologically by measuring only what is directly regulated, while other objectives escape attention and are allowed to get out of control.

Lack of clear evidence that any single cost-containment program is uniformly effective ought not lead one to conclude that there is no hope for an answer to the predicament. It is, perhaps, too much to ask that a single initiative should be found to be the key to cost containment and therefore be forced to assume full responsibility for the policy. Rather, the situation can be likened to an automobile that cannot run on any single wheel, but cannot run without any one of them either. Acting in concert, with each policy covering deficiencies of the others, correct policies might be a *mixture* of several of the programs discussed above.

References

Forsyth, G.
  1975   "Introduction: A British descant on the theme." In Josef van Langendonck, Prelude to Harmony on a Community Theme: Health Insurance Policies in the Six and Britain. London: Oxford University Press.
Fuchs, V.
  1974   Who Shall Live? Health, Economics and Social Choice. New York: Basic Books, Inc.
Fulcher, D.H.
  1973   A Study of Some Aspects of Medical Care Systems in Industrialized Countries. Geneva, Switzerland: International Labor Office

(also published as Committee Print, Subcommittee on Health, Senate Committee on Labor and Public Welfare, U.S. Congress, Washington, D.C.: Government Printing Office, 1974).

forth-   "Research of the International Labor Office into the rising costs
coming   of medical care under Social Security." In S.O. Schweitzer, ed.,
         Proceedings of the International Conference on Policies for the
         Containment of Health Care Costs and Expenditures. Fogarty
         International Center, DHEW.

Gertman, P.H., and J.B. Eagle
forth-   "Utilization review: Its potential as a mechanism for containing
coming   health care costs and expenditures." In S.O. Schweitzer, ed.,
         ibid.

Gibson, R.M., and M.S. Mueller
1977   "National health expenditures, fiscal year 1976." Social Security
         Bulletin 40 (April): 3–22.

Goldberg, L.G., and W. Greenberg
1977   "The effects of physician-controlled health insurance: U.S. v.
         Oregon State Medical Society." Journal of Health Politics, Policy
         and Law (Spring): 48–78.

Hatcher, G.H.
forth-   "Canadian utilization review programs: Their implications for
coming   containment of health care costs." In S.O. Schweitzer, ed.,
         Proceedings of the International Conference on Policies for the
         Containment of Health Care Costs and Expenditures. Fogarty
         International Center, DHEW.

Illich, I.
1976   Medical Nemesis: The Expropriation of Health. New York:
         Random House.

Intersociety Commission for Heart Disease Resources
1972   "Optimal resources for cardiac surgery, cardiac study group." In
         I.S. Wright and D.T. Fredrickson, eds., Cardiovascular Diseases:
         Guidelines for Presentation and Care. Washington, D.C.: Gov-
         ernment Printing Office.

Maronde, R.F., S. Seibert, J. Katzoff, and M. Silverman
1972   "Prescription data processing. Its role in the control of drug
         abuse." California Medicine 117 (September): 22–28.

Maxwell, R.
1975   Health Care: The Growing Dilemma. New York: McKinsey &
         Co. 2nd ed.

Newhouse, J.P.
    forth-   "Medical care expenditure: A cross-national survey." In S.O.
    coming Schweitzer, ed., Proceedings of the International Conference on
                Policies for the Containment of Health Care Costs and Expendi-
                tures. Fogarty International Center, DHEW.
Platt, K.A.
    forth-   "Utilization review programs and their role in cost contain-
    coming ment." In S.O. Schweitzer, ed., ibid.
Pole, J.D.
    1974   "Programs, priorities, and budgets." British Journal of Preven-
                tive and Social Medicine 28 (August): 191–195.
Rosch, G., and S. Sandier
    forth-   "Sharing the cost of health care." In S.O. Schweitzer, ed.,
    coming Proceedings of the International Conference on Policies for the
                Containment of Health Care Costs and Expenditures. Fogarty
                International Center, DHEW.
Smith, D.B., and A.D. Kaluzny
    1975   The White Labyrinth. Berkeley, Calif.: McCutchan Publishing
                Corporation.

The American

Hospital Association Perspective

JOHN ALEXANDER McMAHON
AND DAVID F. DRAKE

Introduction

Some months ago we were completing a paper for inclusion in the
Milbank Memorial Fund's publication, *Health: A Victim or Cause of
Inflation?* We must respectfully contend that this title provided a
more fruitful point of departure for speculation about the direction
of future public policy than does the title of this volume, *Hospital
Cost Containment: Selected Notes for Future Policy.* One of our
objectives is to demonstrate that hospitals themselves are very much
the victims, rather than the cause, of the current round of inflation in
health care costs.

Regardless of their causal relationship to inflation, hospitals have
participated in a broad variety of voluntary programs designed to
contain costs by emphasizing management solutions. Management
programs to contain costs are partially a response to the deleterious
effects of inflation on access to health care services and, in addition,
contribute to the increased efficiency of an institution's operations.
The American Hospital Association (AHA) has sponsored a variety
of programs intended to improve the management of hospitals. The
AHA has urged the creation of hospital committees on cost containment, cost effectiveness, and productivity. The staff has prepared
materials to aid these efforts, and regional discussions have been

held on the subject of cost containment. Various publications and packaged programs have been developed to assist hospitals in both cost containment and operations effectiveness. These programs emphasize methodologies that can be tailored to fit the particular needs of individual institutions. Educational institutes have emphasized departmental contributions to cost control, and management data programs have been designed and implemented to aid the evaluation of departmental and institutional performance. Budget and cost allocation programs and management systems have also been established. Research studies not only provide descriptive data, but also lay a foundation for explanation of cost variables.

Devices such as these intended to sharpen management's ability to contain costs can bring about marginal reductions in prices, depending on the situation of the individual institution. Such management-oriented programs will continue, but are likely to have only a limited impact on the rate of cost increases, because the causes of inflation are beyond the control of individual hospital managers. At most, management decisions can take into account the effects of inflation and respond to changes in price levels. The harmful *effects* of inflation can, to some extent, be minimized by good management, but it is not possible that inflation itself can be alleviated because inflation is not generated solely within hospitals. Any program intended to control the rate of inflation will be inadequate if it addresses only the hospital, and ignores the factors which stimulate and sustain the public's demands for and expectations of medical care.

Our second objective is to demonstrate, through an analysis of the nature of long-run hospital inflation, that the problems of inflation can be successfully approached only if the entire health care system or delivery network is examined for its contributions to and encouragement of inflationary tendencies. Cost-containment strategies directed exclusively at hospitals, therefore, not only are likely to fail permanently to reduce the rate of inflation in health care, but will further discredit mechanisms to control costs.

A third objective is to propose national health insurance (NHI) as a method of addressing the problems of systemic or structurally induced inflation. National health insurance represents a means of reorganizing the health care system through the introduction of a mixture of cost-related incentives and disincentives to consumers and providers alike. This paper thus represents a demurrer to the currently popular position that the enactment of NHI must await the discovery and attainment of effective controls on health care and hospital costs. We believe that the nation has postponed for too long the removal of financial barriers to health care for many of its citizens, and that a carefully constructed NHI plan may represent the only real opportunity for finding the elusive handle on health care costs.

Hospitals and Inflation—The Current Problem

In our earlier contribution to a Milbank publication, we discussed the historical development of inflationary tendencies in the hospital industry.[1] We concluded that the prices of hospital services have traditionally been susceptible to "demand-pull inflation," that is, the demand for health care services grows more quickly than the industry's ability to accumulate, without bidding up prices, the resources necessary to produce the quantity and types of services demanded. The most recent inflationary surge in these prices, however, has been of the "cost-push" variety, that is, the inflationary pressure stems from increases in the prices hospitals must pay for the resources needed to produce hospital services, not from an increase in the quantity demanded.

The situation of the hospital industry in regard to inflation can best be depicted by comparing changes in the prices hospitals must pay for nonlabor inputs with changes in the prices paid by consumers and by other industries for articles they regularly purchase. The AHA constructs annually a Nonlabor Input Price Index (NLIP), consisting of changes in the prices of products purchased by hospitals. The Consumer Price Index (CPI) is regularly issued by the Bureau of Labor Statistics and is the most frequently cited measurement of the impact of inflation on consumer purchases. The Whole-

[1] McMahon and Drake (1976); see also Drake and Raske (1974) and Feldstein (1971)

TABLE 1   A Comparison of Indices
NLIP, CPI, and WPI
1967-1975

Year	Index Values			Percent Change		
	NLIP	*CPI*	*WPI*	*NLIP*	*CPI*	*WPI*
1967	100.0	100.0	100.0	—	—	—
1968	103.6	104.2	102.5	3.6	4.2	2.5
1969	108.1	109.8	106.5	4.3	5.4	3.9
1970	114.0	116.3	110.4	5.5	5.9	3.7
1971	118.8	121.3	113.9	4.2	4.3	3.2
1972	123.5	125.3	119.1	4.0	3.3	4.6
1973	133.8	133.1	134.7	8.3	6.2	12.9
1974	157.1	147.7	160.1	17.4	11.0	18.9
1975	189.7	161.2	174.9	20.8	9.1	9.2

Sources: Bureau of Labor Statistics, Department of Labor; American Hospital Association (1976).

sale Price Index (WPI) is also compiled by the Bureau of Labor Statistics and measures changes in the prices of industrial commodities. Table 1 shows not only that the prices of hospital nonlabor inputs have increased more than consumer and wholesale prices, but also that most of the discrepancy in these rates of growth is of recent origin, specifically arising from the continuing economy-wide inflation. Much of the recent increases in hospital prices can be attributed to increases in the costs incurred by hospitals for nonlabor inputs.

Hospitals have been especially affected recently by increases in the costs of malpractice insurance, fuel, and household and maintenance costs. Almost one-sixth of the 20.8 percent increase in the NLIP in 1975 was due to rising malpractice insurance rates. In 1972, the average premium for basic hospital professional liability insurance was $20,466. By 1974, such a premium had almost doubled in price to $38,583, and during 1975, the cost mushroomed to $118,357.[2] These costs cannot be directly controlled by hospital management, yet they represent inescapable costs of maintaining hospital services.

The experience of hospitals with prices for labor inputs (wages) has been similar, with two-thirds of the inflation of the previous four

[2] Data for 1972 from Survey of Hospital Professional Liability (Malpractice) Insurance; data for 1974 and 1975 from Survey of Selected Hospital Topics. Both surveys were conducted by the Division of Information Services, American Hospital Association.

Table 2   Change in Wage Levels for Hospital and
Total Nonagricultural Workers,
by Dollars and Percent, and Change in CPI, by Percent
1971–1975

| | Average Hospitala Wage | | Total Privateb Wage | | CPI |
Year	$ Amount	% Change	$ Amount	% Change	% Change
1971	2.96	—	3.44	—	4.3
1972	3.08	4.1	3.67	6.7	3.3
1973	3.22	4.5	3.92	6.8	6.2
1974	3.45	7.1	4.22	7.7	11.0
1975	3.83	11.0	4.54	7.6	9.1
Overall increase		29.4		32.0	32.9

aHourly earnings—nonsupervisory workers.
bNonagricultural workers.
Source: Bureau of Labor Statistics, *Employment and Earnings.*

years occurring in 1974 and 1975. The wage levels for hospital workers traditionally have been somewhat lower than those for workers in other nonagricultural sectors of the economy. Despite recent increases in the rate of growth in hospital workers' wages, this differential has been maintained. Moreover, as Table 2 indicates, from 1971 to 1975, average wages for all nonagricultural workers increased more rapidly than did those for hospital workers. The rates of increase in the wages of hospital workers, in fact, failed to keep pace with the rate of inflation as measured by the CPI. In 1972 and 1973, for example, workers in most other industries had a greater chance of minimizing the effects of inflation on their standards of living because of the wage increases they received. In 1975, this situation changed as the average hourly earnings for nonsupervisory workers in hospitals increased 11 percent. The average hourly earnings of workers in all nonagricultural industries rose 7.6 percent. Over the entire period 1971–1975, the percentage increase in wages received by hospital workers was slightly lower than the overall percentage increase for all nonagricultural workers. Wages for hospital workers increased 29.4 percent during this five-year period, but increased 32.0 percent for all industrial workers. Neither group of workers was able to obtain wage increases commensurate with the 32.9 percent increase in the CPI, however.

The year 1975 was the first full year in which wage and price controls were no longer applied to the hospital industry. It is likely that the wage increases achieved then were at least in part a reaction to the prolonged period of economic controls on hospitals, and in part were a response to the historically lower wages paid to hospital workers. The present continuing round of severe inflation, during which hospital workers made considerable gains in wage levels, began after controls on the hospital industry were lifted in April 1974. Unlike prices in earlier periods of inflation in hospital services, this new set of price increases was fueled by rising prices in the rest of the economy, such as those described earlier. This is cost-push inflation, in contrast to the demand-pull inflation that has prevailed historically.

Figure 1 illustrates the relative impact of these types of inflation in 1969—a period of demand-pull inflation—and in 1975, when inflation in hospital prices was cost-push. In 1969, 65.6 percent of the increases in hospital expenses per adjusted patient day[3] was attributable to increased quantity of goods, services, and labor inputs. In 1975, inflation, or increased prices, was responsible for 73.3 percent of the increase in expenses per adjusted patient day.

Although inflation is a persistent phenomenon affecting all sectors of the economy, over the past few years hospitals have been especially severely affected by inflation because hospital purchases are concentrated in many of the commodity areas where inflation has exceeded the average rate of increase. The prices of hospital services have been increased correspondingly to cover the increased costs of providing services. In 1969, for example, expenses per adjusted patient day were $64.26, and by 1974 they were $113.21 (American Hospital Association, 1975: 4). Hospitals have been victims of inflation, but the damage sustained by them is not irreparable. Of greater concern should be the impact of inflation on access to health care.

Inflation counteracts many developments that have rendered health care more accessible to more people. As the prices of health care services rise, those members of society who are least able to afford health care are the ultimate victims. It is true that access to health care services by the aged and the poor has been improved by

[3]Adjusted patient days are an aggregate figure reflecting the number of days of inpatient care plus an estimate of the volume of outpatient services, expressed in units equivalent to an inpatient day in level of effort.

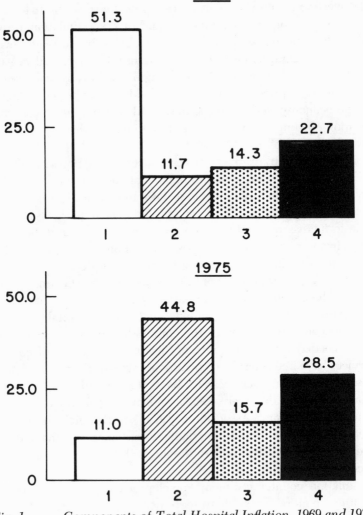

Fig. 1   *Components of Total Hospital Inflation, 1969 and 1975,*
by Percent

Key:
1—Increases in the *quantity* of goods and services purchased
2—Increases in the *cost* of goods and services purchased
3—Increases in the *quantity* of personnel employed
4—Increases in average *wages*

Source: American Hospital Association (1976).

government programs such as Medicare and Medicaid. Inflation has an indirect impact on government funding of these programs, however, because a constant level of expenditures for health care services provides a steadily diminishing amount of care. If public expenditures are increased to maintain a certain level of service, conflicts soon arise with other social programs. One result of such conflicts is that many state Medicaid programs have already been cut back (Taft, 1976). The Ford Administration sought to alter the Medicare program in its budget proposals for FY 1977 by putting a greater share of the cost of illness back onto the very groups the Medicare program was designed to relieve (see Schmeck, 1976, and Taft, 1976). Moreover, even the availability of benefits from such programs has never succeeded in completely eradicating barriers to access. As Karen Davis has written (1975: 480):

> . . . a uniform medical care financing plan has not been sufficient to guarantee equal access to medical care for all elderly persons. Those elderly population groups with the poorest health care are the lowest utilizers of medical care services under the program— the poor, blacks, and residents of the South. Furthermore, differences on the basis of income, race, and location are of sizable magnitude.

Unfortunately, intervention directed at curbing the effects of cost-push inflation cannot be limited to the health care sector alone, because this type of inflation is generated and sustained throughout the entire economy. A decision to combat cost-push inflation necessarily entails government fiscal and monetary intervention. Controls limited to the hospital industry are an inadequate response to inflation of the cost-push variety, as the experience of hospitals with the Economic Stabilization Program illustrates (Ginsburg, 1976). Controls may have postponed price increases, but the retention of controls on hospitals produced the distortions in the marketplace that we experienced in 1974 and 1975. The result was double-digit inflation in the price of hospital services, as the increased costs incurred by hospitals for the purchase of inputs were passed on to consumers and payers. Extensive economy-wide controls, like those of the ESP, distort incentives and lead managers to take a cautious stance because of the uncertainty in the administration of the controls. The development of better fiscal and monetary policies could well have a more important and wider-ranging influence on cost-push inflation than could further experimentation with wage-price controls, either at the health care sector level or at the level of the entire economy. Similarly, political settlement of some of the complex questions about social values involved in the malpractice issue could do a great deal toward reducing the inflationary effects of increasing malpractice insurance premiums.

Hospitals and Inflation—The Long-Run Problem

Even after the momentum of the current cost-push bulge has subsided, most experts agree that the basic inflationary pressures on the hospital will continue to build. Inflation in the prices of hospital and other health care services began in the post-World War II period. Rising incomes, a higher standard of living, and more comprehensive health insurance coverage for a growing proportion of the population all contributed to the growing demand for health care services. Hospitals responded to this increased demand by increasing capacity. Expenditures for hospital care and employment in hospitals became larger. The relatively steady rate of increase in hospital prices was interrupted in the late 1960s after the passage of Medicare and Medicaid (Davis, 1973). The availability of better, more comprehensive, insurance coverage for medical care stimulated demand on the part of two hitherto deprived groups, the poor and the aged. Consequently hospital prices rose sharply in the late 1960s, although the rate of increase abated by the end of the decade (Drake and Raske, 1974).

The unique system of financing health care services through various types of third-party coverage has enabled the industry to provide the sophisticated and expensive types of medical care demanded by the public and their physicians (Feldstein, 1973). Because the *net* costs of hospital care—the single most expensive component of health care costs—have been reduced for consumers through this broad third-party insurance coverage, hospitals have been able to expand their armamentarium of medical technologies.

Without such extensive coverage of otherwise prohibitively expensive care, the demand pressures for increasing health care services would not have distorted supply responses, and rising prices would have served as a rationing device as in other industries. In relation to hospital services, however, rising prices have permitted substantial increases in the intensity, sophistication, and complexity of care.

Demand-pull inflation is partially sustained by this extensive health insurance coverage. In 1950, for example, direct payments were the source of over 68 percent of personal health expenditures. Private insurance benefits covered only 8.5 percent and all forms of public payment about 20 percent of personal health expenditures (Mueller and Gibson, 1976: 17). In 1975, direct payments accounted for only 32.6 percent of personal health care expenditures, while private insurance benefits covered 26.5 percent, and all public sources covered 39.7 percent of such expenditures. Thus, by 1975, private insurers and public sources of payment purchased almost as great a share of personal health care as did direct payments twenty-five years earlier.

Not all health care services are equally covered by third-party payers, however. Hospital care is most heavily covered, with 92 percent of expenditures coming from third-party payments. Physicians' services are also fairly well covered, with 65.5 percent of total expenditures derived from third parties. Only about 15 percent of expenditures for both dentists' services and drugs and drug sundries, however, are derived from third-party payments. About 58 percent of expenditures for other health care services are also covered by third-party payments (Mueller and Gibson, 1976: 15).

Third-party payments directly affect demand because they alter the distribution of resources available for the purchase of health care services. Those types of care that are most extensively covered by insurance or are underwritten by a government program become relatively less expensive to potential consumers as financial obstacles to the receipt of care are lowered. Hospital care is the most expensive single component of health care, and now receives almost 40 percent of all health expenditures. Yet it is also the service most heavily covered by third-party payment, and thus is the service most attractive and financially accessible to consumers. Given a choice between an alternative but less expensive means of receiving care requiring direct payment, and more expensive hospital care covered by some form of third-party payment, the thrifty consumer (and his physician) will choose the latter alternative. At the same time, the availability of funds from these sources of payment and the incentives encouraging greater hospital utilization than might otherwise be required have enabled hospitals to expand the range of facilities and services they offer, including the most up-to-date and advanced technologies.

A second major contributing factor to demand-pull inflation is the unique role of the physician as a primary determiner of demand for health care services (Evans, 1974; Fuchs, 1974). Patients lack information about their illnesses and about alternative modalities of care, and physicians act as their agents in determining the need for and course of care. Physicians are trained to prescribe on the basis of the needs of each individual patient, but they also are trained in the practice of highly technological medicine (Hiatt, 1975). Because of this professional orientation toward the individual case and what Fuchs has called "the technological imperative," physicians have tended to emphasize the results of care without commensurate attention to its cost. This orientation can be seen in the way physicians care for themselves and their families. It has been found that physicians' families have substantially higher rates of surgery than comparable professional groups (Bunker and Brown, 1974).

Medicine is an applied, rather than a pure, science, because of the complexities of diagnosis and the difficulty in controlling all possible factors contributing to an illness. Hiatt (1975: 236) provides a list of once-common procedures which have now been almost abandoned because they were found to be ineffective, not because they were replaced by more adequate therapies. His list includes gastric freezing for peptic ulcer, colectomy for epilepsy, renal-capsule stripping for acute renal failure, lobotomy for mental disorders, and sympathectomy for asthma. Many accepted methods of treatment have never been tested for effectiveness, or compared with alternative forms of treatment (Cochrane, 1972). New technologies and treatments, aisde from drugs, are frequently introduced without testing or evaluation. Not only is effectiveness seldom measured, but the relative cost impact of alternative therapies is similarly ignored. If two procedures were tested and found to produce approximately the same results, that which resulted in lower costs could be encouraged. Few such studies have been undertaken, however. One result is that vast amounts of money can be and have been spent on therapies of questionable value to attain results that, if not dubious, might have been attained at less cost.

A related problem of physician practice is that of variability in the rates at which various procedures are performed. Bunker found that there were twice as many surgeons in relation to population in the United States as compared to England and Wales and that there were twice as many operations (Bunker, 1970; see also Lewis, 1969). A more recent study found that 24 percent of all recommendations for elective surgical procedures were not confirmed when second opinions were solicited (McCarthy and Widmer, 1974). Studies conducted by Wennberg and his colleagues in Vermont and Maine show that the probability of an individual's tonsils being removed ranged from 8 percent to 62 percent among various hospital service areas. Variability existed as well for other surgical procedures, ranging from 24 percent to 52 percent for removal of the uterus, 7 percent to 17 percent for removal of the appendix, and 11 percent to 31 percent for removal of the gall bladder. Hospitalization for bronchitis and upper respiratory infections varied sevenfold (Wennberg, 1976; Wennberg and Gittelsohn, 1973). Thus, in addition to the questions about the value of some types of treatment, considerable discrepancies exist in the rates at which physicians diagnose need and interpret the values of specific modes of treatment. This wide variation indicates considerable professional disagreement about the scope of need for medical and/or surgical intervention. The tendency to recommend elective surgery has implications for health care costs and for patients' health status.

Greater emphasis on peer review, second opinions, and organized group practices may provide one means for creating a professional consensus on appropriate remedies and interventions, with consequences for health care costs and quality of care. To a large extent, such variation in medical practices has been properly viewed as a professional problem. Yet the cost impact of these decisions is on the patient's hospital bill where the facilities for such intervention are housed.

Medical facilities and services reliant upon technology are usually based in hospitals because the general function of hospitals in the health care system is to organize specialized, sophisticated, and complex health care resources for patient care. Modern health care capabilities are best represented by the proliferation of specialists, and as this tendency continues, the integrating function also increases in importance. Services that might otherwise be underutilized or too expensive are affordable in hospitals because of their financial support, because of some of the coverage characteristics outlined earlier, and because of high patient volume.

As new medical technologies increase, the effect is not the more efficient performance of old tasks, but the ability to perform new ones. Innovation is almost always cost-inducing rather than cost-saving in health care because new capabilities are constantly acquired. Some self-proclaimed radical critics of highly technological medicine doubt much of its effectiveness (see Illich, 1976, and Carlson, 1975), but it seems incontestable to us that if technological medical services are to be provided at all, the most appropriate sites for them are hospitals. Not all hospitals should maintain all devices or the ability to perform any type of service, but attempts to apply technologies piecemeal in other locations will only increase inefficiency. Cost increases due to the acquisition of new technologies are likely to be contained only if new technologies are stringently tested and evaluated for their effectiveness before heavy investment is made in them and the technology has proliferated.

With health care expenditures standing at $118.5 billion in 1975 (8.3 percent of GNP), serious questions for public policy have been raised, regarding the need to make social choices among alternative resource deployments. Some have argued that health care expenditures cannot be allowed to continue to increase at their recent rates, or that expensive technologies can be extended to their capacities. Hiatt (1975: 237) cites estimates that the total cost for coronary bypass operations and diagnostic arteriograms could exceed $100 billion per year, an amount almost equivalent to total health expenditures in 1975, if some medical estimates of need were met. Another current example is that of Computerized Axial Tomography (CAT), used to produce head and body scans, a sort of three-dimensional x-ray. At least eleven firms are manufacturing these devices, and over 200 hospitals have already purchased a unit. Body scanners cost between $400,000 and $600,000, plus the costs of maintenance and personnel for staffing the machines (Downey, 1976a; Downey, 1976b; Phillips and Lille, 1976). No consensus has yet been reached on the clinical effectiveness of the body scanner, nor have comparisons been made with other techniques already available to determine the relative diagnostic improvements provided by the more expensive scanners. In short, there has been no determination of the actual benefits to be gained from these sizable investments by hospitals. Physicians collectively must begin to share with hospitals an interest in identifying costly medical procedures which can be reduced without sacrificing the quality of patient care.

As attention shifts from the need to obtain additional resources to the need to make the best use of available resources, not only must new technologies and innovations be carefully evaluated for their cost/benefit effectiveness, but existing technologies and courses of treatments should be similarly evaluated whenever possible. Increasing financial constraints require closer examination of the effectiveness of methods of treatment, but it is not certain that this will actually take place on a systematic basis unless coordinated efforts are made by all segments of the health care system. Greater overall effectiveness of the health care system may then result from efforts to contain health care costs, but a prerequisite for the success of such efforts should be determination of the specific objectives of cost containment.

Demand-pull inflation in the price of hospital services is sustained, then, by the types of choices physicians are trained to make in favoring technological applications of medicine. These decisions are supported by the public despite their cost, because of extensive third-party coverage. Technological medicine is expensive by itself, but costs are increased also by inappropriate or excessive utilization. We feel that many proposals to curb inflation in the price of hospital care are doomed to failure because they fail to address this network of factors that work to maintain a high level of demand for this type of medical care.

Objectives of Hospital Cost Containment

Given the long-run nature of demand-pull inflation in hospital costs, how can a specific policy or policies for containing hospital costs be developed? Frequently, the policy goal is stated in terms of reducing the percentage rate of increases in hospital costs. Should the goal be containment of total hospital costs or expenditures, the costs of units of hospital service, such as per diem or per case costs, or some other measure of relative hospital costs, such as hospitals' share of the Gross National Product or even of total health expenditures? Each of these variables has, at least implicitly, been suggested as the one to minimize in various cost control proposals and there are problems with each as a reasonable goal for public policy.

For example, the goal of minimizing the rate of increase in total hospital costs or expenditures because these are the single costliest component of health care fails to recognize that hospitals provide forms of care other than high-cost, high-technology inpatient acute care. Indeed, the fastest growing hospital service is ambulatory (and presumably, primary) care provided in hospital outpatient clinics and emergency rooms. Between 1965 and 1975, for example, outpatient visits in the nation's community hospitals increased five times more than did inpatient days.[4] Any cost control program directed at total hospital expenditures must recognize that, because ambulatory care is inadequately covered under the current health insurance arrangements, ambulatory care is the first activity that hospitals must curtail when faced with severe financial constraints. The recent New York City financing crisis has vividly illustrated this dilemma.

In addition to the outpatient problem that is ignored in a total expenditure limitation approach, the financial arrangements be-

[4]Calculated from National Hospital Panel Survey Data.

tween the hospital and its medical staff can cause distortions in this overall control approach. Those hospitals that have, or more importantly add, salaried physicians to their medical staffs will report a substantial increase in the level of total hospital expenditures. Cross-national comparisons indicate that there is considerable variation in the share of health expenditures allocated to hospitals in Western industrial nations. Much of this variation stems from the inclusion or exclusion of hospital-based physician services as a component of hospital expenditures. In West Germany, hospital expenditures constituted only 29 percent of total health spending in 1970, as opposed to the nearly 40 percent share in the United States. At the opposite extreme were England and Wales, where the National Health Service allocated 60 percent of its health expenditures for hospitals. France and the Netherlands, on the other hand, each spent about half of their health dollar on hospital services.[5] Until there is greater consensus on the optimum resource allocation and organization of care that defines the appropriate portion and role for the hospital, it would be extremely unwise to set as a goal for hospital cost containment the minimization of the rate of increase in total hospital expenditures or, for that matter, of the relative share of total hospital expenditures in the GNP or in the health care dollar.

In a similar way, the minimization of hospital unit costs as a possible policy goal can be distortive. If we are successful in reducing the use of inpatient hospitalization for dealing with less acute kinds of illness, then we would expect that the remaining patients in hospitals would be acutely ill. Care for these patients would obviously, on a unit basis, be more expensive.

Attempts merely to restrict the amount of money spent on hospital care represent a desire to treat the symptoms of inflation rather than the underlying causes. Limits or caps on the amounts of resources allocated to hospitals simply do not address the problem of providing alternative sources of care to inpatient hospitalization. The appropriate public policy concern is not just to minimize costs or the rate of inflation but to do so without significantly impairing the quality of care available to consumers.

[5] Data from a telephone conversation with Joseph G. Simanis, Office of Research and Statistics, Social Security Administration, July 7, 1976. See also Simanis (1973).

A more appropriate public policy goal than simply limiting the rate of increase in hospital costs is to provide incentives for less costly alternatives to inpatient hospitalization without sacrificing the integrating and coordinating function of the hospital. Such a sacrifice might have to be made if flat and arbitrary limits were imposed on hospital expenditures or unit costs. Recent studies have directed attention to the importance of the organization of medical practice in increasing efficiency and lowering rates of hospitalization (Gaus, et al., 1976; Ellwood, 1976). Physician participation in a group practice, regardless of the type of payment mechanism in effect, and membership on a hospital medical staff are conducive to the development of peer review, coordinated care, better use of resources, and easier access to a broad range of physician services.

If greater organization and rationalization increase the efficiency of physicians' performance, it is quite likely that the efficiency of a health care system in which choices are predominantly made by physicians could also be improved by greater organization. Improved organization should not only include physicians, but also other providers of health care services. The institution best suited by its present role to perform these organizational functions is the hospital. It already deals with similar problems, although on a restricted scale. In order to deal adequately with the inseparable problems of rising costs, especially for inpatient care, and of quality of care, hospitals would have to expand the range of services they provide beyond care for acute illnesses requiring inpatient care. We endorse Freymann's concept (1974) of the "mission-oriented hospital," which not only consists of the traditional facilities and staff, but integrates them with a complex network of interrelated, organized capabilities for providing the whole range of health care services. These include care of the chronically ill, long-term care, home care, nursing home care, outpatient treatment centers, maternity units, and facilities for the terminally ill. Frequently, care of comparable quality can be rendered more efficiently outside the hospital as it is presently constituted. When this is the case, the alternative methods of care should be encouraged. An example is home-based renal dialysis, which can be provided at about one-third the cost of dialysis provided in hospitals (Iglehart, 1976). Alternative means of delivering such services should be welcomed by hospitals because they free resources for other uses. Hospitals themselves should explore the alternatives with regard to both their cost efficiency and their effectiveness and quality.

Experiments and extra-hospital programs will probably operate best when provided in a concentrated and coordinated manner in each community, because each represents a fairly specialized use of resources and manpower that are not readily interchangeable. Isolated or individual units or organizations attempting to provide a similar range and variety of services would be likely to be costly and duplicative. Also, as specialization increases, the need for coordination among specialized units increases. Without it, patients would be unable to receive the appropriate types of care required as their conditions change.

Within a revamped system emphasizing the "mission-oriented hospital," concern would be directed not at hospitals' share of total expenditures or of GNP, but at the ratio of benefits from increased expenditures to their costs. Reorganization of the health care system emphasizing the hospital as an instrument of coordination and integration for a wide variety of services rather than as a site for inpatient care would do away with the issue of the appropriate level of hospital expenditures, because the inflationary inpatient care sector could be reduced in a system making use of complementary methods of care. The problem then becomes one of designing sufficiently attractive incentives to bring about (1) the coordination of services presently provided independently of hospitals; (2) the expansion of hospital responsibilities to encompass a wide range of provider roles beyond inpatient care; (3) the alteration of third-party payment mechanisms to cover sources of care other than inpatient hospital care; and (4) the encouragement of physicians to make use of a variety of coordinated treatment methods rather than to rely so heavily on highly technological diagnostic and therapy regimens.

NHI and Cost Containment

Our analysis of the long-run problem of inflation in the prices of hospital services has emphasized the interrelationship between the preference of physicians for medical treatment dependent on technology and the system of third-party payment which has skewed insurance benefits heavily in the direction of inpatient hospital services. Thus, the most expensive types of health care have been made most accessible to the consumer fortunate enough to be covered by health insurance, while physicians have not been encouraged to explore alternatives to expensive forms of hospital-based care.

We feel that the urgently required changes in the scope of medical insurance benefits and in the delivery system cannot be dealt with in isolation from the issue of equity of access. Policies designed primarily to contain costs are likely to have an unfavorable impact on access, while policies intended to facilitate access alone are likely to be simply more inflationary.

Despite anticipated short-run increases in demand, such as those which followed the inauguration of the Medicare program, we contend that universal, governmentally mandated health insurance provides the only public policy framework sufficiently comprehensive to restructure those components of the health care delivery system that especially support demand-pull inflation. The AHA has long maintained that national health insurance should not simply channel additional funds into a delivery system that remains essentially unchanged. The infusion of these funds should be made conditional on the adoption of structural reforms by providers of health care services. The intentions of these reforms should be specifically mentioned in the NHI statute, although compliance should be initially encouraged through the offering of incentives rather than by the imposition of penalties and sanctions. Providers of health care services should be offered a variety of means to comply with the statutory intent as well, in order to preserve managerial discretion in dealing with particular institutional circumstances.

The salient part of any NHI program will be its schedule of benefits, and the most significant aspect of the benefits will be their contribution to improving access to health care for those currently unable to afford such care. If an NHI plan were to fail to improve access while it successfully contained the rate of inflation, it would ultimately be evaluated as failing to secure its major objectives. Because increased insurance coverage expands utilization and the amounts of resources required to meet greater demand, there is a strong temptation to build into NHI programs devices intended to curb or restrict increased utilization, such as limited benefits or required copayments (McClure, 1975). This curtailment, however, reduces the protection the plan can give, especially to the poor, who are unlikely to be able to afford sufficient care otherwise, and who also may have greater health care needs. Therefore, benefits under NHI must be carefully designed because the potential for conflict between the desire to restrain prices and the desire to improve access is greatest here. It has been proposed that benefits be partially geared to income, to maximize protection for those least able to afford medical care and to minimize the inflationary impact of this protection. Deductibles, copayments, and limits on total out-of-pocket expenditures during a year could all be related to the income of a consumer. Those better able to afford care would be liable for a greater share of their costs, while those with smaller incomes would have a greater proportion of their expenses covered (Donabedian, 1976). A health card mechanism could be established for the collection of these variable copayments.

The determination of the extent of NHI benefits cannot be divorced from consideration of the effect on the system of providers delivering the covered services. Experience with private health insurance plans has driven home this lesson. The present system of benefits provides extensive coverage (and thus incentives) for inpatient hospital care but little coverage for outpatient, long-term, or nursing home care. If NHI benefits are fairly comprehensive and cover a full range of alternate methods of care, one of the artificially imposed causes of inflation in the present health insurance system would be removed, along with the stimulus for overutilization of inpatient hospital care.

Such NHI-mandated financial support for and encouragement of specialized services to supplement traditional inpatient care would be likely to stimulate growth and investment in these services. The primary purpose of such innovations is not simply to shift patients from expensive to less expensive facilities. This would be only one desirable consequence of improved organization within the health care system, intended to maximize the overall amount of care provided in *organized* settings.

We have contended that hospitals, because of their central role in providing health care services to their communities and their historical development, are especially suited to provide this organization. NHI, however, must not go so far as to attempt to mandate centralization of all health care services. Other organizations, such as medical care foundations, health maintenance organizations, and multispecialty group practices, should also be encouraged to participate in integrating and coordinating the health care delivery system. What an NHI plan might encourage through its benefit structure would be growth in the number of group practices of physicians and dentists. This could be done by designing special insurance benefits to cover services provided in these settings, or by covering them more fully than services received from unorganized providers. The provider organization, rather than the delivery site, would then be the requirement for services to be covered by insurance. Hospitals would be only one of several locations at which care covered by insurance would be provided.

Any NHI program should integrate existing regulatory devices intended to contain costs and reduce reliance on uneconomic technology, while monitoring quality. Providing incentives for group practices alone will be insufficient to bring about a reduction in overutilization of expensive sources of care and the full consideration of less expensive alternatives. Health Systems Agencies (HSAs) and Professional Standards Review Organizations (PSROs) have been created across the country for purposes of planning and quality review. These methods of regulation and planning are mandated by federal law, but represent an important departure from previous regulatory policy in the health care sector because they are intended to operate on the local level with guidance from the state and national levels. Dispersal of regulatory authority among a fairly large number of such agencies may be especially important under an NHI plan, but a federal-state regulatory framework should be established to coordinate these decentralized activities. As the federal government becomes increasingly important in creating health insurance benefits, even if it acts through private health insurance carriers, conflicts may develop between government's roles as regulator and as guarantor of benefits for lower income groups, the aged, the disabled, and the unemployed. The separation of government's roles as purchaser and as regulator should be built into the design of an NHI program and the regulatory function decentralized as much as possible.

A deliberate research and development program is an essential feature for NHI. Biomedical research and development may remain relatively unaffected by the transition to NHI because the need for it will continue. General health services research and development should increase markedly in importance, both because there will be a greater need to monitor the costs of care, and because the greater need for coordination in a more unified and tightly organized system will generate a need for feedback information (Wennberg, 1976). Adequate funding for research and development is necessary in order that the new technologies be applied appropriately. The intent should not be to freeze medical technology at its current level or to return to a simpler era, but to apply technology only as it provides positive benefits when compared to alternative therapies at equal or reduced costs. The research and development can be conducted at the level of the individual institution and at the system level, but should be financed as an integral part of the NHI program.

Conclusions

We have contended that the issue of hospital cost containment cannot be successfully approached by means of public policy in isolation from the network of factors that have influenced decisions about the provision of health care over the last thirty years. The system for the delivery of health care is composed of a variety of providers and payment mechanisms, but for policy purposes these institutions are not independent, discrete units. Economic and other incentives have skewed the organization of these components so that sophisticated technologies have been emphasized for treatment of acute illness. Other nonacute health problems have been incompletely recognized by the system because they are less susceptible to these sophisticated medical interventions.

For these reasons we have advocated that public policy responses to the issue of hospital cost containment examine the system of incentives that has made the prices of hospital care prone to inflation. A national health insurance program, we feel, is not only a means for expanding access to care while introducing incentives to redeploy resources for the provision of less costly types of care, but is the only alternative which would not actually imperil the provision of health care services by inappropriate types of controls. Other proposed remedies address only isolated components of the system, such as hospitals, without addressing the reasons for the price increases manifested in those components.

Embarkation on a public policy course of cost containment in the health care field should not be carried to the extreme of repudiating the commitments represented by past national policy— governmental *and* private—to better health care and expanded access. Past health programs, it is now generally conceded, were not designed with cost considerations foremost, but with emphasis primarily on expansion of access, of quality, of manpower, and of facilities. These were program-design flaws, in that the anticipated costs and benefits were not gauged, and in that close monitoring of programs was not often mandated. Yet we believe that lessons can be absorbed by policy makers from these experiences and that trade-offs are not demanded between cost consciousness intended to hold down inflation and the desire to provide good quality health care to all citizens. A national health insurance program should include from the outset a range of services broader than those covered by current health insurance plans to ensure the efficient utilization of health care facilities based on medical suitability rather than on financial accessibility. Contributions by individuals toward the cost of care in proportion to their ability to pay will serve as an inducement for proper utilization of health care services and help defray the cost of care to the public.

Public policy attention to inflation should properly be a concern in all social welfare programs and in all phases of governmental operation. It should never be allowed to become the sole or predominant policy goal of any program, nor should concern about the impact of inflation be made the excuse for postponing badly needed reforms of the health care delivery system. A focus on inflation and the distortions it produces in the economy cannot justify the politically popular step of initiating anti-inflation programs that satisfy political demands but do little either to remove the causes of inflation or to improve the delivery of services.

References and Acknowledgment

The authors wish to thank David M. Kozak, Policy Analyst, Office of Program and Policy Development, for his assistance in the preparation of this chapter.

American Hospital Association
- 1975   Hospital Statistics. 1975 Edition. Chicago: American Hospital Association.
- 1976   The Hospital Economy. Division of Information Services.

Bunker, J.P.
- 1970   "Surgical manpower: A comparison of operations and surgeons in the United States and in England and Wales." The New England Journal of Medicine 282 (January): 135–143.

Bunker, J.P., and B.W. Brown, Jr.
- 1974   "The physician-patient as an informed consumer of surgical services." The New England Journal of Medicine 290 (May): 1051–1055.

Carlson, R.J.
- 1975   The End of Medicine. New York: John Wiley & Sons.

Cochrane, A.L.
- 1972   Effectiveness and Efficiency: Random Reflections on Health Services. London: The Nuffield Provincial Hospitals Trust.

Davis, K.
- 1973   "Hospital costs and the Medicare program." Social Security Bulletin 36 (August): 18–36.

1975 "Equal treatment and unequal benefits: The Medicare program." Milbank Memorial Fund Quarterly/Health and Society (Fall): 449–488.

Donabedian, A.
1976 "Issues in national health insurance." American Journal of Public Health 66 (April): 345–350.

Downey, G.W.
1976a "A scanner for every hospital?" Modern Healthcare (February): 16S–16X.

1976b "Cat fever." The New England Journal of Medicine (April 22): 954–956.

Drake, D.F., and K.E. Raske
1974 "The changing hospital economy." Hospitals, Journal of the American Hospital Association 48 (November 16): 34–40.

Ellwood, P.M., Jr.
1976 "Health delivery in transition: from group practice to HMO to multigroups." Statement before Congress of the United States, House of Representatives, Subcommittee on Health and Environment (February 10).

Evans, R.G.
1974 "Supplier-induced demand: Some empirical evidence and implications." Pp. 162–173 in Mark Perlman, ed., The Economics of Health and Medical Care. New York: John Wiley & Sons, Inc.

Feldstein, M.S.
1971 The Rising Cost of Hospital Care. Washington, D.C.: Information Resources Press.

1973 "The medical economy." Scientific American 229 (September): 151.

Freymann, J.G.
1974 The American Health Care System: Its Genesis and Trajectory. New York: Medcom Press.

Fuchs, V.
1974 Who Shall Live? Health, Economics and Social Choice. New York: Basic Books, Inc.

Gaus, C.R., B.S. Cooper, and C.G. Hirschman
1976 "Contrasts in HMO and fee-for-service performance." Social Security Bulletin 39 (May): 3–14.

Ginsburg, P.B.
1976 "Inflation and the economic stabilization program." Pp. 31–51 in

Michael Zubkoff, ed., Health: A Victim or Cause of Inflation?
New York: Prodist for Milbank Memorial Fund.

Hiatt, H.A.
1975   "Protecting the medical commons: Who is responsible?" The
        New England Journal of Medicine 293 (July 31): 235–241.

Iglehart, J.K.
1976   "Kidney treatment problem readies HEW for national health
        insurance." National Journal 8 (June 26): 895–900.

Illich, I.
1976   Medical Nemesis: The Expropriation of Health. New York:
   .   Random House.

Lewis, C.E.
1969   "Variations in the incidence of surgery." The New England
        Journal of Medicine 281 (October 16): 880–884.

McCarthy, E.G., and G.W. Widmer
1974   "Effects of screening by consultants on recommended elective
        surgical procedures." The New England Journal of Medicine 291
        (December 19): 1331–1335.

McClure, W.
1975   "The medical care system under national health insurance: Four
        models that might work and their prospects." Paper presented to
        the American Political Science Association, Panel on National
        Health Insurance, September 2. San Francisco, California.

McMahon, J.A., and D.F. Drake
1976   "Inflation and the hospital." Pp. 130–148 in Michael Zubkoff, ed.,
        Health: A Victim or Cause of Inflation? New York: Prodist for
        Milbank Memorial Fund.

Mueller, M.S., and R.M. Gibson
1976   "National health expenditures, fiscal year 1975." Social Security
        Bulletin 39 (February): 3–21.

Phillips, D.F., and K. Lille
1976   "Putting the leash on 'CAT'." Hospitals, Journal of the American
        Hospital Association 50 (July 1): 45–49.

Schmeck, H.M., Jr.
1976   "Limiting the cost of major illness would benefit three million
        patients." The New York Times (January 22).

Simanis, J.G.
1973   "Medical care expenditures in seven countries." Social Security
        Bulletin (March): 39–42.

Taft, J.
  1976   "States put scalpel to Medicaid in budget-cutting operation."
          National Journal 8 (May 1): 581–586.
Wennberg, J.E.
  1976   "National health planning goals." Unpublished manuscript
          (March).
Wennberg, J.E., and A. Gittelsohn
  1973   "Small area variations in health care delivery." Science 182
          (December 14): 1102–1108.

The Consumer's Perspective

MARY LEE INGBAR

In the complex market for health care, what do consumers really want to buy? What factors affect their choice? If consumers are more interested in matters of access and equity than in questions of price of service and cost of care, then obviously their interest in containing the costs of medical care will be minimal. Or if, as in buying objects of art, consumers equate higher fees and larger costs with greater value and finer quality, then medical care becomes a "luxury good" and interest in controlling costs of health services will again be minimal.

To deal with these questions, it is first necessary to view the consumer as a *buyer* of service, to discuss the factors influencing demand, and to consider the part price plays. In the health industry, however, this is no simple matter, for the buyer may not be the patient himself, but may be the subscriber or taxpayer who has purchased care in advance, on a contingency basis, or on behalf of others. Furthermore, in paying for services, this buyer no longer acts in isolation, but increasingly negotiates through a corporate entity, public or private. Thus, with the advent of the large third party as the force that mediates demand and pays the bill, the role of the buyer has shifted both in strength and in function.

In this new role, the buyer is increasingly interested in the terms of sale more broadly defined to include not only the prices that the producer charges or the costs that must be paid in the marketplace, but also the quantitative and qualitative aspects of the services that are to be acquired. As a consequence of this broadened concern, the consumer, as represented by employer-employee health programs, third-party carriers, and government programs like Medicare and Medicaid, has increasingly sought to control the product, its producers, and its manner of production. The advent of the institutional buyer has thus provided the consumer with a vehicle through which to become the *regulator*. It is therefore necessary to examine the effectiveness of the consumer in the regulatory role and his success in this capacity in containing the costs of health care.

Finally, as a logical extension of the role of the regulator, there is a need to deal with the problems of the health industry on a prospective rather than on an ex post facto basis. In addition, the emergence of the institutional buyer has created a need to restore strength to individual consumers through the development of planning processes in which such persons will predominate. Consequently, evolving trends are assigning another new role to the consumer, that of *planner*.

The Consumer as Buyer

In order to understand the role of cost containment in the acquisition of medical care, it is necessary to disentangle the complex web of factors that determine the demand for health services. Some of these factors concern the nature of the medical, surgical, or psychological conditions to be treated and the definition of the results to be obtained. Some reflect the sociodemographic characteristics of patients and populations at risk and their expectations about the care they should or will receive. And some involve price, when price is broadly defined to encompass both the monetary and nonmonetary sacrifices that the consumer will incur in seeking care. In the last fifteen years, several econometric studies have sharpened understanding of the effect of these major factors upon the demand for medical care, particularly that for hospital services (see especially Feldstein, 1973, 1976b, and Rosenthal, 1976). The findings of these investigations enable more precise predictions to be made of the effect of incremental shifts in price and of changes in the sociodemographic characteristics of populations at risk. They are obviously not designed to illuminate the dynamics of human behavior at the micro level. For these purposes, it is helpful to review some of the data concerning morbidity and mortality and the epidemiology of disease that underlie consumer behavior in the health field.

Need and Demand—The Problem of Urgency and Range of Consumer Choice

Medical care is currently used by most Americans. In contrast to the early 1960s, when significant proportions of households were reported to have had no medical expenditures (see Huang, 1970; Andersen et al., 1972, 1973), today most of the population expends funds for health care. In fiscal year 1974, apart from premiums paid, only about 15 percent of unrelated individuals and about 7 percent of family units reported no annual out-of-pocket health-related expenses (Wilder, 1975b).

More generally, data for 1974 from the Health Interview Survey conducted by the National Center for Health Statistics indicate that the civilian noninstitutionalized population of the United States experienced about 365 million acute conditions, an incidence rate of 175.7 acute conditions per 100 persons (refer to Table 1). As defined in the Health Interview Survey (Ries, 1975; Wilder, 1975a), these acute conditions are illnesses and injuries of less than three months' duration for which the person either sought medical attention or experienced one or more days of restricted activity.

How much of this utilization of health services ("effective demand") reflects an elective purchase of services by the consumer and how much results from pressured necessity? How much of what the consumer perceives as need for service is in accord with what professionals would perceive? How much stems from the presence of disability and illness, and how much from a desire to maintain health and receive preventive services? How much will this utilization vary with the stage of illness? In other words, to what extent is the consumer able to exercise choice in purchasing health service? And when choice is possible from the medical point of view, will the consumer couple this ability to "elect" service with the power it affords to "bargain" over the costs of care? And if the consumer

**TABLE 1   Incidence of Acute Conditions, Associated Disability
Days, and Persons Injured; Days of Disability;
Limitation of Activity, United States, 1974**

	Number of acute conditions per 100 persons per year
All acute conditions	175.7
Infective and parasitic diseases	19.5
Respiratory conditions	94.4
Upper respiratory conditions	45.8
Influenza	44.8
Other respiratory conditions	3.9
Digestive system conditions	7.8
Injuries	30.4
All other acute conditions	23.5

Days of disability associated with acute conditions	*Days of disability per 100 persons per year*
Restricted activity days	937.7
Bed days	413.0
Work-loss days (ages 17 and over)	
for currently employed population	339.3
School-loss days (ages 6–16 years)	485.9

	Number of persons injured per 100 persons per year
All classes of accident	28.5
Moving motor vehicle	2.1
While at work	4.5
Home	10.3
Other	12.7

Days of disability	*Days of disability per person per year*
Restricted activity days	17.2
Bed days	6.7
Work-loss days (ages 17 years and over)	
for currently employed population	4.9
School-loss days (ages 6–16 years)	5.6

Limitation of activity due to chronic conditions	*Percent of total population*
Limited in all activity	14.1
Limited in major activity	10.6
No limitation of activity	85.9

Source: Ries (1975:2–3).

exerts pressure, will this be applied by directly negotiating over
price or by influencing the amount and type of service to seek and
by selecting from whom and when this care will be received?

The range of choice that the patient might have in acquiring
medical care depends not only upon his perception that something is
wrong, but also upon its apparent urgency and severity. This

evaluation, particularly as regards the appropriate source of care and the speed with which assistance should be sought, need not correspond with the evaluation of professionals. Situations that are painful may not be serious, whereas those without bothersome symptoms may be serious or fatal. In addition to deciding initially whether and when to enter the health care system, the patient must then decide whether to comply with instructions and whether to complete follow-up appointments with the same provider or with others to whom he has been referred. When preventive services, routine evaluations, and dental check-ups are involved, the patient obviously has more time both to explore his possible options and to exercise them in acquiring medical care.

Table 2 presents the principal diagnoses for which ambulatory patients visited their doctors. Nearly one out of five visits are for special conditions and examinations without sickness (17.8 percent) and approximately one out of four visits are either for diseases of the respiratory system (14.1 percent) or diseases of the circulatory system (9.9 percent).

Visits to office-based physicians may also be described in terms of patient problems (DeLozier and Gagnon, 1975: Table 9). Twenty percent of all visits are accounted for by progress visits, pregnancy, and general physical and gynecological examinations. Such scheduled visits together with throat soreness, cold, headache, fatigue, medication visits, and problems of the back and of the lower and upper extremities constitute the fifteen problems accounting for 50 percent of all visits.

Severity and urgency of presenting problems are also evaluated directly as part of the National Ambulatory Medical Care Survey. DeLozier and Gagnon reported that 20 percent of all visits were for problems deemed to be more than slightly serious, but only 3.2 percent were for problems identified as very serious by the physician (refer to Table 3). On the other hand, approximately 50 percent of the visits were for problems that were not serious. Thus, in the majority of their encounters with the health professionals, ambulatory patients are not limited in choosing among alternative sources of care because of the seriousness or urgency of their presenting complaints. At least in theory, they can "bargain" over the terms of

**TABLE 2   Number and Percent Distribution of Office
Visits by Principal Diagnoses, United States,
January–December 1975**

Principal diagnoses classified by major ICDA group (coded) [a]		Number of visits in 1,000's	Percent distribution of visits
All principal diagnoses		567,600	100.0
Infective and parasitic diseases	000–136	22,747	4.0
Neoplasms	140–239	13,332	2.4
Endocrine, nutritional and metabolic diseases	240–279	24,177	4.3
Diseases of the blood and blood-forming organs	280–289	4,744	0.8
Mental disorders	290–315	25,061	4.4
Diseases of the nervous system and sense organs	320–389	44,941	7.9
Diseases of the circulatory system	390–458	56,358	9.9
Diseases of the respiratory system	460–519	80,125	14.1
Diseases of the digestive system	520–577	20,061	3.5
Diseases of the genitourinary system	580–629	37,626	6.6
Diseases of the skin and subcutaneous tissue	680–709	28,564	5.0
Diseases of the musculoskeletal system	710–738	32,732	5.8
Symptoms and ill-defined conditions	780–796	26,177	4.6
Accidents, poisoning and violence	800–999	40,893	7.2
Special conditions and examinations without sickness	Y00–Y13	100,787	17.8
Other diagnoses [b]		3,312	0.6
Diagnosis "none" or unknown [c]		5,963	1.1

[a] Diagnostic groupings and code number inclusions are based on the *Eighth Revision,
International Classification of Diseases, Adapted for Use in the United States*, 1965.
[b] Complications of pregnancy, childbirth, and the puerperium; congenital anomalies; and
certain causes of perinatal morbidity and mortality.
[c] Includes blank, noncodeable, and illegible diagnoses.
Source: Koch and Dennison (1977:8).

acquisition of service, particularly for the nearly 20 percent of the encounters that involve nonsymptomatic conditions.

These data do not, of course, attempt to evaluate the appropriateness of utilization from the provider's point of view, that is in terms of medical need. Likewise, they do not include estimates of the extent to which patients seek advice from different providers in order to verify diagnoses and recommendations for treatment. In an early study of this problem in the hospital setting, Solon and his colleagues (1960) reported that among patients using the outpatient clinics at Beth Israel Hospital, Boston, nearly one-half had been to at least one other clinic of a teaching hospital in the area. To some

**TABLE 3   Number and Percent Distribution of Office Visits
by Seriousness of Patient's Principal Problem,
According to Sex, Color, and Age of Patient
and According to Physician Specialty and Type of Practice
United States, May 1973–April 1974**

Sex, color, and age	Number of visits in thousands	Seriousness of patient's principal problem (percent distribution)			
		Very serious	Serious	Slightly serious	Not serious
All patients	644,893	3.2	16.0	30.4	50.5
Sex					
Male	253,285	3.8	18.1	31.9	46.2
Female	391,608	2.8	14.6	29.4	53.2
Color					
White	575,881	3.1	15.7	30.5	50.6
All other	69,013	3.3	18.2	29.5	49.0
Age					
Under 15 years	125,077	1.5	10.2	29.4	58.9
15–24 years	99,581	1.7	10.7	26.0	61.6
25–44 years	159,551	2.7	14.0	29.4	54.0
45–64 years	160,435	3.9	20.1	32.2	43.9
65 years and over	100,249	6.3	25.1	34.7	33.9
Physician specialty and type of practice					
All specialties	644,893	3.2	16.0	30.4	50.5
General and family practice	260,310	2.3	15.3	32.2	50.1
Medical specialties	169,316	3.6	17.1	32.7	46.6
Internal medicine	74,693	5.1	23.4	33.0	38.5
Pediatrics	53,659	*	7.4	29.9	61.9
Other	40,964	4.8	18.3	35.6	41.3
Surgical specialties	183,787	2.6	13.0	25.4	59.0
General surgery	44,846	3.8	14.7	28.8	52.7
Obstetrics and gynecology	50,715	*	4.1	15.0	80.1
Other	88,227	3.2	17.1	29.6	50.1
Other specialties	31,481	10.5	33.2	32.0	24.3
Psychiatry	20,300	14.9	42.2	28.1	14.9
Other	11,180	*	17.0	39.0	41.4
Type of practice					
Solo	386,208	3.1	16.3	30.3	50.3
Other[a]	258,685	3.3	15.5	30.4	50.8

[a] Includes partnership and group practices.
Source: DeLozier and Gagnon (1975:36–37).

extent, this duplication of services may be wasteful of resources as in
the treatment of what Morris Collen has referred to as the "worried"
well or in what Clifton Meador has called "the art and science of
diagnosing nondisease."

But also this search for confirmation of diagnoses and treatment patterns is an important attribute of the "prudent" buyer that should be encouraged, especially when it results in the avoidance of expensive inpatient procedures. Indeed, some employer-employee health programs and Blue Cross plans have begun introducing coverage for a second medical opinion as either a voluntary or mandatory requirement for covering the cost of specified elective surgical and medical procedures (see Executive Office of the President, 1976a, b, 1977).

For inpatient services, however, the situation is different. Traditional methods of describing illness (see Moien, 1975:4, 5) do not identify urgency and severity of the conditions. Even when patients are not suffering from multiple ailments, the principal diagnoses as defined in terms of the International Classification of Diseases may be insufficient to determine what resources are appropriate and how urgently they are needed, although Rafferty (1971:157) has identified six diagnoses for which hospitalization appears to be at least somewhat discretionary in that admissions decline as the level of occupancy rises. Moreover, 43 percent of the discharges in 1972 involved two or more final diagnoses with an average for all patients discharged of 1.8 diagnoses (Moien, 1975). Finally, an accumulation of seemingly minor conditions may seriously impair the mobility of some patients, such as the elderly, and prevent these persons from seeking care on an ambulatory basis (see Hershey et al., 1975). Consequently, choices in terms of when and where to receive care may be constrained, for reasons that may not appear to relate to the diagnostic condition of the patient.

Nevertheless, some information is available concerning the severity and urgency of the conditions that result in the hospitalization of patients. Whereas the data presented in Table 1 indicate that accidents constitute the cause of approximately 16 percent of all acute conditions reported in 1974, Moien's data indicate that fractures, lacerations, and open wound injuries accounted for nearly 5 percent of the hospital discharges. Complications of pregnancy, childbirth, and the puerperium accounted for nearly another 13 percent of the discharges. In addition a major share of the discharges for heart and cardiovascular disease and for diseases of the respiratory system may also involve the need for immediate hospitalization.

In addition to national data concerning diagnosis, a number of studies have involved detailed analyses of a sample of patients. For example, Kravits and Schneider (1975:179) note that only 11 percent of the surgical procedures involved discretionary admissions once surgery had been decided upon, as compared with 17 percent of the medical admissions (exclusive of the 23 percent for diagnostic purposes). In studying the matter further, Kravits and Schneider (p. 180) found that in a sample of 676 surgical procedures, elective surgery constituted 19.5 percent of the 6.1 procedures per 100 persons per year.

In short, the limited data available concerning reasons for hospitalization suggest that urgency will be more important in these cases than in those treated on an ambulatory basis. This is to be expected. However, these data do not provide precise information concerning the speed with which care must be sought; yet it is this timing that determines the range of facilities and services from which the consumer (or the physician acting in the role of agent for the patient) might seek care. These data also fail to take account of the shift that may occur in the level of urgency between the time of admission and the establishment of the discharge diagnosis; yet it is the admission rather than the discharge diagnosis that determines urgency as viewed initially by patient and physician. Furthermore, were data available concerning the urgency and severity with which conditions must be treated, they would be incomplete without corresponding information concerning the interrelationships between the location of patients and the placement of the resources required to care for their health needs. Fortunately, the fundamental notions of analyzing systems of medical care in terms of their spatial and time relationships are receiving increasing attention (see Ingbar, 1977; Shannon and Dever, 1974; Fox and Fox, 1974; Weiss et al., 1971; and Bosanac et al., 1976).

Assuming that a need for care has been perceived by the consumer, action may not be taken because of lack of information concerning whom to consult in order to obtain service. That neighbors and friends act as advisers in the selection of sources of care attests to the importance of personal information in determining what people do (see Aday and Andersen, 1975:170). The growth in the use of hospitals as a source of outpatient and emergency care also demonstrates the importance of ease of access. The special problem of access to emergency services is explicitly recognized under the new federal programs designed to encourage the development of emergency medical services.

Personal relationships may also serve to constrain consideration of alternatives. Strong allegiance to a particular physician, provider group, or institutional setting may blunt choices. Patients may fear questioning those individuals to whom they regularly turn for assistance lest these questions be viewed as an affront jeopardizing future care. In addition, choosing may have cumulative effects in that selection of a particular doctor may affect the range of choice for hospitals, laboratories, radiology services, and other specialized facilities and services.

There are also subtle attitudinal factors that may influence a patient's willingness to seek treatment and choose sources of care. Among patients with similar symptoms, differences in perceived threats of illness and in beliefs in the efficacy of treatment may determine both how much medical care will be utilized (Kirscht et al., 1976) and where this service will be received. There is increased recognition of the importance of internal psychological factors as well as external factors relating to the social and educational environment (Mechanic, 1972). These influence an individual's perception of health and utilization of services. McKinlay and Dutton (1974) identify the concept of readiness to initiate physician care in terms of a model developed by Hochbaum that involves perceived seriousness of the disease, perceived vulnerability to the disease, and perceived efficacy of medical treatment. The effect of social class on these perceptions is also reviewed by McKinlay and Dutton.

In short, although the process of entering the medical care system is complex, most people in the United States do participate. Once a person is admitted either as an ambulatory or as a hospitalized patient, the odds are better than even that continued care will be obtained. For patients receiving service on an ambulatory basis, probably less than one-third of the encounters involve conditions requiring immediate attention. On the other hand, probably close to one-half of the encounters relate to problems associated with the worried well, the diagnosis of nondisease, and the treatment of minor ailments that will probably cure themselves or be unresponsive to conventional therapy. The probability of drug therapy is particularly striking, as is the frequency of follow-up visits to review progress or to evaluate physical status.

How much of hospital care may be considered to be similarly elective, at least with respect to timing, is difficult to estimate, although a discretionary component is suggested by the variability in surgery rates discussed in the paper by McMahon and Drake. The increasing pressure of utilization review committees is tending to reduce "unnecessary" admissions and to shorten hospital stays, at least if beds are full. Similarly, Professional Standards Review Organizations review the appropriateness of services that have been utilized as part of their monitoring of the quality of care. Payment controls, such as preadmission certification programs, may at least delay the admission of patients who might be treated on an ambulatory basis, just as postadmission certification programs may shorten stays for patients for whom third parties will not pay. As a result of these external forces, it would appear that an increasing portion of hospital admission is nondiscretionary, given the current state of medical knowledge. However, the definition of such admissions is changing. This is indicated by the growing popularity of ambulatory surgery, which it has been estimated could replace nearly one-half of what is now considered to be an appropriate inpatient case-load. On the other hand, evidence that the consumer if left to his own devices will voluntarily choose either the outpatient or the least-cost method of treatment is scant and most of it relates to the maximization of self-interest in choosing between inpatient and outpatient services (Davis and Russell, 1972; Rice and Wilson, 1976; Perkoff et al., 1976; Berki and Kobashigawa, 1976; and Elnicki, 1976).

Need and Demand—Equality and Equity of Access

The patterns of morbidity and mortality that affect the need and demand for services are in turn affected by the socioeconomic and demographic characteristics of the patient. For example, the medical significance of the same physiological symptom, such as a high fever, may depend upon the age of the individual concerned. The interpretation of these symptoms by the patient and his family may also differ according to educational level, ethnicity, urbanization, and other social and cultural elements. These forces have been more fully summarized elsewhere (for example, see Pauly, 1974; Aday and Andersen, 1975; Andersen et al., 1975; and Anderson, 1973a, 1973b), yet a brief review of their effect upon the utilization of services is pertinent. For to the extent that need as perceived by the patient and as corroborated by professionals differs among population groups, equity of access and equality of service in the marketplace imply differing levels of effective demand among consumers.

Variations with age and sex   That age and sex of individuals make a difference in utilization of health services and in patterns of morbidity and mortality is well recognized. As would be expected for short-stay hospitals, for example, the lowest rates of discharge, fewest days of care per 1,000 population, and shortest average length of stay are for patients under fifteen years of age; highest rates are to be found among those sixty-five years and older (refer to Table 4). Differences in these patterns are also evident between males and females, particularly in the age range when women may be child-bearing. Deliveries, of course, exert more influence on discharges than on days of care, since stays tend to be short.

Differences in hospitalization experiences are more marked than those involving ambulatory services. As compared with the average of 4.9 physician visits per person per year for all ages, persons aged sixty-five years and over averaged 6.5 visits per year, or 133 percent of the rate for all ages (Ries, 1975). Children received an average of 4.1 physician visits per year. This compares with a fourfold difference in discharge rates and a nearly threefold difference in length of stay.

The most striking difference among the age groups, however, is in the spending patterns brought about by the extension of health benefits to the poor (Medicaid) and to the disabled and individuals sixty-five years and over (Medicare). Since the inception of these

**TABLE 4   Rate of Discharges and of Days of Care
and Average Length of Stay for Patients Discharged
from Short-stay Hospitals, by Age
United States, 1972**

Age	All regions
	Rate of discharge per 1,000 population
All ages	154.9
Under 15 years	73.7
18–44 years	156.0
45–64 years	177.2
65 years and over	332.9
	Rate of days of care per 1,000 population
All ages	1,199.9
Under 15 years	329.5
15–44 years	886.8
45–64 years	1,642.7
65 years and over	4,076.8
	Average length of stay in days
All ages	7.7
Under 15 years	4.5
15–44 years	5.7
45–64 years	9.3
65 years and over	12.2

Source: Lewis (1975:7).

programs in 1966, per capita expenditures for health care by the elderly have increased dramatically, mainly as a result of the infusion of public funds. In fiscal 1975, these expenditures reached a level of $1,160 for the oldest group as compared with a level of $366 for the group under sixty-five (see Fig. 1). As the data in Table 5 indicate, the aged do not differ markedly in the proportion of spending on health care devoted to hospital care (45 percent) as compared with the group aged nineteen to sixty-four years (49 percent), but their spending on nursing home care (23 percent) is markedly higher.

The differences in utilization and spending patterns of older citizens reflect differences in the ailments from which they suffer. Neoplasms, ischemic heart disease, and cerebrovascular disease, of course, attack those over the age of forty-four much more frequently than the young (Moien, 1975:5-7). In contrast, the only

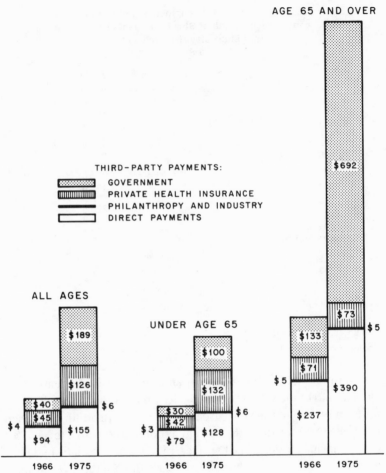

*Fig. 1   Per Capita Expenditures for Personal Health Care Met
by Third Parties and Paid Directly, by Age Group, Fiscal Years 1966
and 1975*

Source: Mueller and Gibson (1976:28).

conditions that yield a discharge rate from hospitals in excess of 100
per 10,000 population are hypertrophy of tonsils and adenoids for
children under fifteen and complications of pregnancy, childbirth,
and the puerperium for women fifteen to forty-four years of age.

Differences in the patterns of care among the age groups also

TABLE 5 Estimated Personal Health Care Expenditures, by Type of Expenditure and Source of Funds, for Three Age Groups, Fiscal Years 1974-1976 [In millions]

Type of expenditure	All ages			Under 19			19-64			65 and over		
	Total	Private	Public	Total	Private	Public	Total	Private	Public	Total	Private	Public
Total	$120,431	$72,013	$48,417	$17,880	$13,190	$4,690	$67,698	$47,576	$20,122	$34,853	$11,248	$23,605
Hospital care	55,400	25,004	30,396	6,461	3,750	2,711	33,164	19,828	13,336	15,775	1,425	14,350
Physicians' services	26,350	19,718	6,632	5,539	4,822	717	14,948	12,509	2,439	5,863	2,387	3,476
Dentists' services	8,600	8,131	469	2,021	1,813	208	5,857	5,638	218	722	679	43
Other professional services	2,400	1,607	793	504	354	150	1,362	1,060	302	534	193	341
Drugs and drug sundries	11,168	10,144	1,023	2,129	1,986	143	6,262	5,774	488	2,777	2,385	392
Eyeglasses and appliances	1,980	1,866	114	329	310	19	1,219	1,133	86	432	424	8
Nursing-home care	10,600	4,744	5,856	159	84	75	2,409	929	1,480	8,032	3,731	4,301
Other health services	3,933	800	3,133	738	71	667	2,478	705	1,773	717	24	693

Source: Gibson, Mueller, and Fisher (1977:4).

reflect the extent to which hospital care is likely to be prolonged and helpful. Once tonsils and adenoids are removed, the job of the surgeon is essentially completed. Although the value of the surgery to the health status of the patient may sometimes be debated, at least the episode of illness and its associated costs end. Likewise, medical expenses associated with maternity are finite because obviously the condition is of limited duration, although it does create further expenses associated with the newborn.

In contrast, care for chronic illness may alleviate but it cannot cure. For the 700,000 people diagnosed as having cancer each year, Holden (1976) has estimated that two out of three will die of their malignancies. Thus, for these people, the question is not whether to be a patient, but where to be treated, and how much of what type of care to consume.

Mushkin with DiScuillo (1974) has illustrated the magnitude of the problem of terminal illness in acute hospitals in the United States. These authors estimate that short-term stays of the dying accounted for approximately 12 percent of all days of patient care in short-term hospitals and for approximately one-fourth of the hospital costs incurred by the Medicare program. For the dying, more-over, expenses are high—under Medicare, hospital payments alone average approximately $1,250 per person who died as contrasted to $861 per person alive at the end of the year. For physicians' services, expenses under Medicare are also estimated to be approximately twice as high for those who died as for those who remained alive at the end of 1968. In the group aged forty-five to sixty-four, which fails to qualify for Medicare and often for other third-party payments, Mushkin and DiScuillo estimate that (in 1973 prices) four out of every ten decedents incurred $2,400 or more in hospital and institutional expenses.

In order to avoid the potentially high-cost no-benefit pattern of caring for the terminally ill, increasing attention is being directed toward the possibility of offering the dying both more appropriate and more "aggressive" care, as in the development of hospices that offer relief from both pain and from the fear of death (see Holden, 1976, and the discussion of St. Christopher's Hospice in London).

Although more humane and less expensive solutions to caring for the aged and terminally ill may be developed, the growing number of individuals in these categories will continue to require more services than younger populations. No matter how generous the funding from public programs and how widely distributed the resources for providing care, on the basis of chance alone it can be anticipated that more of these individuals will find it difficult to obtain the care they need.

Variations with income, race, and education With the advent of better third-party coverage in the United States, it has become increasingly difficult to isolate the effect of socioeconomic factors upon the need for and utilization of health services. It is even more difficult to assign causalities among factors recognized as interrelated, such as poor health, nonwhite status, less education, and lower earnings. Nevertheless, relative to need, differences in utilization persist (Davis, 1976a, 1976b. For a comprehensive review of this literature, see Brook and Williams, 1975, and also Dunlop and Zubkoff, 1976, especially page 86; and Luft, 1972, 1975).

Lando, for example, concluded that "higher levels of educational attainment are correlated with lower levels of disability and that much of the observed racial differences in the relative occurrence of disability can be explained by differences in eductional attainment. . . . Even after accounting for the contribution of age, however, one still finds that years of schooling play a significant role in determining an individual's health status" (Lando, 1975:21–22).

For families who had health insurance and whose household heads were employed, Slesinger, Tessler, and Mechanic (1976) reported that the major difference in utilization was among black adults, who made higher use of preventive medical services than comparable whites for an index of four specific preventive tests and for general checkups in the preceding year. There was, however, no such difference in the overall use of health services by these groups. "Perhaps what is more important in the employed population studied is that all of the respondents had reasonably good insurance coverage and few were burdened with very large out-of-pocket payments. Thus, relatively few barriers existed to the use of preventive and other medical services, and respondents felt that their sources of medical care were accessible and responsive to them" (Slesinger et al., 1976:404).

Just as health insurance has removed barriers to care that were previously associated with income and race of the employed population, so too Medicare and Medicaid may have provided access to care that was previously unavailable to the elderly and the poor. "In just a seven-year period from 1964 to 1971, low-income people made up the gap between their use of medical services and that of others, and for some age groups actually began to see physicians more frequently than middle-income persons" (Davis, 1976a:57; see also Davis, 1976b:126).

As compared with the aged, the poor not covered by Medicaid, as well as Medicaid recipients in many states (Davis, 1976b), have been less fortunate in obtaining improved access to medical care (see Davis, 1974; and Boaz, 1975). Among states, Medicaid programs tend to be least liberal in their benefits where there is the greatest poverty (Cooper and Worthington, 1973, 1974). Such state policies, moreover, are reinforced by federal policies which redistribute wealth from low-income to high-income states. For example, in fiscal year 1969, over 40 percent of federal Medicaid funds went to just two states, California and New York, but these two states bore less than one-fourth of the federal cost burden (Cooper and Worthington, 1973, 1974).

Furthermore, money with which to purchase services will not alone supply the resources to provide care to rural areas (see Heald and Cooper, 1972:4–5), any more than the provision of services in poverty pockets of urban areas has been able to raise the health status of residents from these areas to levels comparable to that of populations in more affluent areas. Ventura, Taffel, and Spratley (1975) have documented this dramatically in analyzing vital and health statistics in poverty and nonpoverty areas of nineteen large cities for the three-year period 1969–1971. The proportion of infants born to unmarried mothers, for example, was slightly more than three times higher in poverty areas than in nonpoverty areas, and the mortality rate for infants residing in poverty areas was also higher than in nonpoverty areas. According to the measures of health used in this study, the health condition of nonwhite persons is generally less favorable than that of the white population, although differences were narrowed by taking account of poverty status for only three indicators (deaths from tuberculosis, proportion of births to mothers with less than twelve years of schooling, and the death rate for violent causes). The proportion of low birthweight infants was consistently higher for nonwhite mothers irrespective of poverty status, however, and race differentials also favored white residents in nonpoverty areas for most of the other measures of health status that were studied. But within the poverty areas, differentials in illegitimacy rates and infant mortality rates between white and nonwhite were not large. Race differentials were also small within the poverty areas for crude birth rates, fertility rates, fetal death rates, and the proportion of births to mothers with no prenatal care. A recent study by Luft (1975) presents even more dramatic evidence that the distinctions in disability that appear in unadjusted data to be associated with race disappear when differences in age, income, and educational level are fully taken into account. Other studies, however, continue to document the fact that irrespective of why these differences in health status arise, sociodemographic factors continue to play a role in explaining why the distribution of health resources and services do not yet mirror the expected patterns of consumer demand and medical need (see Foltz et al., 1975).

The Translation of Need into Effective Demand: The Role of Money Price

In the static world of the classical economist, the price at which an item is exchanged in the marketplace yields revenue to the seller that, in equilibrium, is sufficient to equal the cost of production, including an appropriate allowance for profit. On the demand side, there is likewise a direct connection between market price and the cost of consumption incurred by the buyer. In the acquisition of health care, the situation is complicated by the introduction of third-party payers. These insurance carriers, Health Maintenance Organizations, and governmental programs do not usually receive dollars directly from patients at the time service is rendered. Rather, they receive their revenues from taxpayers when taxes are paid, from employers and employees when wages are earned, and from subscribers when premiums are paid. The third parties then pay the providers of care on behalf of the patients they represent. But the payments may not be paid as service is rendered and may not be based upon market prices of the services as they would be billed to an individual patient. They may reflect institutional costs as determined by past expenditures or prospective budgets, more fully described in the paper by Bauer.

In addition to such third-party payments, providers may receive direct payments from patients. These out-of-pocket expenditures usually reflect market prices and would be incurred by the patient for any services not covered by third parties, except where the provider intentionally offers charitable "free care" or unintentionally suffers nonpayment, that is, bad debts. When co-insurance is involved, however, the out-of-pocket costs incurred by the patient would only be proportional to market price; and when deductibles are imposed, the out-of-pocket costs would depend upon both the level of the deductible and how much service had been previously incurred by the particular subscriber in the period to which the deductible applied. Under these conditions, the complexities of the transactions make it difficult at best to identify who is the buyer and what is the role of the listed price.

In fiscal 1976, national health expenditures reached a level of $139 billion or $638 per person, of which $552 was for personal health care (Gibson and Mueller, 1977). Figure 2 illustrates the distribution of this per capita amount according to source of payments. It is clear that no longer is it usual for the patient to be the payer.

Morgan, Daly, and Murawski (1973) provide a dramatic illustration of the difference between hospital charges and out-of-pocket costs. For eighteen patients and their families, the authors examined the effects of a specific catastrophic illness requiring intensive acute care (acute renal failure following rupture of an abdominal aortic aneurysm). To the authors' surprise and despite the fact that only one patient survived, all the families appeared to be appreciative of the care their relatives had received. In terms of the charges

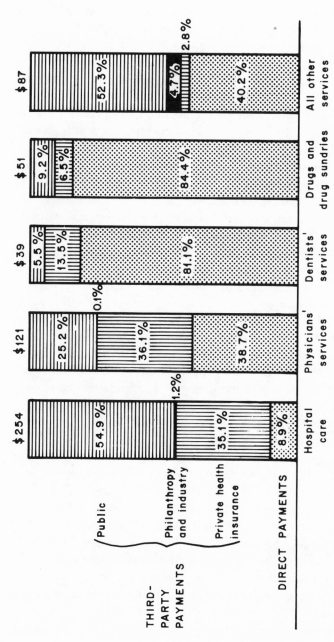

Fig. 2   Percentage Distribution of Per Capita Personal Health Care Expenditures, by Type of Expenditure and Source of Funds, Fiscal Year 1976

Source: Gibson and Mueller (1977).

incurred, this care had cost an average of $539 per day in 1967 and $962 per day in 1971. For the treatment of the group of patients, the total cost as measured by charges was $185,000, or approximately $10,000 per case. In terms of the average out-of-pocket cost incurred by each family, however, the cost of these extraordinary treatment measures had only been $200 to $400.

For the noninstitutionalized population, more precise information concerning out-of-pocket costs of families for health care has been compiled from a study undertaken in 1971 by the Division of Health Interview Statistics of the National Center for Health Statistics. Results as reported by Wilder (1975b) indicate that among the approximately 12,000 households sampled, the average annual out-of-pocket health expense for hospital, doctor, dental, or optical services, prescription medicine, and other medical needs for a family of two or more was $469 (or approximately $805 adjusted to fiscal 1975 levels by applying the 172 percent rise occurring in national health expenditures throughout this period). When expense for health insurance premiums is added, the total in 1970 dollars becomes $628, and when the expense for persons not living with the family unit is included, the grand total of annual out-of-pocket spending for health rose to $648 (Wilder, 1975b:1). By type of expenditure, the average family spent $72 out-of-pocket for hospital bills, including outpatient services as well as inpatient care, compared to $164 per year for doctor bills. Dental bills for the average family amounted to $105, only slightly more than the $93 spent for prescription medicine (Wilder, 1975b:7).

Health insurance premiums (including Medicare premiums) that are paid directly by the family can be isolated from other types of out-of-pocket spending on health care. For all families, these premiums averaged $159 in 1970 or 34 percent of the $469 that was spent by a family of two or more members. The percentage was somewhat greater for unrelated individuals (Wilder, 1975b:10). These data omit health insurance premiums that are paid directly by employers although they may be considered as payments in lieu of wages and thus part of the health spending of the individual as well as part of fringe benefits. Since employer payments for group insurance premiums are not counted as part of the employee's income for tax purposes, income-tax laws create incentives to transfer to the employer responsibility for the payment of health insurance premiums (see Mitchell and Phelps, 1975; and Mitchell and Vogel, 1973). The staff of the Council on Wage and Price Stability (Executive Office of the President, 1976a) estimates that approximately 80 percent of health insurance premiums are paid through employment-related group insurance plans, with another 3 percent being paid through other types of group insurance policies. For such group policies, an average of 67 percent of the total premium is paid by the employer and for 41 percent of the policies the entire premium is paid (Mitchell and Phelps, 1975). Therefore, significant proportions of the cost of health insurance are no longer the direct responsibility of the insured.

Furthermore, for those premiums that remain the responsibility of the employee, one-half (and in some cases, all) of the premium payment will be deductible in the computation of federal income taxes. The same tax advantages would hold, of course, for the nearly 20 percent of payments in which premiums are paid entirely by individuals. In addition, if third-party coverage is inadequate, expenditures for medical care exceeding 3 percent of the taxpayer's adjusted gross income become deductible from taxable income. Thus, federal income-tax policies further reduce the impact of health costs upon the consumer (see Davis, 1975:16, and Feldstein, 1976a). Considering both the income-tax benefits derived from deductions and the tax-free fringe benefits offered by employer-paid premiums, Mitchell and Vogel (1973) estimate that the federal government's subsidy for insurance premiums and medical expenses amounts to $7.6 billion in 1976, compared with $3.8 billion in 1970. However, hearings held in 1976 by the Council on Wage and Price Stability (Executive Office of the President, 1976a, 1977) indicate that even these tax advantages are no longer hiding the importance of the cost of health care in wage negotiations.

The Effects of Shifts in Net Money Price upon Demand

In recent years with the advent of econometric studies of the behavior of the health care industry, it has become increasingly clear that in deciding whether to obtain medical care, patients respond to the net money price that they will have to pay. However, it is less clear how effective price is in influencing demand for service after care has been initiated or when physicians' services are involved.

The sensitivity of demand to shifts in price, that is, the price elasticity of demand, appears to be greatest when price has previously acted as a barrier to receipt of service, as among the poor or in the provision of ambulatory services. Newhouse, Phelps, and Schwartz (1975), for example, estimate that the decrease in out-of-pocket costs that would be associated with an extension, under a national health insurance program, of full-coverage insurance to ambulatory services might increase the demand for outpatient services by as much as 75 percent. In contrast, were a 25 percent co-insurance feature maintained, demand would increase by only 30 percent. The original and ongoing studies by Scitovsky and McCall (1977) expand these findings: a 25 percent co-insurance provision applying to physician services was found both to reduce demand and to reduce enrollment in a prepaid comprehensive plan, particularly for lower-income families as represented by nonprofessional staff at Stanford University. Hopkins and his co-authors (1975), however, observed that for Medicaid patients in California, co-insurance had little effect upon the use and management of services, perhaps because the physicians who acted as the prime generators of demand were unaware of the copayment status of their patients. On the other hand, for this group, regulations placed upon the provider to obtain authorization for reimbursement of services prior to their being rendered had the effect of delaying treatment and reducing follow-up care. Thus, this study concludes that controls should be aimed at the well-defined types of overservicing by providers or the inappropriate use of health care by beneficiaries. The study also points out that the regulations and the prices to which the consumer responds in deciding whether to seek treatment may not be the same as those to which the physician and hospital react in determining how much service to supply.

From the point of view of cost containment, the observed existence of a negative price elasticity of demand is significant (Davis and Russell, 1972). If a 1 percent decrease in price leads to a 1 percent increase in demand, that is, if the price elasticity of demand approaches -1, the decreases in total cost of health care that accompany decreases in price are at least partially offset by the accompanying increases in utilization of services. Thus, it could be argued that the greater the negative price elasticity of demand, the less the consumer is concerned about containing the total costs of health care. This conclusion is consistent with the view that the patient is concerned with maintaining the total cost of health care as a constant, perhaps as a fixed percentage of his income.

It should be pointed out that the traditional hospital bill confronting a patient upon discharge is often both confusing and confounding. Not only does it include an increasing number of individual items, like laboratory services and pharmaceuticals, but also it often lists these only by code number and price. Even though the patient may be fortunate enough to have third-party coverage, and thus prices may play an inconsequential role in determining how much care the patient seeks, nevertheless the "on paper" prices may anger, even outrage, the patient. Moreover, that anger may be heightened by the fact that physicians who act as patients' agents are unaware of price factors or may have reverse incentives to increase the use of ancillary services in order to increase both hospital revenues and their own earnings.

Although listed prices may have little influence on the demand for hospital care, and are only rarely the determinants of consumer costs, they may nevertheless be important in determining the use of physician services and ambulatory facilities. The effect of price on the use of inpatient facilities as compared with use of outpatient services, for example, has been studied by Davis and Russell (1972). They conclude that when the price of ambulatory care is lowered, outpatient services are substituted for comparable inpatient care, particularly if beds are nearly full. The demand elasticity with respect to outpatient price was estimated quite precisely at about -1. (Thus a 1 percent decrease in outpatient price would cause a 1 percent increase in outpatient use, which would be accompanied by a 1 percent decrease in the use of inpatient services.) In their review of the relevant literature, Rice and Wilson (1976) conclude that in the interests of minimizing the costs the patient actually has to pay, the reverse may also be true: high-cost insured services, such as hospital care, may be substituted for low-cost uninsured services, such as ambulatory care. The trade-off between the use of inpatient and outpatient services may be a function of price only if price is defined to be the net out-of-pocket cost that the consumer pays. However, the situation is complicated by introducing concepts of costs of production (Elnicki, 1976) and costs over time. Although ambulatory services may cost less than hospital care in terms of charges per unit of service and for the initial episode of illness, over time these services may be used more frequently and be as costly to provide.

Patterns of consumer choice may be influenced by physicians, both directly and when the doctor acts as the agent of the patient (see Feldstein, 1976b, and Morreale, 1974). The Office of the Assistant Secretary for Health of the Department of Health, Education, and Welfare (Gaus et al., 1976) conducted a study of Medicaid patients receiving care from a variety of providers, including ten different HMOs and fee-for-service physicians. No significant differences were observed in accessibility of care, satisfaction with service, and enrollment selectivity among the groups studied. The only significant difference related to hospital utilization. Group-practice HMOs had significantly lower hospital utilization than the fee-for-service groups; foundation HMOs did not. The authors conclude, "This difference seems to indicate that capitation payment to an HMO alone is not significant enough to produce major changes in utilization and that the organized multispecialty group-practice arrangement with largely salaried physicians may be more significant" (Gaus et al., 1976:3). These findings are supported by Fuller and his colleagues (1975), who reported decreases of 15 percent in ambulatory physician encounters, 18 percent in drug utilization, 30 percent in hospital admissions, and 32 percent in hospital days in the period 1971–1974, among 1,000 Medicaid beneficiaries enrolled in the prepaid group practice plan of the Group Health Association of Washington, D.C., as compared with Medicaid beneficiaries treated under fee-for-service arrangements.

Finally, consumers may be unresponsive to prices because differences among them are slight. Stratmann and his coworkers (1975) were surprised to discover that in deciding where to go for care, consumers were least affected by economic criteria. These authors surmised that, just as insurance coverage decreased the importance of the cost of hospital care to the consumer, lack of variation among the prices charged locally by physicians for office visits made these costs largely irrelevant in selecting among alternative doctors after the decision to seek care had been made by the patient.

Direct studies of consumer willingness to "doctor shop" are rare. Kane and his colleagues (1975) made an exploratory analysis of the extent to which individuals on their own initiative sought advice from a second physician. Among the 634 households interviewed in Salt Lake County, Utah, about 40 percent of the respondents reported that in the last five years they or members of their household had sought a second medical opinion without waiting for a physician referral; another 10 percent expressed a desire to doctor shop, but had not exercised this option. In the final year of the study, 5 percent of the respondents who reported having an episode of illness also reported having doctor shopped. It was interesting to note that shoppers were more likely than nonshoppers to have a significantly higher theoretical knowledge of medical specialties, but a lower practical knowledge. They were also more likely to adopt a sick role and to exhibit less positive attitudes toward physicians.

Time and Opportunity Costs

As money price ceases to act as a barrier to health care because of the advent of third parties, there may be an increase in the impact of other types of cost upon demand. These include the costs associated with scheduling an appointment, reaching the doctor, waiting for care, and forgoing the opportunities that would have been present had there been no time lost in seeking medical care. The latter category, called "opportunity cost," encompasses such factors as wages that cannot be earned and the value of forgone productive activities. In addition, there are the even more intangible costs associated with the anxiety about symptoms and their meaning, as well as with the uncertain consequences of seeking medical care and being ill.

The cost of time spent by patients in reaching hospitals or physicians and in waiting for treatment may be large compared with that spent in receiving medical care. Data from the National Ambulatory Medical Care Survey, for example, indicate that of the nearly 650,000 visits to office-based physicians in the United States between May 1973 and April 1974, nearly one-half were completed in ten minutes or less and only 6.1 percent lasted more than thirty minutes. In most situations, access time will exceed treatment time for ambulatory services.

That minimization of time spent in transit is not in itself a major goal of the patient was observed by Studnicki (1975) in a study of utilization patterns in sixteen selected hospitals in Baltimore City. For obstetrical patients, one out of four of the nearly 4,000 births studied occurred at the most accessible hospital. However, one out of every five births occurred in the four hospitals most distant from the patients in terms of travel time. Particularly for the nonwhite poor, geographical factors were secondary to organizational factors, such as where physicians were located, what hospitals they were affiliated with, and which sources of payment the hospitals would accept.

The importance of factors other than travel time in deciding on sources of care was also noticed in a study of patients utilizing a highly specialized rheumatic diseases clinic at the University of California, San Francisco. Among the patients studied, one-half traveled more than fifty-three minutes to reach the clinic, the average one-way transit time to the clinic being one hour and forty minutes (Henke et al., 1977). Many patients chose to sacrifice convenience for the professional competence of the clinic dealing specifically with their disease.

Although time costs may not be a major factor in deciding where care will be sought, together with transportation costs they may nevertheless play an important role in determining how much care will be utilized. This may be particularly true for individuals under programs such as Medicaid and Medicare (see Acton, 1972, 1973, 1974). Here, the transportation and time costs essentially determine the comparative cost of seeking care. Time costs may also be significant for individuals who place high values on their time, such as students or, more generally, people with higher incomes.

The opportunity cost of receiving medical care depends upon such factors as the value of the productivity and income otherwise created, which in turn is a function of characteristics of the patient, such as age, sex, employment status, occupation, skill level, education, and race. This cost must also be evaluated in the light of the losses that would have arisen from illnesses had medical care not been sought. Consequently, opportunity cost reflects complex and subtle factors, evaluation of which is highly individualized and may reach levels that exceed the money cost of acquiring medical care. Thus, particularly for those patients for whom opportunity cost is high compared with out-of-pocket money cost, opportunity cost may have important bearing upon purchasing patterns.

Information concerning the influence of opportunity cost on the acquisition of medical care is generally lacking. It is, however, possible that the 10 percent higher hospitalization rate (even excluding obstetrical conditions) of women (Moien, 1975:3) is in part a function of their lower opportunity cost compared to that for men. Women may lose less in seeking care because on the average they earn less than men or, as homemakers, have lower imputed earnings. Or, they may lose less because in homemaking and in farm and domestic work, they have more flexible hours. Of course, there are exceptions. The mother with the preschool child might find it more difficult to leave home while the child is awake and this difficulty would increase if the family were larger.

In addition to earnings and hours, another important element in determining the opportunity cost incurred by individuals in seeking medical care is the nature of sick-leave arrangements. Some employers, some industries, and, for that matter, some nations, are more liberal than others. Although the study was undertaken some years ago, Enterline (1966) documented the fact that willingness to be "sick" depends at least in part upon cost in terms of lost wages. In a study of "sick absence rates" in fourteen nations in 1956, the average daily percent of employed persons absent from work owing to illness ranged from 5.7 percent in West Germany to 1.9 percent in the United States and 1.1 percent in Canada. The average number of days of "sick" absence for the employed labor force in these countries increased both with improvements in sick-leave privileges bargained for in union contracts or provided by law and with higher levels of income during covered days of sick absence. Enterline also noted that even within a single country, sickness rates tended to fall as unemployment increased and competition for jobs became more intense. As a corollary, Blue Cross officials have observed that at the initial stages of a cutback in the work force, when lay-offs are first initiated but coverage for health insurance remains in effect, there tends to be an increase in the elective surgery rates among those who otherwise would be idle. Procedures that were postponed because of reluctance to miss work are undertaken when this opportunity cost of illness is removed.

Broader social forces are thus introduced into the evaluation of the opportunity cost of seeking medical care. In national terms, Brenner (1975) reported on the increase in the rates of suicide, mental hospitalization, homicide, alcoholism, automobile accident mortality, cardiovascular-renal diseases, and infant and maternal mortality that has accompanied adverse changes in the national economy, particularly declines in per capita income and employ-ment rates. In terms of the individual, Teeling-Smith, writing about the cost of ill health in England, states: "Studies such as those of Taylor (1968) have shown that the decision to seek medical authori-zation for absence from work can in many cases reflect social discontent—or lack of job satisfaction—rather than medical need" (Teeling-Smith, 1976:63). More generally, Teeling-Smith suggests that morbidity tends always to be rising because of our growing intolerance of less than a state of perfect well-being as our lot as human beings improves.

Some Issues in the Marketing of Health Care

The data presently available for the United States suggest that the consumer's decision to buy medical care is affected by a variety of factors, including the severity of medical need, emotions about illness, attitudes toward treatment, and the relative value of expended time, effort, and money. As third-party coverage is extended, however, prices listed for services by providers become less important to consumers in deciding whether to seek care and how much service to receive. This has already happened for inpatient services for which out-of-pocket direct payments for services by patients are now less than 10 percent of hospital revenues. It can be anticipated that prices for ambulatory services will similarly decrease in importance as insurance coverage expands in these areas.

There appears to be essentially no evidence to support the view that cost determines which of two otherwise identical or comparable services a person will choose, either as a patient or as a subscriber to health insurance plans. There is some evidence from a few studies that consumers will substitute lower cost outpatient care for higher priced inpatient service. Thus, it would appear in general that they are not markedly affected by price in choosing where and from whom they will seek care or how much service they will then receive.

In fairness to both the individual and institutional consumer, however, it should be emphasized that marketing practices in the health industry have traditionally been designed to ignore matters of monetary price or cost containment and to emphasize saving lives, no matter how small the probability. Furthermore, pricing policies emphasize accounting criteria rather than considerations related to utilization. Services are priced on the basis of their average cost, this in turn being derived from the expenses of the cost center. These are defined to include both the direct costs of providing service and the pro rata share of overhead for the operation of the facility *as a whole*. These expenses are converted into the unit cost upon which prices are based by taking into account the quantity of service, expected or past, that the cost center is to render. Price is not considered to be a function of the cost added or removed by changing the quantity of service offered; that is, price is not related to marginal cost, the cost of the last unit of service being produced. In addition, the separate elements of price are not consciously examined. Furthermore, the levels of prices for different types of services are not structured to encourage patients to buy what is medically important, however this may be defined by professionals.

Thus, "price" is not viewed as a tool of market equilibria nor is it utilized to manipulate choice, ration services, and improve health care. It is no wonder, then, that patient and physician alike have until recently shown little interest in price and in containing the costs of the health care they consume or produce.

In addition to the issues surrounding the evolving role of price, the literature suggests that a large portion of health care is elective in nature. Nevertheless, present reimbursement practices assume that all hospitalizations and all services, if they are covered at all, are equally essential. There is little provision for using and purchasing less essential extras. As a consequence of this adoption of the concept of equality among both buyers and services, demands are generated that may threaten the fiscal viability of the health care system. Recognition of the diverse characteristics of needs and the variety of values among consumers might enable a system to be designed that, by limiting coverage to the most essential components, would both preserve the rights of patients to purchase other care they desire and protect against the major costs of illness and injury that cannot be avoided.

The Consumer as Regulator [1]

As the balance of power in determining the demand for service shifts from the individual patient to the third-party payer, new pressures on prices and utilization patterns are emerging. Commercial, nonprofit, and governmental buyers act for the consumer as do a variety of labor and management groups. The governmental buyer, in particular, is becoming increasingly concerned with rising

[1] The presentation in this section is based upon the paper entitled "Controlling Expenditures, Paying for Services, and Improving Health Care: The Role of Mandatory Financial Reports and Statewide Commissions," which was presented to the Medical Care Section of the American Public Health Association at its 101st Annual Meeting in San Francisco, California, November 7, 1973. Work on this paper was undertaken while Dr. Ingbar was Associate Professor of Health Economics in the Division of Ambulatory and Community Medicine of the Department of Medicine as well as a member of the Health Policy Program of the School of Medicine, University of California, San Francisco.

costs. Consequently, federal and state agencies are reviewing and establishing reimbursement rates. Governmental bodies are also controlling the expansion of facilities and limiting the growth in services through the mechanism of certificates of need. Methods of regulation also include PSROs. Health Maintenance Organizations (HMOs), which shift provider incentives away from the treatment of illness toward procedures that maintain health and prevent disease, have also been encouraged in an effort to contain costs from the production side. (For a review of the HMO programs and relevant literature, see McNeil and Schlenker, 1975.)

Federal Rate Review

The most direct approach to control of rising costs is to establish processes for rate review; these may range from mere data-gathering to direct controls on price levels. The latter course was followed by the federal government, with the establishment of the Economic Stabilization Program (ESP) in August 1971. The program began with a nationwide freeze on wages, prices, salaries, and rents. Three months later, Phase II established ceilings on rates of change in the prices of medical care and on total annual provider revenues; in January 1973, Phase III maintained wage and price controls for the health care industry (and other problem areas) while lifting mandatory controls in other sectors of the economy; and finally in the spring of 1974, Phase IV limited charges and expenses per inpatient admission in acute care hospitals to 107.5 percent of the level in the preceding fiscal year although controls were lifted elsewhere in the economy. (For a detailed discussion of ESP see Horowitz, 1973, and Ginsburg's paper in this volume.)

To reinforce the direct controls imposed by the Economic Stabilization Program, the federal government adopted other programs that attempt to curb rising expenditures by encouraging either providers or purchasers of services to review charges and expenditures more carefully. To identify unusual institutional and individual patient expenditures, the Social Security Administration (U.S. DHEW, 1972), itself a major purchaser of service, has adopted the Medicare Analysis of Days of Care (MADOC). PSROs, established as part of the Social Security Act Amendments of 1972, encourage local providers of service to review on a case-by-case basis the appropriateness of both care and charges for each Medicare patient. These programs are continuing although the Economic Stabilization Program has terminated.

Studies of the impact of ESP upon the costs of health care have dealt with the comparative movement over time of different indicators of hospital costs, including national health expenditures, hospital expenditures, hospital expenditures per patient day and per admission, and prices of medical care or hospital treatment. The results of these investigations suggest that increases in *price* of hospital care have been more noticeably curtailed by programs such as ESP than have increases in the *costs* of producing service (Schlenker and Ellwood, 1973; Schlenker and McNeil, 1973). The results may reflect the fact that provider revenues may be increased by alteration in the technological elements of treatment; it is alleged that this is the inevitable consequence of attempting to control prices when the product cannot be well defined (Schlenker and Ellwood, 1973). Thus, the conclusion is reached that it is impossible to examine revenues, costs, and prices of service apart from the quantity of care, mix of service, and technological components of treatment, a viewpoint reinforced by other investigations by Schlenker (1973), Horowitz (1973), Altman and Eichenholz (1973), and Berry (1975). For these and other reasons the performance of ESP in the containment of the costs of health was not noteworthy (Ingbar, 1974; Ginsburg, this volume; Feige and Pearce, 1973; Lanzillotti et al., 1975).

State Rate Review

State legislators have also demonstrated their direct concern with the "price" of health services by supporting the adoption of rate-review legislation. These activities and their goals are the subject of the papers by Bauer, Cohen, and Hellinger (see also Somers, 1973); thus, attention here centers upon these programs as expressions of consumer interests in the containment of hospital costs.

Some of the complexities of the rate-making process are illustrated by its history in Massachusetts (Ingbar and Taylor,

1968:10–11; Ingbar, 1970; Pureka, 1970). The process was initiated on January 1, 1954, with the establishment of the Bureau of Hospital Costs and Finances at the recommendation of a recess study undertaken by the Joint Standing Committee on Public Welfare of the legislature. The bureau's primary purpose was to develop a more equitable and uniform system for reimbursing hospitals, particularly in those cases in which prices paid by the Commonwealth differed among hospitals providing similar services and among public agencies purchasing identical care from the same institution. To rationalize these payment practices, it was necessary to teach hospitals how to maintain the cost records required to calculate more nearly comparable reimbursement rates, develop rules and regulations for uniform accounting, and apply standard audit procedures. The bureau became a division, and then on July 13, 1968, after major reorganization, the Rate Setting Commission was established. This commission retained the authority of its predecessors to: (1) establish reimbursement rates for all governmental units purchasing care for all publicly aided cases; (2) approve contracts and rates of payment between any hospital service corporation, such as Massachusetts Blue Cross, and any provider of services; and (3) approve or establish the rates to be used by governmental units in selling their services to the public or to other governmental users or third-party buyers.

In 1974, the commission was again reorganized, with three full-time members instead of a chairman and four part-time commissioners as in the past. The commission continued to be responsible for establishing "fair" and "reasonable" rates; it was also charged with assuring that these rates be "adequate," a phrase not incorporated in previous legislative directives. To fulfill these obligations, the commission has had to continue to specify, collect, and more important, audit information in order to determine the costs for which hospitals and other health care providers should be reimbursed by the major contactual purchasers of hospital care. Furthermore, the commission approves or disapproves reimbursement rates for individual health care providers in the light of general formulas established for each class of buyers. In 1976, the authority of the commission was again extended by legislative action, this time to include authority to approve any modification in charges associated with any item of service provided by Massachusetts hospitals.

The rate-review experience in Massachusetts, although among the longest in the United States, is not unique. In California a seven-person California Hospital Commission was established as a result of the adoption of the California Hospital Disclosure Act on October 26, 1971 (see Ingbar, 1974). As amended in 1973, the major purpose of the Disclosure Act was to require all hospitals except federal institutions "to file [annually] for public disclosure with the California Hospital Commission . . . uniform reports of hospital cost experience in the provision of hospital services . . . in accord with the systems of accounting approved." Such data were to be used to encourage economy and efficiency in the operation of hospitals as well as to help buyers of service in purchasing care and making fair and reasonable payments to hospitals.

Like its Massachusetts counterpart, the California Hospital Commission has also been undergoing changes. At present it exists as the California Health Facilities Commission, though legislative proposals are pending that would limit its span as an independent agency. Variety and change appear to be almost implicit in the state rate-review process, perhaps reflecting the dynamics of the political process at the state level and the types of regulatory models that are employed—professional, corporate, central planning, or neighborhood (see Kovner and Lusk, 1975). But flux may also reflect the inherent difficulties of containing hospital costs and of arbitrating the diverse goals of the many interested parties. At best, the structure of reimbursement formulas is complex and involves a variety of components. Moreover, to the extent that objective data derived from statistical analyses may be lacking, the precise details incorporated into any particular set of rates may not have been selected on the basis of detailed analysis and explicit design (Ingbar, 1970).

Much as it would be useful to evaluate the performance of rate-review programs, such investigations cannot as yet be readily implemented. Detailed data concerning state expenditures for health services are notoriously inadequate at a national level and have only comparatively recently become available for two years,

1966 and 1969, on a state-by-state basis (Cooper and Worthington, 1973). Until such information is generated more routinely, it will remain impossible to make a state-by-state appraisal of the effect of rate-review legislation upon the distribution of medical services, upon the allocation of health resources, and upon sources of payment. Thus, desirable as this would be, it would appear premature to evaluate the success of these systems of rate review. Whatever their past achievements (described more fully in the papers by Bauer, Cohen, and Hellinger), these systems have not yet satisfied the "consumer." In Massachusetts and California, for example, dissatisfaction has led to consideration of major revision of rate-setting policies.

Before examining other methods of regulating the costs of health care, it should be noted that there are those who remain convinced of the effectiveness of regulation of hospital costs at the state level. Thus, the Health Insurance Association of America (HIAA) (1975) ascribes to the activities of the Connecticut Commission on Hospitals and Health Care a reduced rate of escalation in hospital charges. HIAA notes that between October 1973 and October 1976 the percentage increase in hospital charges was 125.9 in Connecticut while the comparable value for the United States (as measured by the hospital daily service charge of the monthly Consumer Price Index compiled by the Bureau of Labor Statistics) was 145.2 However, the statistics compiled by HIAA do not indicate that all of the states with rate-review systems have been equally successful. Furthermore, the successes in Connecticut might be attributed to the freeze on changes in rates, a tactic that may be effective but that can only be maintained for short periods of time. Consequently, it seems premature for HIAA to ascribe success to the "public/private partnership" in Connecticut.

Federal Control of Capital Expansion

Interest in legislation to curtail the uncontrolled growth of hospitals and proliferation of their services has been increasing (Starkweather, 1975), in the belief that unnecessary duplication of facilities and programs is largely responsible for the rising cost of health care. Certainly, to the extent that hospital costs are fixed, in part because staffed and available beds cost nearly as much when full, the obvious solution is to eliminate beds rather than merely to diminish their use.

Regulation of costs through control of unnecessary expansion of facilities and services has been endorsed by the federal government and is encompassed in sections of the Social Security Amendments of 1972 (P.L. 92-603). In Particular, Section 221 provides that those expenditures incurred through expansions of facilities or programs not approved by local health planning groups or other designated planning agencies are to be excluded from federal reimbursement under programs such as Medicare and Medicaid. These groups must have "a governing body or advisory board at least half of whose members represent consumer interests." Institutional planning as a condition for reimbursement under Medicare is also introduced (Section 234). Other sections of the act include limits on the coverage of costs under Medicare (Section 223), limits on prevailing charge levels (Section 224), and provisions that reimbursement should be on the basis of "reasonable" cost (Section 223).

Because these provisions all refer to the notion of "reasonable," they introduce the possibility that payment will not be made to a particular institution when equivalent services may be purchased at markedly lower unit prices from other sources. Since one reason for high unit prices may be low volumes of service stemming from underutilization of capacity, these provisions of P.L. 92-603 may force institutions to become concerned about the efficiency of their operations and the better use of their facilities. Indeed, provisions relating to the recovery of annual operating costs may prove to be more important in controlling the expansion of health programs than the sections of the act concerning the recovery of capital expenditures incurred initially in modifying and constructing facilities. In this sense, therefore, the Social Security Administration instituted a new approach to the control of hospital costs when it applied the 1972 amendments to impose ceilings under the Medicare program on reimbursement of hospitals for room and board charges. These ceilings on reimbursement rates were determined on an industry-wide basis; when multivariate statistical techniques were applied to define groups of hospitals in which costs were similar, it was found that institutions could be grouped into size categories if they were located in similar economic environments in terms of population density. Because ceilings on reimbursement rates could thus be determined nationally, charges established by providers ceased to be a determinant of maximum prices that the government would pay, even though these charges might be justified on the basis of institutional costs.

State Certification of Need

As discussed in greater detail in the chapter by Salkever and Bice, state legislators have also been eager to initiate programs that would reduce costs by eliminating unnecessary expansions and by promoting more rational planning of health facilities through certification of need. Among states, however, there is variation both in the administrative mechanisms for obtaining such certification and in the magnitude of the shift in facilities and services required to bring these procedures into effect.

The effectiveness of these programs is increasingly being questioned, both on practical grounds (Ingbar, 1974) and in terms of their past performance. Hellinger (in this volume) reports from an empirical investigation that certificate-of-need legislation has not significantly lowered hospital investment, and Salkever and Bice (also in this volume) note that hospitals have exhibited a tendency to circumvent certificate-of-need requirements by expanding services, facilities, and equipment in lieu of their bed capacity, for which specific authorization is required. These studies are summarized by Rosenthal (1976; see also California Hospital Association, 1974).

Although there is a conceptual difference between regulating an industry by controlling reimbursement rates and regulating expansion and entry, it may prove as difficult in practice to segregate these methods at the state level as at the federal level (Havighurst, 1973; Cohen, 1973). Authorization for changes in capitalization may become a condition for recovery of the expense of operating new facilities and services. Additionally, the development of reimbursement rates from target occupancy levels, rather than from actual utilization data, melds the two approaches. For example, in developing per diem rates for payment of hospitals under the Medicaid program, New York state divides an institution's expenditure by the actual quantity of services provided only if actual occupancy is greater than 80 percent for medical and surgical services, 70 percent for maternity services, and 60 percent for pediatric services. In Maryland, the use of target occupancy for proprietary and relatively low capital-intensive firms has been proposed as a substitute for the direct control of reimbursement rates (Cohen, 1975).

Labor and Management Controls

The growing concern over the escalating costs of employee health care benefits has resulted in a recent surge of innovative efforts by management and labor to deal with the problem. These efforts have been identified in a study just completed by the Council on Wage and Price Stability (Executive Office of the President, 1976b, 1977). The investigation describes at least briefly 126 projects, 93 of which began in 1965 or thereafter, 82 implemented since January 1, 1970, and 63 started after 1973. As discussed in the report, the most common mechanisms of cost containment utilized by the employer-employee groups are shown in Table 6. Although all of these mechanisms are designed to encourage the containment of costs, only a few regulate the behavior of patients and providers or control the prices, quantities, or types of services covered by employees health benefit plans.

Of particular interest are the health plans of the United Storeworkers Union and District Council 37 of the American Federation of State, County and Municipal Employees in the New York City area. In both cases prospective review of elective surgery by board-certified specialists is offered without cost to the member of the Health Security Plan, albeit in the first case such review is mandatory, whereas in the second it is voluntary. As reported by the Council on Wage and Price Stability (1976b), the cost incurred in rendering 3,721 second opinions from February 1972 through March 31, 1976 was approximately $300,000, including both consultant fees and diagnostic tests; but the cost of undertaking the 1,099 surgical

TABLE 6   Cost-Containment Mechanisms Utilized by Employer-Employee Groups

	Number of projects[a]
Alternative delivery systems (HMOs)	32
Preventive care	26
Concurrent or prospective peer review	17
Alternative methods of provider reimbursement	16
Coverage of less costly care	15
Claims review	12
Health education	8
Miscellaneous	6
Health planning	5

[a]Some of the 126 projects in the report are counted more than once in this table because they involve more than one mechanism of cost containment.
Source: Executive Office of the President (1976b).

procedures that were thereby prevented would have reached an estimated $2.4 million. Thus, although surgery may eventually be required in a proportion of these cases (estimated at approximately 16 percent) despite the fact that initially this need was not confirmed by the second opinion, significant savings seem to result from the voluntary and mandatory prospective review of the need for elective or nonurgent surgery. For 2,373 members of District Council 37 and other participating health funds who voluntarily had recommendations for surgery reviewed by a board-certified specialist, nonconfirmations appeared to be particularly high (38–44 percent) for certain elective procedures, such as hysterectomy, dilatation and curettage, and surgery of the knee, prostate, and varicose veins. Although comparable detail is not reported for other employee benefit plans that offer similar prospective surgical review, such programs are in fact sponsored by Blue Cross–Blue Shield in Massachusetts, Michigan, New Hampshire, Pennsylvania, New York City, and Albany, New York.

Unlike the programs designed to reduce inappropriate utilization through the imposition of controls upon the covered services of physicians, dentists or hospitals, certain other union-management programs are lowering costs by influencing prices directly. The leverage upon price that stems from the ability to purchase in large quantities, for example, is the basis of the mail-order prescription service offered to members of the nationwide Health Services Plan of the International Ladies' Garment Workers Union. Not only does their size permit the four pharmacies from which members may order prescriptions to obtain the lowest possible wholesale prices for the drugs they will resell, but in addition they are each large enough to achieve significant economies by utilizing partially automated processes in filling prescriptions as well as in mailing them to members. In contrast, the United Federation of Teachers Welfare Fund in New York City uses a program that is becoming increasingly prevalent in New York City and is expanding elsewhere: a fixed "professional fee" for the dispensing service is negotiated with thousands of retail pharmacies which then agree to accept this fee for providing prescription drugs at wholesale prices. Such contractual arrangements retain for members the advantage of maximum convenience and speed—they can purchase the whole range of prescription drugs at almost any pharmacy in the New York City area. By virtue of having controlled the retail mark-up, the United Federation of Teachers is able to provide these drugs at savings that are estimated to average 15 to 20 percent of the usual retail market price (Executive Office of the President, 1976b). However, it has been suggested that this level of savings may not be retained if pharmacists find a legal way to negotiate as a group with the union.

In addition, as described by the Council on Wage and Price Stability, some labor and management groups have initiated claims review systems that substitute for or supplement peer and utilization review mechanisms that intervene more explicitly in the delivery systems. Like their counterparts in programs financed from federal, state, or other private funds, these claims review systems are customarily primarily designed to identify unwarranted charges and to prevent their payment. As used by Rockwell International, however, such data are the basis of an information management system designed to identify the cost of employee benefits at each of the hundreds of plants owned by the company. This information is presented to the management of every plant in a quarterly trend report that forces management to consider the costs of health care as part of its corporate thinking. The quarterly trend report not only quantifies the costs and emphasizes their significance, but also permits costs in each plant to be compared with those in every other. By identifying those plants with high claims experience, the report triggers investigations of causes, including possible explanations such as unreasonable fees, unnecessary hospitalizations, inappropriate treatments, epidemics, and high average age of employees. Thus, claims data become the basis of a system for controlling the costs of health care as well as reviewing the appropriateness of payment.

The Health Industry as a Public Utility

Despite these varied attempts to control the costs of health services both directly and indirectly, there is growing dissatisfaction with the performance of the health industry. In an attempt to deal with this disenchantment, new forms of organization are being encouraged by federal and state governments in the hope of providing incentives to both producers and consumers to control costs of service without detriment to the quality of care (for a review of these trends, see Ellwood, 1975, and Starkweather, 1975). These efforts are exemplified at the federal level by the Health Maintenance Organization Act of 1973 (P.L. 93-222). This legislation, of course, did not initiate interest in prepaid group practice offering comprehensive coverage of services, both inpatient and outpatient. The Kaiser Foundation, for example, which originated in the early 1940s as a health plan for Kaiser's own employees, now serves three million members and is the largest multicommunity prepaid group practice in the United States. But the new HMO legislation encouraged consumers and employees or employers to consider such alternative methods of delivering health care, particularly when experience with their performance has been favorable. Illustrative of this process is the growth of the Genesee Valley Group Health Association, which in 1974 succeeded in reducing the medical-surgical inpatient days of its members by 7 percent at a time when patient days were rising by 5 percent for beneficiaries who retained traditional indemnity plan coverage (Roghmann as quoted in the report of the Council on Wage and Price Stability, Executive Office of the President, 1976b:138). Employers in cities such as Winston-Salem, North Carolina, Albuquerque, New Mexico, and Minneapolis–St. Paul are also encouraging prepaid group practice. The United Automobile Workers, the Amalgamated Clothing Workers of America, the Hotel and Restaurant Employees, and Bartenders International Union are among the labor organizations that offer direct service programs to members and R.J. Reynolds Industries and Scott Paper Company are among the employers (for a complete list, see Executive Office of the President, 1976b:149–152).

Demands are growing, however, for more stringent regulation to control all aspects of the production of health services, including the number of facilities, location of resources, and prices to be charged to consumers, both individual and third party. This "do something" approach to regulating the health industry culminates in the notion that the hospital sector at least should be regulated as a public utility (Cohen, 1975; Ellwood, 1975; Noll, 1975). Support of the public utility approach stems not only from frustration and impatience, but also from the implicit assumption that present failures of regulation in the health industry reflect the pursuit of piecemeal approaches, the inadequacies of which would be overcome by the adoption of more global arrangements that integrate control of prices, expenditures, capital expenditure, and entry and exit into the health care industry.

The Effectiveness of Regulation

Is the notion of the consumer as a regulator sound? Can governments or third parties acting in their role as purchasers of service establish "fair" and "reasonable" rates which serve to contain the overall costs of medical services?

As previously described, the effectiveness of regulatory programs may be questioned. There appears to be a lack of any consistent and major difference between the performance of the hospital industry in the states with active rate-review programs and in those without them. It may be argued that this apparent lack of impact reflects the paucity of relevant data, the associated inapplicability of multivariate statistical techniques, and the inexperience of some states with rate-review programs. By the same token, the vicissitudes and uncertainties associated with ESP's short-lived policies may explain why the national program failed to override interstate differences in the performance of the industry. At best, the impact of ESP would not have been expected to become apparent until the year ending September 30, 1972, by which time there was little chance for the benefits to reach fruition before the program was terminated.

The apparent failure of regulatory activity to contain the costs of care may be explained by the underlying characteristics of the hospital industry. As tools of regulatory activity, rate review and rate setting may be ineffective because the hospital industry lacks the traditional economic characteristics that respond favorably to regulation. The three conventional justifications for introducing regulatory activity, as commonly defined in the literature (Noll, 1975; Bothwell, 1973), are not evident in the health industry; the health industry is not a natural monopoly with declining unit costs, it does not rely on nonmarketable scarce resources, and it is not engaged in ruinous price competition which threatens the quality of service.

Another possible explanation for ineffectiveness relates to the characteristics of the regulatory process. Economists have argued that, in contrast to the supply considerations mentioned above, there are demand considerations that lead to regulation. Stigler (1971), for example, supports the notion that regulation is both acquired and designed by an industry and operated primarily for the benefit of the regulated by virtue of political processes that allow relatively small groups to control. Thus an industry "captures" (Noll, 1975) the control enabling it to exercise the power of the state, including "the 'power' to prohibit or compel, to take or give money, . . . [to] help or hurt a vast number of industries" (Stigler, 1971). Control over entry, prices, employment, and other aspects of industrial activity is used to preserve the self-interest of the powerful forces within the industry. According to the "capture" theory, therefore, there is no reason to expect regulation to benefit the public or the consumer; rather it will favor the economic position of the regulated groups.

Finally, it should be noted that the seeming ineffectiveness of rate-review processes may, in fact, reflect the inapplicability of traditional economic theory to the market for health. After the consumer adopts the role of the patient, the producer—that is, the doctor—determines demand for services. Furthermore, at least for hospital care, the consumer is frequently not the purchaser of service since payment may be via third-party carrier, whether public or private. The goals of the producer are also difficult to define (see Davis, 1972). The institutional authority may be a not-for-profit corporation and may exercise little control over the physicians and other professionals who actually provide the service. Together these traits may create a situation in which monetary incentives lack their usual impact. This may explain why Bauer and Densen (1973) observed from their review of fourteen incentive reimbursement plans: "In sum, the incentive plans may have made a difference in cost containment, but for the most part one can't be sure how much, or why." This may also explain why after its extensive analyses of the problem, the staff of the Council on Wage and Price Stability (Executive Office of the President, 1976a:iv) ". . . remain convinced that the goal of quality health care, at reasonable costs, is attainable within the context of a largely privately disciplined system. Indeed, we feel it is only within the context of the private system that it is attainable. . . . It [private incentive] is the key ingredient in bringing about the much-needed change in the system."

In summary, in view of the particular characteristics of the health services industry and the questionable effectiveness of regulatory activities in the past, agencies concerned with the regulation of hospitals and other health providers should reevaluate their roles and develop more imaginative methods of influencing market behavior. Certainly, the marketplace for medical care encompasses a tangled web of facilities and utilization patterns in which needs of populations and demands of consumers are not necessarily the only determinants of either the quality of services or the prices at which the care is produced. It may be inappropriate, therefore, to apply to the health industry the static regulatory concepts implicit in attempts to establish allowable limits and fix appropriate levels for prices, capacity, and utilization rates. Rather, the pace of medical progress, the variety of appropriate services, the diversity of patient preferences, and the flexibility of the production process may require a dynamic approach—one that stresses the thoroughness and appropriateness of the procedures and processes used to set rates and build capacity.

The Consumer as Planner

As part of the broad national trend toward self-realization, increased emphasis has been placed upon the rights of individuals to select and receive the kind of medical care they prefer. It has therefore been recognized that individuals must be involved in the early phases of developing facilities and programs so that these can be planned to suit their individual preferences as well as their medical needs. In addition, the consumer is being assigned more responsibility for sponsoring and controlling health policies as they are being applied in the delivery of medical care (see Sheps, 1972). It is as yet too early to assess whether these attempts to place the individual at the fulcrum of the market will succeed. Nevertheless, it is necessary to discuss briefly the potential for cost containment that this new role for the consumer may offer.

The Consumer Role in the Administration of Health Planning Legislation

On November 3, 1966, President Lyndon B. Johnson signed into law the Comprehensive Health Planning and Public Health Services Amendments of 1966 (P.L. 89-749). Better known as the "Partnership for Health or Comprehensive Health Planning," this legislation created both statewide "A" and local "B" Comprehensive Health Planning (CHP) agencies (named for the sections of the act under which they were created) to provide a means through which consumer preferences and priorities could be implemented. Although the effectiveness of these groups may be questioned (see O'Connor, 1974), the legislation unquestionably succeeded in introducing consumers into the establishment of providers that had hitherto been able to provide health service without the necessity of conducting an ongoing forum with the users of their services.

Commenting upon this process, O'Connor notes that the influence of consumers was not proportional to their numerical majority, perhaps reflecting that fact that ". . . the reward for the considerable amount of work and controversy necessary to become a well-informed consumer representative is relatively meager. Few people in today's society have either the leisure or the motivation to fulfill such an important role in a truly adequate fashion" (O'Connor, 1974:403–404). In addition, the limited powers of health planning agencies and their reliance upon community support further restricted their potential impact. Nevertheless, at least in certain areas of the country, these groups claimed success in helping to bring about the consolidation of underutilized hospital facilities and the prevention of unnecessary hospital expansion. They have also helped in bringing about the regionalization of special services such as renal dialysis, cancer therapy, and family planning (see O'Connor, 1974:410; and various studies cited in *Weekly Government Abstracts—Health Planning*, compiled by the National Health Planning Information Center, DHEW).

On January 4, 1975, President Ford signed the National Health Planning and Resources Development Act of 1974 (P.L. 93-641). This act signaled the demise not only of the Partnership for Health, but also of the regional medical programs, and of the Hill-Burton facilities construction authorities. The new act established state health planning and development agencies and local Health Systems Agencies (HSAs). As defined in the legislation, these groups are responsible for:

1. Improving the health of residents of a health service-area;
2. Increasing the accessibility (including overcoming geographic, architectural, and transportation barriers), acceptability, continuity, and quality of the health services provided them;
3. Restraining increases in the cost of providing them health services; and
4. Preventing unnecessary duplication of health resources. (P.L. 93-641, sec. 1513(a)).

This legislation provides federal grant funds for the support and operation of state and local planning and development agencies; includes a new program for health facilities construction and modernization; and authorizes funds to HSAs for developing health resources to implement these plans. The HSAs are responsible for areawide health planning and development throughout the service areas designated by the Secretary of Health, Education, and Welfare on the recommendation of the state governors. Each HSA is required to prepare a health systems plan and an annual implementation plan; to provide technical and financial assistance for the development of health resources, to preview proposed federal health project grants; to assist states in review of health services and facilities needs; and to coordinate with appropriate planning and regulatory entities for the purpose of improving the health of the area's residents, increasing accessibility, acceptability, continuity, and quality of health services in the area, restraining increases in the costs of providing health services, and preventing unnecessary duplication of health resources.

The administrative process required for the implementation of this act is just beginning to proceed beyond the stage of designating geographic areas and selecting specific agencies for planning. Thus, it is obviously premature to evaluate the effectiveness of the HSAs. It is also too soon to know whether consumers will function any more effectively when they constitute the 51 to 60 percent majority on local HSA boards than when they constituted the majority in CHP agencies. The hope is that the greater reliance on the federal funding of HSAs as compared with CHP groups will, when funds are eventually made available, provide a more solid financial base from which consumers will be able to implement their responsibilities under the act.

Furthermore, under the provisions of P.L. 93-641, individuals are to be chosen to represent consumer interests which in turn are representative of the diverse groups within the constituent population of each HSA. Such individuals are disqualified if they are associated with providers, either directly via their own work or indirectly via marital arrangements or representation (even as consumers) on the governing bodies of hospitals or other organizations delivering health care. Under these new definitions, therefore, many individuals who have devoted years of effort to serving the public through their memberships on boards of nonprofit health agencies and hospitals will no longer qualify as *consumer* representatives in terms of health planning activities. Conversely, any board member from an HSA who accepts an appointment on the governing board of a health care organization—even though this might arise because the person had been articulate in representing the viewpoint of consumers—would automatically cease to be a *consumer* if the additional appointment were accepted. Thus, the new legislation rigidifies and compartmentalizes the definition of who may participate in the planning process and in governing board activities of the HSA on the basis of criteria that have no necessary association with competence in and contribution toward the stated objectives of improving the health of all residents of the geographic area to be served. At the same time, however, those individuals that meet the requirements as consumers under the new legislation are not formally accountable to the constituencies they are supposed to serve: they are neither elected representatives nor official appointees.

The Objectives of the Consumer

Who then is this "consumer" who is to be designated a "planner" and how will his goals differ from those of the "regulator" and the "buyer"? Will this consumer be more aware of quality and cost or will this consumer be more interested in medical care as the source of political power and jobs? (See National Health Council, 1975:76.) These and many similar questions concern the potential impact of the consumer as a planner.

Although it is too soon to answer these questions in regard to P.L. 93-641, there appears to be no obvious reason why the record should improve because individuals are members of the HSAs rather than of CHP bodies. More to the point, the complexity of the health industry itself and the elective and nonurgent nature of much of the medical care that is acquired suggest that pluralism in structures and in values will persist. Under these conditions, attempts to establish uniform objectives are doomed to failure because what is one person's preference is another's anathema. Such differences in objectives may encompass predilections for pain and risk-taking as well as for medical outcomes.

Not only do individuals differ in the benefits they seek but they also vary in the costs they will incur. As the expansion of third-party coverage decreases the importance of dollar price, there is a compensating increase in the relative importance of time costs and opportunity costs. Since these by definition vary greatly among individuals, it would appear that some mechanism is required to enable patients to continue to exercise their options in acquiring their medical care. Traditionally money price has served this purpose. Whether this function of price should be reinstated for at least those medical services that are least essential is a question that requires reinvestigation. If costs are to be contained at the same time that consumers are to be offered maximum choice, a revitalized and revamped pricing structure is required. Such a system would encourage all consumers to seek "necessary" treatment at the same time that it would stimulate all appropriate providers to supply those services that best meet these needs as efficiently as possible. It should be feasible to devise for this purpose a new series of "global" fees and retainer rates that would relate payment to specific conditions, diagnoses, episodes of illness, procedures, surgery, or time periods. Such prices would encompass more than a fee for a service but less than the annualized capitation rate of prepaid comprehensive Health Maintenance Organizations. They might be based upon treatment requirements as gleaned from studies such as those identifying AUTOGRPS (Thompson et al., 1975; Mills et al., 1976). Above all, however, such rates would bring self-interest into line with system requirements. They would not penalize doctors and hospitals for providing cheaper services that do the job as well, and they would not stimulate patients into seeking the most expensive services because payment is at someone else's expense. Rather, such rates would encourage all groups to be interested both in good medicine and in containing the costs of this care.

References

Acton, J.P.
  1972   Demand for Health Care Among the Urban Poor, with Special Emphasis on the Role of Time. Santa Monica, Calif.: The RAND Corporation, R-1151-OEO/NYC, October.
  1973   Demand for Health Care When Time Prices Vary More Than Money Prices. Santa Monica, Calif.: The RAND Corporation, R-1189-OEO/NYC, May.
  1974   Non-Monetary Factors in the Demand for Medical Services: Some Empirical Evidence. Santa Monica, Calif.: The RAND Corporation, P-5021-2, November.

Aday, L.A., and R. Andersen
  1975   Development of Indices of Access to Medical Care. Ann Arbor, Mich.: University of Michigan, School of Public Health, Health Administration Press.

Altman, S.H., and J. Eichenholz
  1973   "Control of health care costs under the Economic Stabilization Program." A paper presented to the American Economic Association and the Health Economics Research Organization, New York, December 30.

Andersen, R., R. Greeley, J. Kravits, and O.W. Anderson
  1972   Health Service Use: National Trends and Variations 1953–1972. DHEW Publication No. (HSM) 73-3004, October.

Andersen, R., J. Kravits, O.W. Anderson, and J. Daley
  1973   Expenditures for Personal Health Services: National Trends and Variations 1953–1970. DHEW Publication No. (HRA) 74-3105, October.

Andersen, R., J. Kravits, and O.W. Anderson
  1975   Equity in Health Services: Empirical Analyses in Social Policy. Cambridge, Mass.: Ballinger Publishing Company.

Anderson, J.G.
  1973a   "Demographic factors affecting health services utilization: A causal model." Medical Care 11 (March–April): 104–120.
  1973b   "Health services utilization: Framework and review." Health Services Research 8 (Fall): 184–199.

Bauer, K.G., and P.M. Densen
  1973   "Some issues in the incentive reimbursement approach to cost containment: An overview." Boston, Mass.: Harvard University,

Center for Community Health and Medical Care, Program on Health Care Policy, Discussion Paper No. 7, May.

Berki, S.E., and B. Kobashigawa
1976 "Socioeconomic and need determinants of ambulatory care use: Path analysis of the 1970 Health Interview Survey data." Medical Care 14 (May): 405–421.

Berry, R.E.
1975 "Perspectives on rate regulations." Pp. 105–122 in Controls on Health Care. Papers of the Conference on Regulation in the Health Industry, January 7–9, 1974. Washington, D.C.: National Academy of Sciences, Institute of Medicine, 1975.

Boaz, R.F.
1975 "Equity in paying for health care services under a national insurance system." Milbank Memorial Fund Quarterly/Health and Society 53 (Summer): 337–352.

Bosanac, E.M., R.C. Parkinson, and D.S. Hall
1976 "Geographic access to hospital care: A 30-minute travel time standard." Medical Care 14 (July): 616–624.

Bothwell, J.L.
1973 "The economics of regulation: A review of the literature" (MS). San Francisco: University of California, San Francisco, Health Policy Program; and Department of Economics, University of California, Berkeley.

Brenner, H.M.
1975 "Impact of the economy on health status and utilization." A paper presented to the 103d Annual Meeting of the Medical Care Section of the American Public Health Association, Chicago. Baltimore, Md.: The Johns Hopkins University, November.

Brook, R.N., and K.N. Williams
1975 Evaluating Quality of Health Care for the Disadvantaged: A Literature Review. Santa Monica, Calif.: The RAND Corporation, R-1658-HEW, November.

California Hospital Association
1974 Effective Health Facility Regulation for California. Report to California Hospital Association's Board of Trustees of CHA Economic Stabilization Program Study Task Force. Sacramento.

Cohen, H.
1975 "State rate regulation." Pp. 123–135 in Controls on Health Care. Papers of the Conference on Regulation in the Health Industry,

January 7-9, 1974. Washington, D.C.: National Academy of
Sciences, Institute of Medicine.

Cohen, H.S.
1973   "Regulating health care facilities: The certificate-of-need process
        re-examined." Inquiry 10 (September); 3-9.

Cooper, B.S., and N.L. Worthington
1973   Personal Health Care Expenditures by State: Volume I, Public
        Funds 1966 and 1969. DHEW Publication No. (SSA) 73-11906.
        Washington, D.C.: Government Printing Office.
1974   Comparison of Cost and Benefit Incidence of Government
        Medical Care Programs, Fiscal Years 1966 and 1969. U.S. Staff
        Paper No. 18, DHEW Publication No. (SSA) 75-011852. Wash-
        ington, D.C.: Government Printing Office.

Davis, K.
1972   "Economic theories of behavior in non-profit private hospitals."
        Economic and Business Bulletin 24 (Winter): 1-13.
1974   "National health insurance." Pp. 207-246 in Setting National
        Priorities: The 1975 Budget. Washington, D.C.: The Brookings
        Institution.
1975   National Health Insurance: Benefits, Costs, and Consequences.
        Washington, D.C.: The Brookings Institution.
1976a   "The impact of inflation and unemployment on health care of
        low-income families." Pp. 55-69 in M. Zubkoff, ed., Health: A
        Victim or Cause of Inflation? New York: Prodist for Milbank
        Memorial Fund.
1976b   "Medicaid payments and utilization of medical services by the
        poor." Inquiry 13 (June): 122-135.

Davis, K., and L.B. Russell
1972   "The substitution of hospital outpatient care for inpatient care."
        Review of Economics and Statistics 54 (May): 109-120.

DeLozier, J.E., and R.O. Gagnon
1975   National Ambulatory Medical Care Survey, 1973 Summary,
        United States, May 1973-April 1974. Data from the National
        Health Survey, Vital and Health Statistics Series 13, Number 21.
        DHEW Publication No. (HRA) 76-1772, October.

Dunlop, D., and M. Zubkoff
1976   "Inflation and consumer behavior in the health care sector." Pp.
        84-114 in M. Zubkoff, ed., Health: A Victim or Cause of
        Inflation? New York: Prodist for the Milbank Memorial Fund.

Ellwood, P.M., Jr.
1975   "Alternatives to regulation: Improving the market." Pp. 49–72 in Controls on Health Care. Papers of the Conference on Regulation in the Health Industry, January 7–9, 1974. Washington, D.C.: National Academy of Sciences, Institute of Medicine.

Elnicki, R.A.
1976   "Substitution of outpatient for inpatient hospital care: A cost analysis." Inquiry 13 (September): 245–261.

Enterline, P.E.
1966   "Social causes of sick absence." Archives of Environmental Health 12 (April): 467–473.

Executive Office of the President, Council on Wage and Price Stability
1976a   The Complex Puzzle of Rising Health Care Costs: Can the Private Sector Fit It Together? A summary of hearings held in New York, Chicago, San Francisco, Philadelphia, Boston, and Miami. A Compendium of Labor-Management Innovations in Reducing Health Care Costs. Washington, D.C., December.
1976b   "Employer health care benefits: Labor and management sponsored innovations in controlling cost." Federal Register 41:182:40298–40325 (September 17).
1977   The Rapid Rise of Hospital Costs: Staff Report. Washington, D.C., January.

Feige, E.L., and D. K. Pearce
1973   "The wage-price control experiment—Did it work?" Challenge 16 (July–August): 40–44.

Feldstein, M.S.
1973   "Econometric studies of health economics." Cambridge: Harvard University, Harvard Institute of Economic Research, Discussion Paper No. 291, April.
1974   "Econometric studies of health economics." In M.D. Intriligator and D.A. Kendrick, eds., Frontiers of Quantitative Economics II. Amsterdam: North-Holland Publishing Company.
1976a   "How tax laws fuel hospital costs." Prism (January): 15–19.
1976b   "Quality change and the demand for hospital care" (MS). Washington, D.C.: Executive Office of the President, Council on Wage and Price Stability.

Foltz, A.M., M. Chen, and A. Stoga
1975   "Socio-economic indicators, health resources, and health status: A statistical analysis and its policy implications" (MS). A paper

presented to the 103d Annual Meeting of the Medical Care
Section, American Public Health Association, Chicago. Yale
School of Medicine, Department of Epidemiology and Public
Health, November.

Fox, R.T., and D.H. Fox
  1974   "The use of central place theory for the location of maternal and
            infant care projects." American Journal of Public Health 64
            (September): 898–903.

Fuller, N.A., M.W. Patera, and K. Koziol
  1975   "Report on a study of Medicaid utilization of services in a
            prepaid group practice health plan" (MS). A paper presented to
            the 103d Annual Meeting of the Medical Care Section, American
            Public Health Association, Chicago. Washington, D.C.: National
            Capital Medical Foundation, Inc.

Gaus, C.R., B.S. Cooper, and C.G. Hirschman
  1976   "Contrasts in HMO and fee-for-service performance." Social
            Security Bulletin 39 (May): 3–14.

Gibson, R.M., and M.S. Mueller
  1977   "National health expenditures, fiscal year 1976." Social Security
            Bulletin 40 (April): 3–22.

Gibson, R.M., M.S. Mueller, and C.R. Fisher
  1977   "Age differences in health care spending, fiscal year 1976." Social
            Security Bulletin 40 (August): 3–14.

Havighurst, C.C.
  1973   "Regulation of health facilities and services by 'certificate-of-
            need.'" Virginia Law Review 59 (October): 1143.

Heald, K.A., and J.K. Cooper
  1972   An Annotated Bibliography on Rural Medical Care. Santa
            Monica, Calif.: The RAND Corporation, R-966-HEW, April.

Health Insurance Association of America, Consumer and Professional
Relations Division
  1975   "A public/private partnership for effective regulation of hospital
            costs: Connecticut Commission on Hospitals and Health Care."
            Viewpoint (December).

Henke, C.J., E.H. Yelin, M.L. Ingbar, and W.V. Epstein
  1977   "The university rheumatic diseases clinic: Provider and patient
            perceptions of cost." Arthritis and Rheumatism 20 (March):
            751–758.

Hershey, J.C., H.S. Luft, and J.M. Gianaris
   1975   "Making sense out of utilization data." Medical Care 13 (Oc-
            tober): 838–854.
Holden, C.
   1976   "Hospices: For the dying, relief from pain and fear." Science 193
            (July 30): 389–391.
Hopkins, C.E., M.I. Roemer, D.M. Procter, F. Gartside, J. Lubitz, G.A.
Gardner, and M. Moser
   1975   "Cost-sharing and prior authorization effects on Medicaid ser-
            vices in California: Part I. The beneficiaries' reactions." Medical
            Care 8 (July): 582–594; (August): 643–647.
Horowitz, L.A.
   1973   "Medical care price changes under the Economic Stabilization
            Program." Social Security Bulletin 36 (June): 28.
Huang, Lien-fu
   1970   "Measurement of the effect of health insurance on the demand
            for medical care." Ph.D. thesis, University of Rochester, Depart-
            ment of Economics.
Ingbar, M.L.
   1970   Report on the Rate Setting Commission of the Commonwealth
            of Massachusetts: Its Problems and Prospects. Boston: Common-
            wealth of Massachusetts, Office of Comprehensive Health Plan-
            ning, Research Report No. 1, August.
   1974   "Controlling the expansion of health care facilities in a state: The
            prediction dilemma." In Proceedings of the Public Health
            Conference on Records and Statistics meeting jointly with the
            National Conference on Mental Health Statistics, June 12–15,
            1972. DHEW Publication No. (HRA) 74-1214. Washington,
            D.C.: Government Printing Office.
Ingbar, M.L., with the assistance of C.J. Henke and E.H. Yelin
   1977   "Economics and politics as instruments for improving the deliv-
            ery of medical care and the health status of populations."
            Chapter 9, pp. 91–117, in R.L. Kane, ed., The Behavioral
            Sciences and Preventive Medicine: Opportunities and Dilem-
            mas. Proceedings of the Fogarty International Center Confer-
            ence on the Behavioral Sciences in Preventive Medicine, Be-
            thesda, Maryland, December 5 and 6, 1974. Washington, D.C.:
            Government Printing Office.

Ingbar, M.L., and L.D. Taylor
  1968   Hospital Costs in Massachusetts. Cambridge: Harvard University Press.

Kane, R.L., J. Kasteler, C. Thetford, and D.M. Olsen
  1975   "Doctor shopping: An exploratory study" (MS). A paper presented to the 103d Annual Meeting of the Medical Care Section, American Public Health Association, Chicago. Salt Lake City, Utah: University of Utah, College of Medicine, Department of Family and Community Medicine.

Kirscht, J.P., H. Becker, and J.P. Eveland
  1976   "Psychological and social factors as predictors of medical behavior." Medical Care 14 (May): 422–431.

Koch, H.K., and N.J. Dennison
  1977   "Ambulatory medical care rendered in physicians' offices: United States, 1975." Advance data from the National Center for Health Statistics, Vital and Health Statistics Number 12. DHEW, Public Health Service, Health Resources Administration, Division of Health Resources Utilization Statistics.

Kovner, A.R., and E.J. Lusk
  1975   "State regulation of health care costs." Medical Care 13 (August): 619–629.

Kravits, J., and J. Schneider
  1975   "Health care need and actual use by age, race and income." Chapter Ten, pp. 169–187, in R. Andersen, J. Kravits, and O.W. Anderson, eds., Equity in Health Services: Empirical Analyses in Social Policy. Cambridge, Mass.: Ballinger Publishing Company.

Lando, M.
  1975   "The interaction between health and education." Social Security Bulletin 38 (December): 16–23.

Lanzillotti, R.F., M.T. Hamilton, and R.B. Roberts
  1975   Phase II in Review: The Price Commission Experience. Washington, D.C.: The Brookings Institution: Studies in Wage-Price Policy.

Lewis, W.F.
  1975   Utilization of Short-Stay Hospitals: Summary of Nonmedical Statistics. Data from the National Health Survey, Vital and Health Statistics, Series 13, Number 19. DHEW Publication No. (HRA) 75-1770, June. Washington, D.C.: Government Printing Office.

Luft, H.S.
1972   "Poverty and health: An empirical investigation of the economic interactions." Unpublished dissertation. Cambridge, Mass.: Harvard University, Department of Economics.
1975   "The probability of disability: The influence of age, race, sex, education and income" (MS). A paper presented to the 103d Annual Meeting of the Medical Care Section, American Public Health Association, Chicago. Stanford University School of Medicine, Department of Community and Preventive Medicine, November.

McKinlay, J.B., and D.B. Dutton
1974   "Social-psychological factors affecting health service utilization." Pp. 251–303 in S.J. Mushkin, ed., Consumer Incentives for Health Care. New York: Prodist for Milbank Memorial Fund.

McNeil, R., Jr., and R.E. Schlenker
1975   "HMOs, competition, and government." Milbank Memorial Fund Quarterly/Health and Society 53 (Spring): 195–224.

Mechanic, D.
1972   "Social psychologic factors affecting the presentation of bodily complaints." The New England Journal of Medicine 286 (May 25): 1132–1139.

Mills, R., R.B. Fetter, D.C. Riedel, and R. Averhill
1976   "AUTOGRP: An interactive computer system for the analysis of health care data." Medical Care 14 (July): 603–615.

Mitchell, B.M., and C.E. Phelps
1975   Employer-Paid Health Insurance and the Costs of Mandated National Coverage. Santa Monica, Calif.: The RAND Corporation, R-1509-HEW, September.

Mitchell, B.M., and R.J. Vogel
1973   Health and Taxes: An Assessment of the Medical Deduction. Santa Monica, Calif.: The RAND Corporation, R-1222-OEO, August.

Moien, M.
1975   Inpatient Utilization of Short-Stay Hospitals, by Diagnosis, United States—1972. Data from the National Health Survey, Vital and Health Statistics Series 13, Number 20. DHEW Publication No. (HRA) 76-1771, November. Washington, D.C.: Government Printing Office.

Morgan, A., C. Daly, and B.J. Murawski
    1973   "Dollar and human costs of intensive care." Journal of Surgical
            Research 14 (May): 441–448.
Morreale, J.C.
    1972   "The role of the physician in the demand for medical services: A
            microeconomic approach" (MS). Kalamazoo, Mich.: Western
            Michigan University, College of Arts and Sciences, Department
            of Economics, September.
Mueller, M.S., and R.M. Gibson
    1976a   "National health expenditures, fiscal year 1975." Social Security
            Bulletin 39 (February): 3–21.
    1976b   "Age differences in health care spending, fiscal year 1975." Social
            Security Bulletin 39 (June): 18–31.
Mushkin, S.J., assisted by A. DiScuillo
    1974   "Terminal illness and incentives for health care use." Pp. 183–216
            in S.J. Mushkin, ed., Consumer Incentives for Health Care. New
            York: Prodist for Milbank Memorial Fund.
National Health Council
    1975   Making the Health Care System More Accountable: Report of
            the Western Regional Health Forum. San Francisco, Calif.,
            December 1–3, 1974. New York.
Newhouse, J.P., C.E. Phelps, and W.B. Schwartz
    1975   "Policy options and the impact of national health insurance."
            The New England Journal of Medicine 290 (June 13): 1345–1359.
            Reprinted in R. Zeckhauser et al., eds., Benefit-Cost and Policy
            Analysis, 1974. Chicago: Aldine Publishing Company.
Noll, R.C.
    1975   "The consequences of public utility regulation of hospitals." Pp.
            25–48 in Controls on Health Care. Papers of the Conference on
            Regulation in the Health Industry, January 7–9, 1974. Washing-
            ton, D.C.: National Academy of Sciences, Institute of Medicine.
O'Connor, J.T.
    1974   "Comprehensive health planning: Dreams and realities." Mil-
            bank Memorial Fund Quarterly/Health and Society 52 (Fall):
            391–413.
Pauly, M.
    1974   "Economic aspects of consumer use." Pp. 219–250 in S.J. Mush-
            kin, ed., Consumer Incentives for Health Care. New York:
            Prodist for Milbank Memorial Fund.

Perkoff, G.T., L. Kahn, and P.J. Haas
 1976 "The effects of an experimental prepaid group practice on medical care utilization and cost." Medical Care 14 (May): 432–449.
Pureka, P.T.
 1970 "Evaluating effectiveness in a government agency: A case study of the Commonwealth of Massachusetts Rate Setting Commission." Unpublished dissertation. Cambridge, Mass.: Massachusetts Institute of Technology, June.
Rafferty, J.A.
 1971 "Patterns of hospital use: An analysis of short-run variations." Journal of Political Economy 79 (January/February): 154–165.
Rice, D.P., and D. Wilson
 1975 "The American medical economy—problems and perspectives." Chapter 3, pp. 23–53, in Teh-Wei Hu, ed., International Health Costs and Expenditures. DHEW Publication No. (NIH) 76-1067. Washington, D.C.: Government Printing Office.
Ries, P.W.
 1975 Current Estimates from the Health Interview Survey, United States—1974. Data from the National Health Survey, Vital and Health Statistics, Series 10, Number 100. DHEW Publication No. (HRA) 76-1527, September. Washington, D.C.: Government Printing Office.
Rosenthal, G.
 1976 "Statement by Gerald Rosenthal, Director, National Center for Health Services Research, Health Resources Administration, Department of Health, Education and Welfare before the Subcommittee on Interstate and Foreign Commerce, House of Representatives" (MS). DHEW, Health Resources Administration, National Center for Health Services Research, February 10.
Schlenker, R.E.
 1973 Notes on Medical Care Price Controls under the Economic Stabilization Program. Minneapolis: InterStudy, February 26.
Schlenker, R.E., and P.M. Ellwood, Jr.
 1973 Medical Inflation: Causes and Policy Options for Control. Minneapolis: InterStudy, March 12.
Schlenker, R.E., and R. McNeil
 1973 Phase II and Phase III: Controls on the Hospital Sector. Minneapolis: InterStudy, April.

Scitovsky, A.A., and N. McCall
   1977   Changes in the Cost of Treatment of Selected Illnesses
           1951–1964–1971. Research Digest Series, NCHSR, DHEW Publi-
           cation No. (HRA) 77-3161.
Shannon, G.W., and G.E.A. Dever
   1974   Health Care Delivery: Spatial Perspectives. New York:
           McGraw-Hill.
Sheps, C.G.
   1972   "The influence of consumer sponsorship on medical services."
           Milbank Memorial Fund Quarterly/Health and Society 50 (Oc-
           tober): 41–69.
Slesinger, D.P., R.C. Tessler, and D. Mechanic
   1976   "The effects of social characteristics on the utilization of preven-
           tive medical services in contrasting health care programs."
           Medical Care 14 (May): 392–404.
Solon, J.A., C.G. Sheps, and S.S. Lee
   1960   "Patterns of medical care: A hospital's outpatients." American
           Journal of Public Health 50 (December): 1905–1913.
Somers, A.R.
   1973   "State regulation of hospitals and health care: The New Jersey
           Story." Blue Cross Reports, Research Series 11, July.
Starkweather, D.B.
   1975   "Hospitals: From physician dominance to public control." Public
           Affairs (Bulletin of the Institute of Government Studies, Univer-
           sity of California, Berkeley) 16 (October): 1–6.
Stigler, G.J.
   1971   "The theory of economic regulation." The Bell Journal of
           Economics and Management Science 2 (Spring): 3–21.
Stratmann, W.C., J.A. Block, S.P. Brown, and M.V. Rozzi
   1975   "A study of consumer attitudes about health care: The control,
           cost, and financing of health services." Medical Care 13 (Au-
           gust): 659–668.
Studnicki, J.
   1975   "The minimization of travel effort as a delineating influence for
           urban hospital service areas." International Journal of Health
           Services 5: 679–693.
Taylor, P.G.
   1968   "Personal factors associated with sickness absence." British
           Journal of Industrial Medicine 25: 105.

Teeling-Smith, G.
1976   "The cost of ill health." Royal Society of Health Journal 96 (April): 62–66.
Thompson, J.D., R.B. Fetter, and C.D. Mross
1975   "Case mix and resource use." Inquiry 12 (December): 300–312.
U.S. Department of Health, Education, and Welfare, Social Security Administration, Office of Research and Statistics
1972   The MADOC Report: Medicare Analysis of Days of Care, July–December 1970. Washington, D.C.
Ventura, S.J., S.M. Taffel, and E. Spratley
1975   Selected Vital and Health Statistics in Poverty and Nonpoverty Areas of 19 Large Cities: United States: 1969–1971. Data from the National Health Survey, Vital and Health Statistics, Series 21, Number 26. DHEW Publication No. (HPA) 76-1904, November. Washington, D.C.: Government Printing Office.
Weiss, J.E., M.R. Greenlick, and J.F. Jones
1971   "Determinants of medical care utilization: The impacts of spatial factors." Inquiry 8 (December): 50–57.
Wilder, C.S.
1975a   Acute Conditions: Incidence and Associated Disability: United States: July 1973–June 1974. Data from the National Health Survey, Vital and Health Statistics, Series 10, Number 102. DHEW Publication No. (HRA) 76-1529, October. Washington, D.C.: Government Printing Office.
1975b   Family Out-of-Pocket Health Expenses: United States—1970. Data from the National Health Survey, Vital and Health Statistics, Series 10, Number 103. DHEW Publication No. (HPA) 76-1530, December. Washington, D.C.: Government Printing Office.

The Hospital
Cost Containment Act of 1977:
An Analysis of the
Administration's Proposal

WILLIAM L. DUNN
AND BONNIE LEFKOWITZ[*]

Introduction

The Administration's proposed Hospital Cost Containment Act of 1977 (S. 1391 and H.R. 6575) would sharply reduce projected increases in the operating revenues and capital expansion of most short-term care hospitals. Title I of the bill would limit to about 10.6 percent the total increase in hospital operating revenues from inpatient care in 1978; Title II would reduce capital spending for the year to $6.5 billion, with greater decreases in the future. Without these controls, hospital revenues are expected to rise by about 15

[*]This analysis was prepared by William L. Dunn and Bonnie Lefkowitz of the Congressional Budget Office in response to a request from Senator Edward M. Kennedy, Chairman of the Subcommittee on Health and Scientific Research of the Senate Committee on Human Resources. The cost estimates were prepared by Jeffrey C. Merrill. Throughout the text the years referred to are fiscal years unless otherwise noted.

percent and capital spending to total about $8 billion. While the provisions of Title I are labeled "transitional," Title II is intended to provide permanent amendments to existing regulatory efforts.

Short-term hospitals have been singled out for strong regulatory action because of sustained growth in the total amount paid for their services and because the annual increase in the cost of an inpatient hospital day continues to be double the rate of overall inflation. The amount spent for hospital care has increased as a proportion of total health expenditures from about 30 percent in 1950 to almost 40 percent today. By 1981 hospital care costs are expected to account for over 43 percent of total health expenditures.

The amount spent for hospital care has risen because of increases in cost per patient day and in the number of hospital days. The former factor is much more important, accounting for about 90 percent of the increase. Over the past twenty-five years, the cost of the average day in a hospital has gone up tenfold. Nevertheless, the demand for hospital care has not abated. A major reason for this is the growth in health insurance payments, which now account for 91 percent of all hospital revenues. This high level of third-party payments has created a situation in which none of the participants involved in determining the level and type of hospital care—the patient, insuring agent, physician, or hospital administrator—has an overriding interest in or need to control either per unit costs or total expenditures.

The patient has limited ability to distinguish necessary from unnecessary care. Once in a hospital, he has a strong interest in receiving the best care available. The pervasiveness of insurance coverage has meant that the cost of treatment is of little concern. The insuring agent has usually chosen not to question the value of or need for the services provided. The physician, who acts on the patient's behalf, is inclined to use all the services that will improve his diagnosis and therapy or reduce the possibility of malpractice suits. The hospital administrator is concerned that the quality of care be of a high standard and that his facilities and equipment be such as to attract physicians to the hospital. The administrator is therefore willing to meet physicians' requests to expand the scope and complexity of the services that their institutions provide. This entails little financial risk for the administrator because the majority of hospital insurance payments are based on the costs incurred. If costs rise because of new or more intensive testing, more complex procedures, or more staff, higher reimbursements will be forthcoming.

This unique set of characteristics has encouraged the following hospital and communitywide inefficiencies in the use of resources:

- *Uneconomic hospital operation.* Inefficiency occurs when the combination of resources used to provide hospital services is more costly than necessary.
- *Uneconomic provision of services.* Inefficiency occurs when services are provided that cannot reasonably be expected to have a medical value that justifies their cost.
- *Excess community capacity to provide general care.* Even a carefully operated hospital may be relatively uneconomical if demand is low relative to capacity.
- *Excess community capacity to provide various forms of special-purpose care.* An otherwise economically run hospital may have a special facility that is underutilized because other hospitals in the area have developed the same capability.
- *Excessive utilization resulting from the existence of excess hospital facilities or equipment.* Unnecessary hospital admissions and utilization of procedures and equipment may be stimulated by the availability of capacity because no participant is motivated to be cost-conscious.

To remedy these problems hospitals must be induced by statute, financial incentives, or public pressure to behave differently. In general, the first two problems show promise of responding to changes in the reimbursement system since both are internal to the hospital. On the other hand, reimbursement pressures on hospitals to correct for underutilization may induce an increase in unnecessary care; therefore, reimbursement practices need to be coordinated with communitywide planning and investment decisions if the last three problems are to be addressed.

The Administration's proposal would place a limit on the operating revenues of hospitals, with the effect that hospital administrators could no longer expect a level of revenues equivalent to costs. The extent to which hospitals would be able to keep their costs in line with the revenue limits would depend on the decision-making process within hospitals and on how effective administrators were in gaining the cooperation of physicians, who decide on the level and complexity of care. There is nothing in the Administration's proposal that would necessarily induce physicians to alter their current behavior in the utilization of resources. If physicians did not cooperate, hospital administrators might be forced to cut back on expenditures for community services, which they do control, to stay within the revenue limits.

The Administration's proposal would also impose two new types of capital controls—a nationwide dollar limit on new capital expenditures and standards for the number of hospital beds and their rate of occupancy. The expenditure ceiling, which would be distributed among states for allocation to individual hospital projects, would significantly reduce hospital capital outlays and, thereby, could lower future hospital costs. The response of the state and local agencies that would allocate the ceiling among hospital projects would determine whether the types of investments made within the ceiling are beneficial.

This paper analyzes the two elements of the proposed Hospital Cost Containment Act of 1977. Part one describes Title I, the revenue limitation proposal, evaluates its major features, and presents possible alternatives to the Administration's approach. These alternatives include the approach proposed by Senator Herman Talmadge in the Medicare-Medicaid Administrative and Reimbursement Reform Act of 1977 (S. 1470 and H.R. 7079), which would deny federal reimbursements for unusually high routine hospital costs.[1] Part two discusses Title II, the limitation on new investments, evaluates its major features, and presents some alterna-

---

[1] For a more thorough analysis of alternative reimbursement reforms and the growth of health expenditures, see *Federal Programs and Their Impact on Health Expenditures*, CBO Background Paper (forthcoming).

tive approaches. Part three discusses the reasons for considering Titles I and II together rather than as separate proposals.

The Administration's Proposal to Limit Hospital Revenues (Title I)

The Administration has proposed in Title I of the Hospital Cost Containment Act of 1977 to place a growth ceiling on the total inpatient revenues received by short-term care hospitals (those with an average length of stay of under 30 days) beginning October 1, 1977. Revenues of federal hospitals, hospitals that derive over 75 percent of their patient care revenue from Health Maintenance Organizations (HMOs), and hospitals that are less than two years old would not be limited by the growth ceiling. The proposal is viewed as transitional and would require the Secretary of the Department of Health, Education, and Welfare (DHEW) to submit his recommendations for a permanent remedy by March 1, 1978.

The revenue limit would be applied separately to each type of payer: cost payers such as Blue Cross, Medicare, and Medicaid; and a single class known as charge payers that includes commercial insurers and self-paying patients. This would avoid disadvantaging patients of cost payers, who have traditionally negotiated a lower rate with hospitals. The proposal would also require that hospitals maintain their share of charity patient admissions.

For 1978 the growth ceiling for individual hospitals would be 8.7 percent. The growth ceiling for each year would be determined by a formula containing both an inflation component and a separate allowance for real growth. Because the proposal is intended to deter increases in the number of patients treated, this growth component is considered to be an allowance for increases in the intensity or real level of services provided per admission. The inflation component would be based on the annual percentage change of the Gross National Product (GNP) deflator over the 12 months prior to the end of June in the year in which the control period starts. The intensity component would be equal to one-third of the difference between the percentage increase in total hospital expenditures and the increase in the GNP deflator for the two calendar years prior to the year in which the control period begins. The computation for fiscal year 1978 is shown as follows:

	Inflation Component	*Intensity Component*
Growth Ceiling 1978	= GNP deflator	$+ \frac{1}{2}$ (Total hospital expenditures minus GNP deflator)
	(Percentage change 1976–III through 1977–II)	(Percentage change from Jan. 1975 through Dec. 1976)
8.73	= 5.52	+ 3.21

If the Secretary of DHEW determined that the rate of increase in the GNP deflator during the control period would be more than 1 percent greater than that computed in the inflation component of the formula, the growth ceiling could be increased.

The limit on total revenues would not be a substitute for existing reimbursement systems; rather, it would be imposed on the existing structure. Hospitals would still be reimbursed on the basis of costs or charges depending upon the method used by the payer. However, both the hospital and intermediaries would be restricted from increasing total hospital revenues by more than the growth ceiling. For example, in the case of reimbursement from a cost payer, if a hospital's costs rose 7 percent, it would get 7 percent greater revenues from the payer but could carry forward the unused 1.7 percent from the 1978 revenue limit. if costs rose 11 percent, the hospital would receive only an 8.7 percent revenue increase from that payer and revenues in excess of the limit would have to be returned to the payer. In the case of charge payers, excess revenues would have to be set aside in an escrow account and applied against the following year's allowable level. Failure to follow these procedures could result in a 150 percent excise tax on the excess revenues.

For increases up to 2 percent and decreases up to 6 percent in the number of patients admitted to a hospital during the year, there would be no change in the revenue limit. However, to allow for more substantial changes in the number of patients admitted, a volume adjustment to the total revenue limit is included in the proposal. For each increased admission between 2 and 15 percent, a hospital's total revenue could be raised by 50 percent of the base period's average revenue per admission.[2] Increases over 15 percent would not be reimbursed in large hospitals; in smaller hospitals, the allowance would continue without a cutoff because admissions to such hospitals are subject to more variation.[3]

A similar type of volume adjustment would be applied to decreases in admissions. For each decreased admission between 6 and 15 percent, a hospital's total revenue would be reduced by 50 percent of the base period's average revenue per admission. In large hospitals, decreases beyond 15 percent would mean a reduction of the full average revenue per admission. The revenue limit for small hospitals would not be changed for decreases in admissions of less than 10 percent; beyond 10 percent, total revenue would be reduced by 50 percent of the average revenue per admission.

Hospitals could elect to have their limits on revenue increased to the sum of the actual percentage increase of nonsupervisory personnel wages weighted by this input's share of total costs, plus the formula-determined growth ceiling weighted by the remaining share of total costs. Therefore, for 1978 if nonsupervisory workers accounted for 25 percent of total costs and their wages rose by 16 percent, the revenue limit would be 10.5 percent (.25 × 16.0% + .75 × 8.7%) rather than 8.7 percent.

In addition to the fairly automatic adjustments that have been described, a federal review board could increase a large hospital's revenue limit if admissions increased or decreased more than 15 percent, or if there were changes in hospital capacity or services that increased costs by more than the intensity component of the growth ceiling (3.2 percent in 1978). Changes in admissions, capacity, or services would have to have been approved by the state certificate-of-need or Section 1122 review agency. In order to appeal, the appellant hospital's ability to pay its current liabilities after the change (as measured by the ratio of its current assets to liabilities) would have to be in the lowest 25 percent of all hospitals included in

[2]Fifty percent of average revenue is believed by the Administration to be an adequate measure of the added cost per admission.

[3]Smaller hospitals are defined as those with fewer than 4,001 admissions annually in the base period.

the revenue limit.[4] Financial distress alone would not be a sufficient basis for appeal.

A successful appeal based upon admission changes alone would result in treatment of the large hospital as a small hospital in calculating the volume adjustment. A successful appeal based on changes in service or capacity would result in raising the revenue limit, but only by the amount needed to increase the hospital's asset to liability ratio to a level where it is no longer in the lowest 25 percent of hospitals included in the revenue limit.

The proposal would not preclude states or payers from operating their own cost control programs concomitantly with the federal controls. However, nonfederal programs could be substituted for the federal program only in certain situations.

State cost-containment programs could be substituted if the state's governor ensured that the federal revenue limit would be met and that procedures for recovering excess hospital revenues and returning them to the payers would be established. The state cost-containment program would have to have been in operation for at least one year before the application for a waiver from the federal program and would have to have included 90 percent of the hospitals in the state and 50 percent of all hospital inpatient revenues. The state would have to include 100 percent of inpatient revenues once it received a waiver to substitute its own controls for the federal program. Hospitals in prospective reimbursement demonstrations approved by the federal government—whether or not all the hospitals in the state participate—could be exempted without meeting these conditions.

---

[4]This ratio is the sum of cash notes and accounts receivable (less reserves for bad debts), marketable securities and inventories held by the hospital divided by the sum of its liabilities falling due in the accounting year for which the exception is requested. A preliminary estimate, derived by the Administration from American Hospital Association data, is that this ratio is higher than 2 to 1 for 75 percent of the hospitals subject to the revenue limit.

The Administration has not determined whether the standard would be a fixed ratio or a ratio that declines over time as the financial condition of hospitals worsens as a consequence of the revenue limit. In the latter case, the criterion would be increasingly stringent.

Impact of the Administration's Proposal

There are a number of major advantages to the Administration's proposal, the most important being that it would result in substantial savings in the amount paid for care in nonfederal short-term hospitals as early as 1978. These savings would grow rapidly in subsequent years, with an increasing proportion coming from reduced growth in the intensity of services. Growth in hospital admissions would probably decline as well, because the proposal contains strong incentives for most hospitals to treat fewer patients.

The Administration's approach would be simple to administer and could be implemented immediately. In many ways it is the proposal's very simplicity that creates some of its shortcomings. While a great deal of the following discussion concentrates on describing these disadvantages it should be noted that most of them could be addressed through modifications in the Administration's proposal. In addition, an approach similar to that taken by the Administration, placing a growth ceiling on the amount paid for care, may be the only way of significantly reducing the rapid rise in hospital costs.

Among the proposal's disadvantages are the following: First, it would do little to reward efficiency, and in some cases, would penalize past efficiency. Second, the proposal would not distinguish well among types of hospitals and the mix of patients they serve. Third, the exceptions process would be quite restricted and its remedies fairly limited. Fourth, the ceiling could be applied too abruptly for hospitals to cut back on growth commitments. Fifth, the optional wage pass-through may raise costs and may not be an effective way to protect hospital workers. Sixth, the measure chosen to reflect inflation in the growth ceiling formula is not a good index of the price increases facing hospitals. Both the advantages and disadvantages of the Administration's proposal are discussed in greater detail below.

If existing policies continue, total expenditures for nonfederal short-term hospitals are expected to be $61.3 billion in 1978 and $104.0 billion by 1982 (refer to Table 1). If the Administration's proposal were implemented in 1978, including expected adjustments for admission increases, wage pass-throughs, and exceptions,

TABLE 1   Estimated Impact of the Administration's Proposed Growth Ceiling
on Nonfederal Short-term Care Hospital Revenues,
Fiscal Years 1978–1982
(dollars in billions)[a]

	Current Policy		Under Administration's Proposal			
Fiscal Year	1. Rate of Growth	2. Expenditures for Hospital Services[b]	3. Growth Ceiling	4. Growth Ceiling + Expected Increases[d]	5. Expenditures for Hospital Services	6. Savings due to Growth Ceiling
1978	15.1%	$61.3	8.7%[c]	10.6%	$58.9	$2.4
1979	14.0	69.8	9.3	11.2	65.5	4.3
1980	14.1	79.7	7.6	9.5	71.8	7.9
1981	14.0	90.8	7.1	9.0	78.2	12.6
1982	14.5	104.0	7.0	8.9	85.2	18.8
1978 to 1982	14.3%	$405.1	7.9%	9.8%	$359.6	$46.0

[a] Congressional Budget Office estimates. Entries do not sum to totals because of rounding.
[b] These figures are for only those hospitals that would be covered by the Administration's proposal. Total expenditures for hospital care without any new cost-containment initiatives are estimated at $55.4 billion for 1976, $64.3 billion for 1977, and $73.9 billion for 1978.
[c] The growth ceiling for 1978 differs from the Administration's 9 percent projection because, at the time the Administration made its estimate, figures for calendar year 1976 hospital expenditures were not available.
[d] Column 4 is column 3 plus a 1.0 percent allowance for increases in admissions plus a 0.9 percent allowance for revenue increases due to the pass-through of wage increases and to the exceptions process.

these expenditures would be limited to $58.9 billion, a 10.6 percent increase over the 1977 level. The nation's hospital care bill would be $2.4 billion lower than otherwise expected and federal payments for Medicare and Medicaid would be reduced by $1 billion.

By 1982, under the Administration's proposal, expenditures for nonfederal short-term care hospitals would rise to $85.2 billion, $18.8 billion lower than otherwise expected. Federal payments for Medicare and Medicaid would be reduced by about $8.2 billion. The total reduction in hospital revenues or savings expected from the Administration's proposal during the five-year period 1978–1982 would be about $46 billion.

The Administration's proposal would probably have its most profound impact on the real growth (increases net of inflation) in hospital revenues because the intensity component of the limit is designed to decrease over time.[5] This component depends each year

[5] If admissions did not decrease, or if the inflation component underestimated the rate of increase in prices hospitals must pay for goods and services, very little would actually be left of the limit for increased intensity or real growth per admission.

TABLE 2   Estimated Components of Annual Growth in the
Administration's Proposal
Fiscal Years 1978–1982 [a]

	Intensity Component (For Two Calendar Years Before Fiscal Year)			Inflation Component (12 Months Prior to June of Previous Fiscal Year)	
Fiscal Year	1. Total Hospital Expendi- tures [b]	2. GNP De- flator	3. Allowance for Intensity [c]	4. GNP De- flator	5. Growth Ceiling [d]
1978	15.51	5.87	3.21	5.52	8.73
1979	14.91	5.55	3.12	6.22	9.34
1980	12.65	6.00	2.22	5.40	7.62
1981	11.50	5.39	2.04	5.02	7.06
1982	10.98	5.12	1.95	5.06	7.01

[a]Congressional Budget Office estimates.
[b]Those hospitals not included in the cost-containment program are assumed to increase their expenditures by 14 percent per year. While the proposal excludes new hospitals and those whose primary source of revenue is from HMOs, these estimates did not adjust for their exclusion because of their insignificant effect.
[c]Column 3 is one-third of the difference between Column 1 and Column 2.
[d]Column 5 is the sum of Columns 3 and 4.

on the two prior years' increase in total hospital expenditures. Since such expenditures are expected to be reduced by the proposal, subsequent allowances for increased intensity will also be smaller.

Since 1965, real growth in expenditures by hospitals has occurred at an average rate of almost 8.4 percent annually. Approximately 2.3 percent of the growth has been attributable to additional admissions and 6.1 percent to increased intensity. Under the Administration's proposal, the noninflation component would be about 3.2 percent in 1978 and would be reduced to less than 2 percent by 1982 (refer to Table 2).

Because revenue per admission increases as the volume of admissions is cut back, a strong incentive to treat fewer patients would be created by the Administration's proposal. If a large hospital reduced the volume of patients treated up to the threshold of 6 percent, total revenues allowed would remain the same and revenues per admission would be increased (refer to Table 3). If volume were reduced between 6 and 15 percent, the hospital's income would be decreased by only 50 percent of the base period's average revenue per admission. Therefore, at 85 percent of the base year's volume, a hospital could receive 123 percent of the base period's revenue per admission. Even reductions in admissions

TABLE 3   Total Revenues and Revenue per Admission under the
Administration's Proposal at Varying Levels of Admissions
(All figures expressed as percents of the base year)

Annual Admissions	Potential Total Revenue	Potential Revenue Per Admission
Hospitals over 4,000 Admissions		
60	79	132
85	104	123
94	109	116
100	109	109
102	109	107
115	115	100
150	115	77
Hospitals under 4,001 Admissions		
60	94	156
90	109	121
94	109	116
100	109	109
102	109	107
115	115	100
150	133	88

beyond 15 percent would allow for an increase in revenues per admission.

Small hospitals could reduce volume by 10 percent without lowering their total revenue limit, and further reductions in volume, no matter how great, would result in a decrease of 50 percent of the base period's average revenue per admission. Thus a small hospital would be eligible to receive up to 121 percent of revenue per admission when it is at 90 percent of the base period's volume and 156 percent of revenue per admission at 60 percent of the base period's volume.

These incentives would of course be limited not only by the hospital's operating costs, but also by its desire to maintain its patient volume relative to other hospitals, its concept of service to the community, and the behavior of its physicians. Most hospitals would probably attempt to reduce admissions slightly or to avoid increases in admissions.

A major problem with the Administration's approach is that it does not significantly recognize different levels of efficiency among hospitals. The only way the proposal would reward efficient behavior would be to let a hospital whose revenues were less than those allowed add the difference to its next year's limit. Other types of efficiency incentives would require more reliable and uniform reporting of hospital costs than is currently available.

The revenue ceiling should force many hospitals to operate more efficiently. However, without more specific incentives, hospital administrators might not be able to withstand pressure from physicians to continue inefficient practices. Moreover, fast-growing hospitals would be most affected by the Administration's proposal, whether or not they were efficient. Because efficient hospitals may have already sought the obvious economies, they could find it more difficult to reduce their growth rates than would inefficient hospitals with a lot of slack in their operations.

The Administration's proposal could induce some hospitals to admit more patients that are inexpensive to treat, such as simple surgery cases and candidates for diagnostic testing, and to direct expensive cases elsewhere. Some expensive cases might be referred to teaching hospitals, and others might end up in county and municipal hospitals that have no choice in the patients they accept. While there would be some protection in the Administration's proposal against a hospital's "dumping" charity patients and patients whose insurance pays less relative to other types of payers, there is no provision to prevent adverse selection by type of diagnosis.[6] Neither would the proposal recognize this tendency by allowing higher growth rates for the hospitals that must treat additional expensive cases.

The volume adjustment provided in the Administration's proposal could also affect patient mix under certain circumstances. While most hospitals would tend to decrease the number of admissions or maintain their current volume, some of those already at 102

[6]Approximately 200 Health Systems Agencies established nationwide by the Health Planning and Resources Development Act of 1974 would be responsible for enforcing the maintenance of the charity patient provision when complaints were received from hospitals, presumably mostly county and municipal, which would have to treat those refused by the others. However, the hospitals that might be expected to complain are those that pay less attention to the insurance status of their patients. Moreover, Health Systems Agencies have little experience in such enforcement.

percent of their base year's volume might attempt to increase admissions further. This would occur if they could find cases that cost less to treat than the amount by which their revenue limits would increase—50 percent of the base period's average revenue per admission. To the extent that volume was increased by patients who would not have otherwise been hospitalized, the Administration's proposal would encourage behavior that increases expenditures.

Under the Administration's proposal, the exceptions process would be limited to those hospitals with substantial changes in admissions or services that can also demonstrate financial distress. The process would clearly simplify federal administrative procedures, but it would be difficult to deal with problems specific to a particular hospital or with unanticipated price increases that are not systemwide. The stringency of the exceptions process might also lead to undesirable behavior on the part of hospitals. For example, a hospital might choose to cut back on services needed by the community, such as an emergency room or an outpatient clinic, rather than using up most of its reserves, which it would have to do before applying for an exception.

In addition to the fact that only a limited number of hospitals could apply for an exception, the remedies available under the Administration's proposal are not likely to be attractive to hospitals. The remedy for an increase in admissions greater than 15 percent, without an increase in capacity, would be to allow the hospital to receive 50 percent of average revenue per admission. When a hospital is operating close to capacity, this is probably substantially less than it costs to care for an additional patient. The remedy for a change in capacity or a change in the character of services would be to increase the hospital's revenue limit just enough to bring its current ratio of assets to liabilities up to the level where it would be disqualified from applying for an exception. Such remedies may provide relief that is less than the added costs incurred by the hospital.

The Administration's proposal might impose a particular hardship on hospitals that have already committed themselves to growth in capacity or intensity of services. The lead time for such commitments is often as great as three years. With only nine months' notice of a growth ceiling, hospitals may not be able to extricate themselves from commitments they would have avoided with more notice.

The wage pass-through option offered in the Administration's proposal could undermine hospitals' resistance to large wage increases for nonsupervisory personnel in two ways. First, the existence of the growth ceiling could lead unions and workers to expect wage increases equal to the limit. This would be greater than most past raises for such workers, which averaged 7.2 percent annually between 1969 and 1976.

Second, hospitals and unions could collaborate to escape the growth ceiling by arranging to have large wage increases every second or third year. In the year in which the wage increase was given, the hospital could request a pass-through, making it indifferent to an increase that might be as great as 15 or 20 percent. In the other year or two when no wage increase was given, the hospital could select the standard method for calculating its growth limit and could use its entire revenue increase for nonlabor purposes.

Under the Administration's proposal, hospitals may not be well protected from increases in the cost of the goods and services they need to maintain their existing level of care because these increases are not well measured by the GNP deflator. Moreover, the use of past rates of inflation in the Administration's formula does not reflect current price increases. An adjustment could be made only if the most recent annual rate of increase reported for the GNP deflator is more than 1 percentage point greater than the rate used in the formula.

Alternatives to the Administration's Proposal

Both incremental changes and more distinct alternatives to Title I of the Hospital Cost Containment Act of 1977 exist. Those that represent minor modifications of the Administration's proposal could address most of the problems that have been raised above without delaying implementation. However, they would do little to promote efficiency, since the proposal is structured to control growth rather than to affect present hospital operations.

A distinct alternative is the Medicare-Medicaid Administrative and Reimbursement Reform Act recently introduced by Senator Herman Talmadge. The Talmadge proposal is directed at eliminating operating inefficiencies rather than containing the growth of hospital services. It would take several years to implement and would result in much smaller savings than the Administration's proposal. Approaches that combine the advantages of the Administration's proposal and the Talmadge approach could also be formulated.

Modifications in the Administration's proposal include grouping hospitals as to size and case mix before applying growth ceilings, broadening the exceptions process, combining allowable increases over the first two years, either making the wage pass-through mandatory or eliminating it entirely, and using a more precise indicator of hospital costs than the GNP deflator.

Varying the Growth Limit among Hospital Types   The Administration's proposal would create incentives for further concentration of patients with illnesses that are expensive to treat in teaching hospitals and those operated by county and municipal governments. It might therefore be desirable to recognize that such hospitals may need to grow at a faster rate. Hospitals could be classified according to the services they provide and different growth limits applied to each class. A further modification would require a more refined classification system but might also provide some incentives for effieicncy by allowing each member of a class the same dollar increment rather than the same percentage increase in revenues. For example, if the average revenue for a specific class were $1,000 per admission and the growth limit were set at 9 percent, all hospitals in that group would be permitted a $90 increment per admission over their previous year's revenues. For a hospital whose revenues were only half that of the average, this would represent an 18 percent increment; for a hospital whose revenues were 50 percent greater than the group average, it would be only a 4.5 percent increase. This approach would require a sufficient number of hospital classes so that those in each class were reasonably alike. It might also be necessary to group hospitals by region of the country to avoid imposing hardships on hospitals in high-cost regions.

Broadening the Exceptions Process The proposed exceptions process would be accessible only to those institutions that are expanding admissions, services, or capacity and are, at the same time, in relatively poor financial shape. There may be ways of making the exceptions process more flexible, although this would entail more staff, either at the state or federal level. A more flexible exceptions process could delete the present proposal's financial distress requirement. In addition to restricting access to the process, this requirement may not be an appropriate screening device for determining whether expanded services should be reimbursed.

Broadening the exceptions process would not necessarily decrease anticipated savings. Since a more flexible and accessible exceptions process could reduce the danger of imposing hardship on individual hospitals, a revenue ceiling lower than that arising from the proposal's current formula could be set. For example, the revenue ceiling could be set at the inflation rate plus 1 percent (6.5 percent for 1978). Three percent could be set aside for exceptions, rather than the less than 1 percent the Administration has estimated for its proposal. Such a procedure might be more acceptable to the hospital industry since it would be less arbitrary.

Combining Allowable Increases over the First Two Years The imposition of a growth ceiling would penalize all high rates of growth, whether sustained or temporary. This may not be undesirable if capital outlays that the cost-containment proposal seeks to discourage are responsible for sudden spurts in expenditures. However, if the growth in hospital outlays expected in 1978 reflects obligations and decisions that have already been made, hospitals may have very little ability to control immediate growth. A modification would be to combine the growth allowed in hospital revenues over the next two fiscal years, achieving the same savings but giving hospitals a longer period in which to adjust.[7]

Making the Wage Pass-Through Mandatory or Eliminating It The growth ceiling could be calculated for each hospital on the basis of its actual wage increases, thus making the wage pass-through

---

[7] The compound rate of growth for the two-year period that would be allowed under the present proposal is about 18.8 percent.

mandatory. With this modification, a hospital could not squeeze wage increases in order to maintain other spending as it could with the standard method of calculation in the Administration's proposal. Thus a mandatory pass-through would be more likely to protect nonsupervisory hospital employees. It would also eliminate the possibility that hospitals might cooperate with unions to avoid the growth ceiling by alternating large wage increases in one year with none in the next. If annual wage increases continued to average less than the growth ceiling, anticipated savings would be greater with a mdndatory wage pass-through than under the Administration's proposal. However, if the pass-through were mandatory, there would be little reason for hospitals to resist wage increases and there could be a danger of larger increases. Some concern about future hospital wage levels could be retained by making it clear to hospitals that permanent reforms of hospital reimbursement might use a wage index based on area wages or average hospital wages rather than the hospital's actual wage level. Since the Administration's proposal would allow the Secretary of DHEW to consider eliminating the wage pass-through after eighteen months, statements to unions that wage increases would have to remain in line with those for comparable employees in other industries to preserve the pass-through might encourage restraint.

Alternatively, the pass-through could be made mandatory only for those hospitals that choose it initially. Those hospitals not selecting the wage pass-through would not have to report labor and nonlabor costs separately, and, as with the first alternative, the possibility of union-hospital collaboration to evade the growth limit would be eliminated. However, nonsupervisory hospital employees would be no more protected than with the present proposal.

Finally, the wage pass-through could be eliminated. This would not protect hospital employees, particularly in geographic areas where wages are still low. However, the elimination would recognize that the wages of hospital workers in other geographic areas may no longer be out of line with nonhospital workers.

Improving the Measure of Inflation   While the Consumer Price Index (CPI) would seem to be a better indicator of prices that a hospital must pay then the GNP deflator, the best alternative would be the construction of a separate hospital cost index. Such an index could be designed to reflect most accurately the price changes for the types of goods and services purchased by hospitals. Rate-setting commissions in some states currently use a hospital price index in determining allowable increases in revenues.

The problem of using past rather than current measures of inflation could be remedied by using projected rates, such as those used in the President's budget. An adjustment could be made at the end of the year or could be added to the next year's ceiling to compensate for any difference between the projected and the actual rate.

The Talmadge Proposal

The proposal introduced by Senator Talmadge in May 1977 is a distinct alternative to the Administration's proposal to control hospital costs. It would apply limits only to Medicare and Medicaid reimbursements and only to the 30 percent of those reimbursements attributable to room and board and some salaries which the proposal labels as routine. Under the Talmadge proposal, hospitals would be grouped by number of beds and type (short-term general, teaching, and specialty hospitals). The average routine operating cost for each hospital group would be determined, and reimbursements to any hospital would be limited to 120 percent of its group's average cost. Bonus payments of up to 5 percent of routine costs would be awarded to a hospital that is below the average cost for its group.

The changes in hospital reimbursement called for in the Talmadge proposal would not take effect until 1981, when a uniform cost-reporting system would be in place. The total reduction in federal expenditures for hospital care under Medicaid and Medicare might range from $0.1 to $0.4 billion in 1982.[8] While the Talmadge

[8]The range is wide because hospitals would have three years to prepare for implementation and it is difficult to predict changes in their behavior. The data on hospital costs used to estimate the savings were collected in 1973 during the Economic Stabilization Program and thus may not represent 1982 hospital costs very well.

proposal would reward operating efficiency quite well, it would not assure reduction in the growth rate of expenditures by hospitals, even for routine services. If all the hospitals in a class became less cost-conscious, the group average for routine costs of operation and the reimbursement limit would increase together.

If the Talmadge approach were applied to total hospital costs rather than to routine costs, savings might be lower because bonuses might increase more than penalties.

The savings generated by the Talmadge proposal could be increased if the limit on unusual costs were moved closer to the average cost. For example, if reimbursements were disallowed for routine costs in excess of 110 percent of the group average, rather than 120 percent, the cost savings might range from $0.2 to $0.8 billion in 1982. A limit set this close to the average cost for the group might cause substantial losses for some hospitals unless it were phased in even more slowly than anticipated by the Talmadge proposal.

Another option that could increase savings using the Talmadge approach would be to reduce or eliminate the bonus payments. Alternatively, the bonuses could be retained for hospitals with below-average costs and only a part (perhaps a third) of that portion of hospital costs above the average could be reimbursed. There would then always be an incentive for a hospital to cut its costs. Under the current proposal, hospitals above the group's average but below 120 percent have no such incentive.

Still another way of comparing hospitals' costs rather than limiting their growth would be to have hospitals submit bids in advance for providing care. The bids would include all costs, not just routine costs, and could be implemented fairly quickly without a uniform cost-reporting system. The only information required from hospitals would be the hospital's past volume and its estimated operating costs for the next fiscal year. Hospitals would be grouped as under the Talmadge proposal but their bids, rather than their actual costs, would be averaged and compared. A hospital with a bid below the group average would receive more than 100 percent of its bid for its interim payment; in other words, it would receive a bonus payment. Conversely, a hospital with a bid above the norm would receive a reimbirsement rate below its bid—or be penalized.

As with the Talmadge approach, the savings from this alternative would be quite low but efficiency incentives would be introduced. To assure that bids reflected actual costs, a retrospective adjustment of the reimbursement rate could be made at the end of the fiscal year. This adjustment could also be varied according to the extent to which the hospital's actual cost differed from its original bid.[9]

The Administration and Talmadge proposals could be integrated to retain the advantages of both. If the Administration's revenue controls or a similar program were implemented in 1978, immediate savings would result. As soon as there were sufficient data to differentiate among types of costs, the Talmadge approach could be applied to routine costs for all payers, rather than just for Medicare and Medicaid. The efficiency incentives of the Talmadge proposal are best applied to routine hospital operations, over which the hospital administrator has the greatest authority. The Administration's approach, which is directed at reducing growth in the intensity of services, could continue to be applied to nonroutine costs, for which the hospital administrator shares authority with the hospital's medical staff. In general, expenditures by hospitals for nonroutine services are the principal source of growth in the industry. Thus, both problems of hospital operation—uneconomic hospital operation and uneconomic provision of services—would be addressed by a combined approach.

---

[9]The formula for determining the reimbursement rate could have two components, one which rewards hospitals for bidding low and penalizes high bids and another which rewards hospitals that hold their costs below their bid and penalizes those that do not.

$$\text{Reimbursement} = \text{Cost} \times \left[1 + \frac{(\text{Avg. Bid} - \text{Bid})}{\text{Avg. Bid}}\right] \times \left[1 + \frac{(\text{Bid} - \text{Cost})}{\text{Bid}}\right]$$

Bid Adjustment   Cost Adjustment

This option is discussed in more depth in *Federal Programs and Their Impact on Health Expenditures*, CBO Background Paper (forthcoming).

The Administration's Proposal to Limit
Hospital Capital Expenditures (Title II)

Background

Rising capital expenditures are an important—some believe the most important—source of hospital cost increases. These expenditures comprise about 13 percent of all spending by nonfederal short-term hospitals. If there is no change in current policy, they are expected to reach $8.0 billion in 1978 and $14.1 billion by 1982. The annual increases in capital expenditures have been slightly higher than those of total hospital spending, averaging 15.5 percent between 1970 and 1975. Approximately half of this increase, or 8.2 percent, is attributable to rising prices; the remainder reflects real growth in capital spending.

Most new capital spending is not considered a cost in itself; rather, it raises hospital costs in two ways. First, more than 80 percent of capital expenditures are paid for by borrowing, which adds to the hospital's annual debt service burden. Second, and more important, capital spending affects operating costs. While the precise relationship is not known, in the aggregate every dollar invested is thought to raise annual operating costs very roughly by 50 cents in subsequent years.

There are two types of capital expenditures—those that change the type of service provided each patient, usually measured by plant assets per bed, and those that increase the capacity of the facility, usually measured by number of beds. Plant assets per bed in community hospitals increased from $21,300 to $34,500, or an average of 10.1 percent annually between 1970 and 1975. This first type of expenditure can either lower or raise operating costs. For example, better insulation could lead to lower fuel bills, or new laboratory apparatus could reduce the need for more costly manual analyses. On the other hand, new technology is often more expensive to operate than existing equipment and adds to the services provided each patient. A frequently cited example is the Computerized Axial Tomography (CAT) scanner, a diagnostic device that costs roughly $500,000 to buy and can be expected to cost a hospital another $300,000 annually to run.

The second type of expenditure, an increase in bed capacity, almost always raises total operating costs. Nearly 100,000 community hospital beds were added between 1970 and 1975, increasing the total supply by an average of 2.2 percent annually and bringing the nationwide bed-to-population ratio to 4.4 beds per 1,000 persons. Many health planners believe that a ratio of 4.0 beds, or less, per 1,000 would be sufficient. If capacity is idle because it is greater than the demand for care, hospitals will operate inefficiently. This inefficiency is particularly pronounced in the hospital industry, where fixed costs represent approximately 60 percent of total costs.

Additional capacity can raise costs in another way because the number of days spent in the hospital and the volume of hospital-based procedures performed often increase with availability. This is related to the fact that physicians and their patients do not face the cost constraints found in most industries. Although individual hospitals may operate at a more efficient occupancy level in the presence of this induced demand factor, total hospital costs will be higher and the population may receive unnecessary care.

While additional costs to hospitals tend to be passed on in some form to consumers, hospitals may also use their assets or reduce their spending in an unrelated area to pay for a cost increase attributable to capital expenditures. Thus, a one-to-one relationship does not exist between capital expenditure-related cost increases and patient payments. A good case in point is debt service, which is not included directly in reimbursement rates. Reimbursements do include interest and depreciation, but the latter is often calculated on a larger base than that for which debt principal is owed, and it is figured over a longer period of time than the term of the debt.

In the past, the federal government supported expansion of hospital capacity directly through construction grants (the Hill-Burton program). Expansion is still supported indirectly through guaranteed loans and the tax-exempt nature of some bonds issued in behalf of nonprofit hospitals. Money raised through tax-exempt bonds paid for more than 50 percent of all hospital construction outlays in 1976.

Only recently have steps been taken to control capital growth and reallocate resources. The primary regulatory mechanism is the National Health Planning and Resources Development Act of 1974, which requires every state to have a certificate-of-need program satisfactory to the Secretary of HEW no later than September 30, 1980, if the state is to continue to receive most federal health grants. Certificate-of-need agencies have approval power over proposals for new beds, services, and other capital expenditures in excess of $150,000. Thirty-two of the fifty states now have certificate-of-need statutes. Only five of these, all initiated before 1969 by the states themselves, appear to be at all effective. That is, available evidence indicates that they may reduce capital expenditures 5 percent annually, at the most, from otherwise anticipated levels.[10]

Another mechanism for controlling hospital capital expenditures was established by a 1972 amendment to the Social Security Act (Section 1122). This amendment provided for a similar state review process but with a $100,000 threshold and a federal sanction. If a capital expenditure is not approved, the amount attributable to depreciation and interest for that expenditure is disallowed from Medicare and Medicaid reimbursements. Seventeen of the eighteen states that do not have certificate-of-need statutes have Section 1122 agreements.

Despite current efforts to control hospital capital expenditures, the following five types of problems remain:

- Growth is not being curbed rapidly or effectively enough because of the long lead time needed to establish a properly functioning review process and the political pressures on states to approve new projects.
- Excess capacity and maldistribution of hospital resources persist, primarily because most current programs control only new projects and cannot close or reduce existing facilities. Only a few states have moved tentatively to eliminate existing unneeded beds.

---

[10] Congressional Budget Office, *Federal Programs and Their Impact on Health Expenditures* (forthcoming).

- In the absence of need and effectiveness criteria for new technology, state agencies have found it especially difficult to control nonbed expenditures.
- Many expenditures are under the $150,000 or $100,000 threshold and are therefore too small to be reviewed by certificate-of-need or Section 1122 agencies. Only a complementary system of reimbursement controls could affect these expenditures, and such a system is not yet in place.
- Hospital-type procedures performed outside a hospital are not controlled.

The Administration's Proposal

In an effort to deal with some of these remaining problems, the Administration has proposed in Title II of the Hospital Cost Containment Act of 1977 two new types of permanent federal controls: a capital expenditure limit and bed and occupancy standards. New sanctions would be provided to help ensure implementation.

The Administration has proposed that no more than $2.5 billion in new capital expenditures by nonfederal short-term hospitals be approved by review agencies nationwide in any year beginning with 1978. This limit would be allocated among the states on the basis of population during the first two years of the legislation. In subsequent years other factors, such as need for new facilities, construction costs, and condition of existing hospitals, might be considered in the allocation.

A state would specify the maximum expenditure by a hospital under each certificate of need issued and the total of these could not exceed the state's portion of the limit. Expenditures supported by charitable contributions and those made in nonhospital premises leased by the hospital would be included in the limit. Any part of a state's limit that was unused at the end of the year would be added to its limit in the subsequent year. A state's limit could be increased by the amount of unrealized depreciation on beds or facilities it closes. That is, if a hospital facility valued at $10 million when new were to close down after it had received $7 million in depreciation payments, the remainder, or $3 million, would be added to the state's capital expenditure limit.

The Administration's proposal would also establish a standard of no more than 4.0 beds per 1,000 persons and at least 80 percent aggregate bed occupancy for each of the nation's 212 health service areas.[11] For hospitals in areas meeting both criteria, a certificate of need resulting in additional beds could be issued only if the area would be in compliance with the criteria after the new project was completed. In areas not meeting both criteria, a certificate of need resulting in additional beds for an individual hospital could be issued only if twice as many existing beds were eliminated in the area as a whole. However, the two-for-one requirement would not apply to an individual hospital if no net increase resulted from its proposal to eliminate some beds and add others.[12]

The Administration has proposed that in states without a certificate-of-need program, and in those where the certificate-of-need program does not yet include dollar limits on investment approvals, the limits would be enforced through Section 1122 of the Social Security Act, but with greatly expanded penalties. Unapproved capital expenditures would result in a penalty of ten times the amount attributable to depreciation and interest for those expenditures, applied against Medicare and Medicaid reimbursements. If the state has neither an acceptable certificate-of-need program nor a Section 1122 agreement, the Secretary of HEW would apply the Section 1122 sanctions directly. In all states, bonds would no longer be tax-exempt if they supported bed increases that would force an area out of compliance with the standards, or for which a certificate of need had not been issued.

Impact of the Administration's Proposal

The Administration's proposal would address the first and probably most pressing problem—continued growth in capital spending—with a substantial but partially delayed cut in allowable

[11]The proposal does allow for the possibility that different ceilings and standards could be established for areas with special characteristics. Presumably places such as the health service area in Minnesota containing the Mayo Clinic would be included.
[12]It has not yet been determined whether the beds would have to be eliminated during the year that the certification is awarded, or at the time that the new beds were ready for occupancy.

expenditures. The proposal would only partially address the problem of excess capacity and maldistribution, and it might exacerbate the third problem—difficulty in reviewing nonbed expenditures. The proposed controls would not deal with the problem of hospital-type procedures performed outside the hospital. Neither would they cover small investments, although the revenue controls in Title I could do so.

If hospitals continued their current policies and the Administration's proposal were not adopted, capital expenditures requiring certificate of need or Section 1122 review would amount to $6.8 billion in 1978 (refer to Table 4). Additional capital expenditures that are too small to require review would raise total capital spending in 1978 to roughly $8 billion. If the Administration's proposal were adopted, the $2.5 billion ceiling would be applied to certificate-of-need and Section 1122 applications in 1978. However, its full impact would not be felt until 1981, because much of the capital spending during the next few years will be related to construction projects that were approved before 1978 but are not yet completed and in use. Thus, actual 1978 capital expenditures would be about $6.5 billion even with the Administration's limit in place. In 1981, when the full impact of the ceiling would be felt, capital spending would be $4.3 billion, $7.9 billion below the $12.2 billion anticipated without such controls. In 1982 spending would be $4.6 billion of an otherwise anticipated $14.1 billion.

One criticism that might be leveled against the Administration's proposal is that the magnitude of the cut is rather arbitrary, since it is not based on an evaluation of need for new capital expenditures. Once few or no new beds are being added, there may be an unmet need for modernization of outmoded facilities that exceeds the capital spending limit.

A second criticism that might be leveled is that allocation of the $2.5 billion ceiling among states on the basis of population is arbitrary, bearing little relation to differences in costs or to the states' relative need for replacing or improving facilities. Nationwide, the $2.5 billion would represent a reduction of about 70 percent from an anticipated level of $8.1 billion that would have been approved by state review agencies in 1978. With a distribution based on popula-

TABLE 4   Components of Hospital Capital Expenditures under Current Policy and the Administration's Proposal, Fiscal Years 1978–1982 (dollars in billions)

	Current Policy						Administration's Proposal				
	1975	1978	1979	1980	1981	1982	1978	1979	1980	1981	1982
New beds[a]	$1.2	$1.8	$2.1	$2.4	$2.8	$3.2	$1.8	$2.1	$2.4	—	—
Other construction and modernization[b]	2.6	4.0	4.6	5.3	6.1	7.0	3.0	2.0	2.0	$2.0	$2.0
Equipment[c]	.6	1.0	1.2	1.3	1.5	1.8	.5	.5	.5	.5	.5
Total requiring certificate of need or 1122 review	4.4	6.8	7.9	9.0	10.4	12.0	5.3	4.6	4.9	2.5	2.5
Not requiring certificate of need or 1122 review	.8	1.2	1.4	1.6	1.8	2.1	1.2	1.4	1.6	1.8	2.1
Total capital expenditures[d]	$5.2	$8.0	$9.3	$10.6	$12.2	$14.1	$6.5	$6.0	$6.5	$4.3	$4.6

[a]Spending attributable to new beds is assumed to have been approved and initiated three years previously; the total expenditure is recorded for the year the project is completed.
[b]Spending for construction and modernization not attributable to new beds is assumed to take place as follows: one-half of the projects are assumed to have been approved one year previously, with all of the expenditures for a particular project recorded the year the project is completed. The other half of the projects are assumed to have been approved in the same year that they are completed and recorded.
[c]Spending for equipment and technology is assumed to have been approved in the same year it is completed and recorded.
[d]All components of capital expenditures are based on 1975 estimates compiled by the Office of Research and Statistics, Social Security Administration. All components under current policy, and those components not controlled by the provisions of the Administration's proposal, are assumed to increase at the average annual rate of 15.5 percent that occurred between 1970 and 1975.

TABLE 5   Hospital Capital Expenditures Expected to be Approved by Certificate-of-Need and Section 1122 Agencies under Current Policy, and Administration' Proposal Fiscal Year 1978, by State (dollars in millions)

	Current Policy[a]	Administration's Proposal[b]	Percentage Change
Total U.S.	$8,100.0	$2,500.0	−69
Alabama	136.7	42.3	−69
Alaska	55.0	4.1	−93
Arizona	67.6	26.0	−62
Arkansas	53.4	24.8	−54
California	570.3	247.9	−57
Colorado	103.7	29.7	−71
Connecticut	165.0	36.2	−78
Delaware	34.6	6.8	−80
District of Columbia	99.0	8.4	−92
Florida	355.0	97.8	−73
Georgia	212.1	57.7	−73
Hawaii	23.6	10.1	−57
Idaho	14.1	9.6	−32
Illinois	535.7	130.4	−76
Indiana	92.7	62.2	−33
Iowa	92.7	33.6	−64
Kansas	94.3	26.5	−72
Kentucky	56.6	39.7	−30
Louisiana	158.7	44.4	−12
Maine	37.7	12.4	−67
Maryland	44.0	48.0	+9
Massachusetts	259.2	68.2	−74
Michigan	446.2	107.2	−76
Minnesota	132.0	45.9	−65
Mississippi	67.6	27.5	−59
Missouri	333.0	55.7	−83
Montana	40.8	8.8	−78
Nebraska	81.7	18.1	−78
Nevada	12.6	6.9	−45
New Hampshire	15.7	9.6	−39
New Jersey	237.2	85.6	−64
New Mexico	25.1	13.4	−47
New York	923.7	212.1	−77
North Carolina	80.1	63.8	−20
North Dakota	70.7	7.4	−90
Ohio	487.0	125.9	−74
Oklahoma	265.5	21.7	−88
Oregon	75.4	26.8	−65
Pennsylvania	419.5	138.4	−67
Rhode Island	28.3	10.8	−62
South Carolina	34.6	33.0	−5
South Dakota	23.6	8.0	−66
Tennessee	125.7	49.0	−61
Texas	328.3	143.2	−56
Utah	15.7	14.1	−10
Vermont	15.7	5.5	−65
Virginia	165.0	58.1	−65
Washington	138.2	41.5	−70
West Virginia	78.5	21.1	−73
Wisconsin	166.5	53.9	−68
Wyoming	11.0	4.4	−60

tion, the amounts that could be approved by individual states would be very uneven in relation to anticipated levels. One state would be allowed to increase approved spending slightly despite the nation-wide cut of 70 percent (refer to Table 5). Several others would be forced to cut back on approved spending by over 80 percent. While the population distribution might be replaced by a more judicious formula after two years, the shifts in levels resulting from changing formulas might pose a further problem to state agencies.

A ceiling of 4.0 beds per 1,000 persons used alone would permit a total of seventy-two health service areas to expand capacity.[13] These areas would be distributed fairly widely around the nation. The concomitant use of the 80 percent occupancy standard would curtail the number of areas allowed to expand capacity to only seventeen. The use of the occupancy standard would also have the effect of maintaining existing geographic disparities in supply and utilization. The seventeen areas would be in nine eastern and two midwestern states, where occupancy rates are relatively high (refer to Table 6). While high occupancy rates are a measure of individual hospital efficiency, high rates for an area may also mean excess hospitalization for the population as a whole. Some indication of this may be found in the fact that the number of hospital days per 1,000 persons also tends to be higher in eastern states.

The use of an occupancy standard would be a greater problem if the capital expenditure title were approved by the Congress and the revenue control title defeated. If this occurred, there would be no

[13] 1974 data on number of beds and occupancy rates in health service areas from DHEW, Health Resources Administration. The number of areas affected by the standards could change if more recent data were available.

---

[a] Includes only those expenditures requiring certificate-of-need or 1122 review. The total of $8.1 billion is for sums expected to be approved in 1978 rather than those expected to be spent, and was derived from the current policy figures in Table 4 as follows: $2.8 billion for new beds is expected to be spent in 1981 and therefore would have been approved in 1978. One-half the spending for construction and modernization expected to occur in 1979, or $2.3 billion, would have been approved in 1978. One-half the spending for construction and modernization expected to occur in 1978, or $2.0 billion, would have been approved the same year. All the spending for equipment expected in 1978, or $1.0 billion, would have been approved the same year. Distribution among states is based on each state's proportion of estimated capital expenditures in 1975 (data from American Hospital Association, *Hospital Statistics*, 1975 and 1976 editions).
[b] Assumes imposition of $2.5 billion ceiling on sums approved by certificate-of-need or Section 1122 agencies. Distribution based on relative population of states, July 1975.

TABLE 6   States and Number of Areas Permitted Expansion of Hospital Beds

(Using bed ceiling of 4.0 beds per 1,000 plus 80% occupancy standard)

Connecticut	(1)	North Carolina	(1)
Delaware	(1)	Ohio	(1)
Illinois	(1)	Pennsylvania	(1)
Maryland	(3)	Rhode Island	(1)
New Jersey	(2)	Virginia	(1)
New York	(4)		

countervailing pressure to decrease admissions, and areas with excess hospitalization would be encouraged to maintain current levels. There would be less tendency to actually increase admissions, since incentives to do so would exist at the level of the health service area rather than for individual hospitals.

A total of 195 health service areas would be held to the requirement of eliminating two beds before approving construction of, or actually adding, one new bed. If states intended to eliminate beds, they would probably have to establish decertification statutes and procedures and criteria by which to choose the targets for elimination. It would be especially difficult in a political sense to close hospitals or parts of hospitals if such institutions served not only a geographically defined area but particular religious, ethnic, or racial groups.

The two-for-one approach would assure control of expansion and, assuming that any new construction is to take place, savings would result fairly quickly from the closings. However, there is no assurance that beds would be eliminated. States might simply be unable to eliminate a sufficient number of beds, and do nothing. If no beds were eliminated, no additional cost savings or needed reallocations of resources would occur. A second problem with the two-for-one approach is that no allowance is made for areas that do not now meet the criteria but might in the future because of population growth. For example, a rapidly growing area might have 4.1 beds per 1,000 persons now, but by the time an approved expansion of capacity is in operation, the area would have 3.8 beds per 1,000.

Because only seventeen of the nation's 212 health service areas would be allowed to expand bed capacity, nearly all of the newly allocated capital limit would be spent on modernization and equipment. State agencies would be required to make decisions of the kind they have found most difficult in the past: choices between improvements needed to maintain an adequate level of service and increases in intensity that raise costs. An example of such a choice would be an inner city hospital's proposed modernization, on the one hand, and a suburban hospital's purchase of a CAT scanner, on the other.

Under the Administration's proposal, the revenue controls of Title I would be relied upon to limit small capital expenditures. If these revenue controls were not enacted, reimbursements, including depreciation and interest payments in excess of debt service, could continue to generate slack in hospital budgets. In the presence of capital expenditure controls alone, hospitals could not spend this slack on major investments. Thus there would be strong incentives to increase smaller expenditures which, taken individually, are not large enough for certificate-of-need or Section 1122 review. It could be especially difficult to identify larger equipment purchases that were split into parts to keep them below the review threshold.

Strict controls on new services within hospitals could force some services (for example, diagnostic procedures and simple surgery) outside the hospital. To the extent that a particular service could be provided more economically in a nonhospital setting, this would be a positive development. However, the absence of volume controls outside the hospital might lead to a proliferation of unneeded services. It would be more difficult to control the quantity of such services if they were performed in the offices of 250,000 physicians rather than in 6,000 hospitals.

Estimated Savings in Costs to Hospitals from the Administration's Proposal

The costs incurred by hospitals would be reduced in a number of ways by the Administration's proposal. First, the amount they spend from their own assets or on debt service for capital expenditures would be lower. Second, subsequent operating costs attributable to capital expenditures would also be decreased. It is important to note that these cost savings would not necessarily be passed on to consumers on a one-to-one basis. A third type of savings can result from decreases in the bed-to-population ratio, but this is not very likely to occur under the Administration's proposal.

Cost savings to hospitals would occur to the extent that they did not spend their own assets on investments. Such assets are the source of roughly 8 percent of all capital spending. Cost savings would also occur to the extent that hospitals' debt burden is reduced in future years. These savings could be substantial because debt financing is the source of roughly 80 percent of capital spending.[14] The combined savings in capital spending would be approximately $410 million in 1978 and would increase to $4.35 billion by 1982 (refer to Table 7).

It is more difficult to predict accurately the savings in operating costs that would result from reducing capital expenditures, especially since so little is known about the types of nonbed investments that would be made. If one assumes that the aggregate average ratio of hospital capital expenditures to annual operating costs remains at roughly 2 to 1, savings would be approximately $370 million in 1978 and $10.77 billion by 1982 (refer to Table 7). Total savings from reduced capital spending and operating costs would amount to $780 million in 1978 and $15.1 billion by 1982.

Further savings, in addition to those already estimated from reduced capital expenditures and operating costs, would result if enough beds were eliminated. If no beds were eliminated but a minimal number of new beds were approved, there would be no reduction in the bed to population ratio before 1985 and no additional savings would occur before that time. However, if beds were eliminated, and the bed to population ratio were reduced to 4.0 per 1,000 in all areas by 1982, additional savings of roughly $6.95 billion would result (refer to Table 7).[15]

---

[14] Estimates of the savings from capital spending do not include the 12 percent of such spending that originates outside the hospital but is not debt financed—primarily philanthropy. However, estimates of savings from reduced operating costs do include this 12 percent because all capital spending, whatever its source, can be expected to influence the subsequent level of operation.

[15] The beds already under construction will bring total beds to approximately 1,050,000 in 1980. If there were no elimination of beds but minimal new beds after

TABLE 7   Estimated Cost Savings to Hospitals Resulting from
Administration's Proposal to Control Hospital Capital Expenditures,
Fiscal Years 1978–1982
(dollars in billions)

	1978	1979	1980	1981	1982
Savings in capital expenditures[a]	$.41	$1.11	$1.84	$3.04	$4.35
Savings from reduced operating costs[b]	.37	1.57	3.42	6.42	10.77
Total anticipated savings	$.78	$2.68	$5.26	$9.46	$15.12
Additional savings if bed to population ratio were reduced 2 percent each year[c]	$.83	$1.89	$3.22	$4.88	$6.95

[a]Assumes that debt financing accounted for 80 percent of capital expenditures and was amortized as follows: new beds, 25 years at 8.5 percent interest; other construction, 10 years at 10 percent interest; equipment, 3 years at 12 percent interest.
    Assumes that hospitals' own assets accounted for 8 percent of capital expenditures that would have been spent in the year the project was completed.
    Assumes that outside but not debt financed sources, primarily philanthropy, accounted for 12 percent of capital expenditures and were not part of the hospital's costs.
[b]Assumes that for each dollar of decrease in total capital expenditures for a particular year, hospital operating costs in subsequent years would be reduced 50 cents. Also assumes that half the capital expenditures in a particular year would result in savings in operating costs that same year.
[c]Assumes increases in occupancy rate with resulting decreasè in cost per patient day; also assumes reduction in hospital utilization from more taut supply. Estimates from W. McClure, *Reducing Excess Hospital Capacity* (Excelsior, Minnesota: InterStudy, October 1976).

Alternatives to the Administration's Proposal

The Administration's hospital capital expenditure proposal is a major step toward a highly controlled system that could run many of the risks of regulation, such as inflexibility and the freezing out of new competition. However, such an approach may be the only way substantially to reduce and redirect new capital investment. There are a number of possible incremental changes in the Administration's proposal that might deal with some of the unresolved problems.

If one believes that the proposed limit of $2.5 billion on capital expenditures is arbitrary, a ceiling related to some measure of need could be devised. One method for doing this would be to assume

that, population growth would not begin to lower the bed to population ratio until 1985 or 1986.
    To reduce the bed to population ratio to 4.0 per 1,000 by 1982, it would be necessary to eliminate roughly 130,000 beds, bringing the total number down to 920,000.

that current commitments reflect need more accurately and therefore to freeze nonbed capital expenditures at their 1977 level with
adjustments for expected price increases. If this approach were
applied in 1978, the ceiling would be $4.6 billion instead of $2.5
billion; construction projects already in the pipeline would bring
actual capital expenditures to nearly $8.0 billion, the level antic-
ipated without a limit.

Another method might be to impose a ceiling of $2.5 billion in
1978 but to let the limit grow over time. The full impact of the
Administration's capital expenditure limit is expected to be felt in
1981 when, for the first time, there would be almost no new beds
under construction. Thus an increase in the 1980 ceiling would let
nonbed expenditures rise at a time when replacement and modernization may be most needed.

Neither an inflation nor a time-based method of adjustment
would reflect specific needs for additional investment. A third
method might be to establish an exception system for proposals in
excess of the $2.5 billion ceiling. States could be granted permission
to raise their limits only to the extent that they could demonstrate a
pressing unmet need to modernize existing capacity. Other justifications for exceptions might include proposed use of federal energy
funds to improve insulation, or other improvements that would
clearly save money in future years. The exception system would
require more information and staff to administer but would control
types of spending and could be used to indicate federal priorities.

State review under the conditions of a ceiling could also be
facilitated by establishing a multifactor formula for distribution
among states immediately, rather than relying on population alone.
While it would be difficult to establish quickly a formula reflecting
health care needs, some simple measures of construction cost and
need for renovations such as lack of compliance with life safety
codes, could be included. The average of several years' hospital capital expenditures in each state might also be considered as
one of the factors if it were believed to have some relationship
to need.

Problems arising from the use of an occupancy standard could
be dealt with by eliminating it, thus allowing the seventy-two areas

that meet the bed to population standard to expand capacity. If fewer new beds are desired, this could be achieved by a more restrictive bed to population ratio without adding a second criterion such as an occupancy standard. For example, the use of a 3.5 beds per 1,000 persons ratio, without an occupancy standard, would permit twenty-nine areas to expand capacity. These areas would be distributed slightly more widely across the nation than the seventeen areas that could expand under the Administration's proposal.

Certain changes in the Administration's proposal would make decreases in the number of beds more likely and facilitate the reallocation of resources. For example, each area could be required to establish a year by year plan to reach a target bed to population ratio in five years. Population growth rates could be considered and penalties imposed on hospitals and areas whose bed numbers were out of compliance with the plan.

Additionally, a plan for decreasing the number of beds could be implemented more easily if incentives were provided to individual hospitals for eliminating or converting beds. The Administration's proposal would allow a state to increase its capital expenditure limit when beds are eliminated. However, no incentive would be provided a hospital to eliminate beds in the capital expenditures title. In the revenue controls title, a slight incentive to hospitals would be provided by allowing revenue from unneeded facilities that are closed to be included in the base year calculation. This would have the effect of maintaining a higher level of revenue for a smaller number of beds. The Talmadge proposal would provide direct payments for eliminating beds, but only on a limited experimental basis to not more than fifty hospitals.

The problems involved in reviewing proposals for nonbed expenditures suggest the need for additional staffing and technical assistance for state agencies. Additionally, accurate projections of savings or increases in future operating costs attributable to a proposed capital expenditure could be required as a condition for certificate of need or Section 1122 approval. Incentives could also be provided or priority required for modernization as opposed to technology-intensive changes. This would be complemented by the type of targeted exception system suggested above.

The Interrelationships Between Titles I and II

The Administration's proposal would assure substantial reductions in hospital revenues in 1978 and beyond. Because of the compounding effect of the annual growth ceilings in hospital revenues and the lowering of the ceiling over time, the amount that the nation spends for hospital care could be almost $19 billion lower than currently projected for 1982 if the proposal were enacted. This estimate represents a minimum savings from the proposal. The capital controls and restrictions on the construction of new beds included in Title II could add significantly to these long-run savings under certain conditions. The reduction in capital expenditures should bring more hospitals' costs below the revenue ceiling. To the extent that savings attributable to reduced capital expenditures are not spent elsewhere, costs, and therefore revenues, would be reduced below the level specified in Title I. However, even if the capital restrictions did not add to the total savings generated by the revenue ceiling, the restrictions on new investments would make it easier to maintain the revenue limits over time by lowering operating costs and thus reducing some of the pressure to raise the revenue limit.

The approaches included under Titles I and II of the Administration's proposal for constraining future hospital costs are, therefore, integrally related. This fact should be taken into account in working out changes in the specifics of the proposals as well as in their administration. In establishing the level of new investments permitted, care must be taken to assure its consistency with future allowable increases in operating revenue. States, which will administer the capital restrictions, should know the current asset to liability ratio of the hospitals that seek permission to make investments, as well as how capital purchases will affect hospital operating costs.

Moreover, the ability of states to eliminate excess capacity and reallocate resources would be much greater if they were allowed to determine the level of revenues received by hospitals. One way to involve states in a federal revenue control program would be to require state approval of exceptions.

There is some danger in accepting only one of the titles of the

Administration's proposal. Controls on large capital purchases without a revenue ceiling could result in an increase in the purchase of less expensive capital equipment, thus maintaining growth in hospital costs. Conversely, a ceiling on revenues without capital controls might allow hospitals to cut back on services needed by the community rather than on duplicative capacity that adds to their prestige.

Summary

In the Hospital Cost Containment Act of 1977, the Administration has proposed to limit both the revenues and capital expenditures of nonfederal short-term hospitals.

Hospitals have been singled out for strong regulation because the total amount paid for hospital care has grown steadily and because the cost per patient day has been increasing at double the rate of overall inflation. Under current policy, the amount paid for care in the hospitals covered by the Administration's proposal is expected to total $61.3 billion in 1978 and $104 billion by 1982.

Excessive increases in the amount paid for hospital care are thought to be caused by operating inefficiencies, unnecessary growth in the intensity of services provided each patient, and duplicative facilities. These problems result, in turn, from a lack of cost consciousness by physicians and patients and from the fact that the federal government and private insurance plans most often reimburse hospitals on a cost basis. There are no existing federal controls on the total amount paid for hospital care.

Capital spending by hospitals has been singled out along with total revenues because it increases the amount of care delivered and the cost per patient day. Under current policy, capital expenditures by the hospitals covered by the Administration's proposal are expected to total $8.0 billion in 1978 and $14.1 billion by 1982.

Currently, the primary mechanism to control hospital capital expenditures is the National Health Planning and Resources Development Act of 1974, which requires that by 1980 each state establish a certificate-of-need program to ascertain the need for major new hospital investments. Of the thirty-two states that have so far passed certificate-of-need laws, only five seem to be operating programs that are at all effective.

Proposal to Limit Hospital Revenues (Title I)

The temporary authority in Title I of the act would place a ceiling on total inpatient revenues of nonfederal short-term hospitals. Including expected adjustments in the ceiling for admission increases, wage pass-throughs, and exceptions, the growth in total revenues would be limited to 10.6 percent in 1978 and 8.9 percent by 1981. Revenues in excess of the limits would have to be returned or, in the case of commercial insurers and self paying patients, set aside for use in the following year; they would otherwise be subject to a 150 percent excise tax. Some states would be allowed to continue operating their own hospital cost control programs. The bill specifies that recommendations for permanent reform of hospital financing shall be made by the Secretary of DHEW by the beginning of March 1978.

Adjustments in the revenue ceiling could be made fairly automatically for small to moderate changes in the volume of admissions. Those hospitals with substantial changes in admissions or major changes in capacity or type of service approved by the state agencies that review capital spending, could apply to a federal board for exceptions to the ceiling. A hospital would have to show that the increase in its costs would, without an exception to the revenue ceiling, force it into the lowest 25 percent of all hospitals in terms of ability to pay current liabilities. Upon a hospital's request, increases in the wages of nonsupervisory employees could be passed on automatically to payers. In this case the limit would be calculated only for revenues attributable to other costs.

The Administration's proposed revenue controls offer a number of major advantages. First, and most important, they would produce substantial cost savings as early as 1978, when total anticipated spending would be reduced $2.4 billion. These savings would grow rapidly in subsequent years, reaching $18.8 billion by 1982. Federal expenditures for Medicare and Medicaid would be reduced $1 billion in 1978 and $8.2 billion by 1982.

Second, the majority of savings would come from greatly reducing the growth in services, which is thought by many to be excessive and the most important source of increases in the amount paid for hospital care. Third, growth in admissions would also tend to decline since the proposal's volume adjustments are structured to encourage hospitals to treat fewer patients. This might address the problem of unneeded hospitalization, another source of cost increases.

Among the other advantages of the Administration's proposal are that it would be simple to administer and could be implemented immediately. In many ways it is the proposal's lack of complexity that leads to some of its shortcomings. While much of the following discussion concentrates on describing these disadvantages, it should be noted that all but one could be addressed by modifications that need not delay the proposal's implementation. Moreover, an approach similar to that taken by the Administration, placing a growth ceiling on the amount spent for care, appears to be the only way of significantly reducing the rapid rise in hospital costs.

The first problem with the Administration's proposal is that, while the growth ceiling should force many hospitals to become more efficient, there would be few specific incentives for efficiency. The only way efficiency would be rewarded would be to let hospitals whose revenues were under the ceiling carry over the surplus to the next year's limit. Because the Administration's proposal would restrict relatively fast growing hospitals, whether or not they are efficient, efficient hospitals might find it more difficult to live within the limit than rapidly growing inefficient ones.

Second, while there would be protection against a hospital's "dumping" patients because their insurance pays less relative to other types of reimbursements, there is no provision to prevent adverse selection by type of diagnosis. A hospital hard pressed by the limit could be tempted to admit more short-term cases that are inexpensive to treat and to direct expensive cases to other hospitals.

Third, the exceptions process would be limited to few hospitals in order to simplify federal administrative procedures. Thus it would be difficult to deal with problems specific to a particular hospital or with unanticipated price increases that are not systemwide. Faced with such a situation, a hospital might cut back on services, including those needed by the community, such as emergency rooms and outpatient clinics, rather than run down its reserves so as to be eligible for the exceptions process.

Fourth, with only nine months' notice of the imposition of a growth ceiling, some hospitals might experience difficulty early in the proposed program because they will have already committed themselves to expenditures they would have avoided with more notice.

Fifth, hospitals and unions could cooperate in evading the growth limit by alternating a high wage increase that would be passed through in one year with no increase the following year. The second year hospitals could apply the full growth allowance for all revenues to nonlabor purposes.

Alternatives to Title I

Incremental changes can be made in the Administration's proposal or more distinct alternatives could be considered.

Incremental changes in the Administration's proposal would not deal with the issue of efficiency incentives directly, but could address the four other problems discussed above. Such changes include:

- Dividing hospitals into different classes based on their size and services provided and applying different growth ceilings to each. These changes would recognize the different roles of hospitals and help prevent adverse case selection.
- Broadening the exceptions procedure to increase its accessibility and relative sensitivity among hospitals. If it were assumed that more hospitals would apply for and receive exceptions, it might be appropriate to adjust the legislated limit downward. For example, instead of an 8.7 percent growth limit and an estimate of less than 1 percent for exceptions, there could be a 6.5 percent growth limit and an estimated 3 percent for exceptions. A broader exceptions procedure would permit the specific needs of individual hospitals to be treated more judiciously.

- Combining allowable growth levels for the first two years. For example, using the proposed formula, the legislated limit would be 18.8 percent over two years rather than 8.7 percent in the first year. This would allow hospitals that have already made plans for expansion to better prepare for the revenue ceilings.
- Making the wage pass-through option mandatory for all hospitals. This would prevent hospitals and unions from cooperating to evade the growth ceiling. Alternatively, the pass-through could be eliminated.

A major alternative to the Administration's approach is the Medicare-Medicaid Administrative and Reimbursement Reform Act of 1977 proposed by Senator Talmadge, which includes an attempt to improve basic hospital efficiency rather than to impose a growth ceiling on the industry. Only Medicare and Medicaid reimbursements would be affected, rather than all hospital revenues, and the proposal would focus only on routine costs—the 30 percent of total hospital costs attributable to room, board, and some salaries. An average for routine costs would be established for each type of hospital; hospitals would be paid bonuses if they were below the average, and any routine costs in excess of 120 percent of the average would be disallowed.

Since the Talmadge proposal would require a uniform cost reporting system, it could not be implemented before 1981. Medicare and Medicaid savings from these provisions of the Talmadge proposal would be between $100 and $400 million in 1982. Cost savings under this approach are low compared to the Administration's proposal but they could be increased by reducing the bonus payments or the 120 percent limit.

The Talmadge and Administration proposals could be integrated so as to retain the advantages of both. If the Administration's revenue controls or a similar program were implemented in 1978, immediate cost savings would result. As soon as there were sufficient data to differentiate among hospitals and types of costs, a method similar to that of the Talmadge proposal could be used to control routine costs of all payers. Routine costs are believed to be most susceptible to efficiency incentives because they are under the control of hospital administrators. A growth ceiling could then be applied to nonroutine costs, in which the greatest growth is occurring.

Proposal to Limit Hospital Capital Expenditures (Title II)

Title II of the Hospital Cost Containment Act of 1977 would provide permanent limits on both capital expenditures by hospitals and beds per 1,000 population. Beginning in 1978, no more than $2.5 billion could be approved nationwide each year for capital expenditures. For the first two years, this limit would be allocated among the states on the basis of population; in subsequent years, other factors could be considered. A standard of no more than 4.0 beds per 1,000 persons and at least 80 percent aggregate bed occupancy would be established for each of the nation's 212 health service areas. In areas meeting both bed and occupancy criteria, no certificate of need could be issued for a project that would force the area out of compliance. In areas not meeting both criteria, a certificate of need resulting in additional beds could be issued only if twice as many existing beds were eliminated from the area as a whole.

In states without a certificate-of-need program, the limit would be enforced through Section 1122 of the Social Security Act. The federal government—with the advice of states—could disallow Medicaid and Medicare reimbursement for 10 times the amount attributable to depreciation and interest for a disapproved expenditure.

The Administration's proposal would address the overall problem of continued growth in capital spending by means of a substantial but delayed cut. Because previously approved construction projects will continue to affect capital outlays for up to three years, the ceiling would result in reducing the $8.0 billion in 1978 capital spending anticipated under current policy to only $6.5 billion. By 1982, however, a level of $4.6 billion could be expected instead of the $14.1 billion that would otherwise occur. Very roughly, these reductions in capital spending would translate into cost savings to hospitals of $780 million in 1978 and $15.1 billion by 1982.

While the Administration's capital expenditure controls would be quite successful in reducing future investment, five problems would remain.

First, the $2.5 billion limit is not based on an evaluation of need and could restrict necessary and possibly cost saving improvements in future years. Similarly, distribution of the limit by population, though used only in the first two years, might not reflect states' relative need for spending.

Second, while only seventeen of the nation's 212 health services areas could build additional hospital beds, the proposal would be less successful in addressing existing excess capacity—estimated by some at close to 100,000 beds—or maldistribution. The areas that could expand capacity would nearly all be in the east, primarily because of the effect of the occupancy standard. The other 195 areas that would have to eliminate two beds to add one might simply maintain the status quo. In that case, no shrinkage of the existing system would occur and it would be difficult to reallocate resources.

Third, with tight restrictions on new beds, nearly all new spending would be for plant modernization and equipment, for which it has been difficult to determine need and ultimate cost.

Fourth, strict controls on new services could force some in-hospital procedures outside the hospital, where they could proliferate in volume.

Fifth, small investments under the review threshold of $100,000 would not be controlled and, especially if revenue controls were not enacted, could begin to grow at a faster rate.

Alternatives to Title II

In view of the record of current efforts to control hospital capital expenditures, the Administration's proposal, or similar steps, may be the only way to substantially reduce and redirect the system. However, such actions would entail many of the risks of regulation, including inflexibility and the elimination of new competition. The following incremental changes could minimize some of the unresolved problems.

- If one believes that the dollar amount of the proposed ceiling is arbitrary and not related to need, it could be increased now or in the future. Alternatively, an exceptions system could be established that would allow any expenditures in excess of the $2.5 billion ceiling to be targeted on needed renovation and investments that offer future cost savings.

- The imposition of any ceiling would be facilitated by establishing a multifactor distribution formula immediately, rather than relying on population alone in the first two years.
- Excess capacity and maldistribution might be addressed more effectively by requiring a lower bed to population ratio in five years and penalizing hospitals and health service areas for any excess capacity. Direct payments could be provided to relieve hospitals of the costs of eliminating beds.

Relationship of Revenue Controls and Capital Expenditure Controls

Titles I and II are integrally related and reinforcing. Reductions in capital investment would result in lower operating costs, which should make it easier for hospitals to live within the revenue limit. Because of this interrelationship, the specific limits of the proposal must be consistent. The administration of Titles I and II must also be coordinated. Because states would be the primary administrators of the capital expenditure controls, it may be desirable for them to participate more actively in the federal revenue control program. Even if states did not operate their own cost control programs, they could administer an expanded exceptions process similar to that described as an incremental change in Title I.

Addendum

In the paper presented above, the Congressional Budget Office calculated the savings that would accrue as a result of this plan to the federal government and all hospital care purchasers. If the proposed revenue limit were effective for five years, those savings would be $46 billion.

It has recently become evident that the Administration plans to implement the revenue limit in a different manner than was assumed in the CBO estimate. In the first place the base period revenues will be lower than was assumed by CBO, thus reducing the revenue increases permitted in future years. Using the Administration's method of determining base year revenues the five-year savings estimated for the proposal would be $50 billion rather than $46 billion.[16] Second, to determine the revenue limits for future years the Administration plans to add rather than compound the percentage increases in revenues permitted for preceding years. This procedure raises the five-year savings of the proposal from $50 to $61 billion.

The Effect of the Definition of the Base Year

The future revenue limits under the Hospital Cost Containment Act of 1977 are calculated relative to each hospital's revenues during the base period—the twelve months ending on September 30, 1977 (fiscal year 1977). Because the actual revenues received during the base period would not be available in time to implement the Hospital Cost Containment Act in fiscal year 1978, the act calls for these revenues to be estimated. This is done by taking the revenues received by each hospital during its accounting year ending in 1976 and projecting these revenues forward to the base period using a growth rate equal to the average annual growth in revenues experienced by the hospital during its two previous accounting years (1974 to 1976). In calculating this average, rates of growth above 15 percent are set equal to 15 percent and those below 6 percent are set equal to 6 percent. Because the average hospital is expected to experience a revenue growth of greater than 15 percent during 1977, this method of estimating base year revenues is likely to result in many hospitals being assigned base year revenue figures that are below those that they will actually receive during the base year. For the hospital industry as a whole the base year revenues, as calculated under the act, are estimated to be about $1 billion less than those that will actually be received during the base year.

For the first year the growth ceiling plus other allowed increases

[16]The original CBO estimate of $46 billion was based upon data which did not adequately exclude hospital outpatient revenues. When these revenues are removed, savings under the original estimate drop to $43 billion. Thus the effect of changing the definition of base revenues is $7 billion (from $43 to $50 billion) rather than $4 billion.

An Overview of Perspectives

TABLE 1A   Projected Growth Ceilings for Hospital Cost Containment Act of 1977

Fiscal Year	Growth Ceiling	Growth Ceiling + Expected Increases[a]
1978	8.7%	10.6%
1979	9.3	11.2
1980	7.6	9.5
1981	7.1	9.0
1982	7.0	8.9
1978 to 1982	7.9	9.8

[a]Includes a 1.0 percent allowance for increases in admissions plus a 0.9 percent allowance for revenue increases due to the pass-through of wage increases and to the exceptions process.

are estimated to total 10.6 percent (refer to Table 1A). However, 10.6 percent of the base year revenues as calculated under the act will amount to only 8.2 percent of the actual revenues that hospitals are projected to receive in fiscal year 1977. The effect on the Medicare program will be even more pronounced because that program is growing more rapidly than total hospital revenues. As a consequence, the actual Medicare revenue growth the industry will be permitted in 1978 will be less than that allowed in the second, third, and fourth years of the cost-containment program (refer to Table 2A).

The Effect of Calculating Future Revenue Limits by Adding rather than Compounding the Percentage Revenue Increases

The Administration plans to calculate a hospital's revenue limit by adding together, rather than compounding, the allowable percentage revenue increases for each year since the program's inception and multiplying this sum by the base year's revenues. This procedure ignores the effects of compound growth, reduces allowable revenue increases, and weakens the relationship between the growth limit and the rates of inflation and service increases experienced by the hospital industry. Using a compounding approach and the growth ceilings projected by CBO, hospital revenues would be permitted to increase by 44.7 percent from 1978 to 1982. Under the Administration's additive procedure the allowable increase would only be 34.9 percent.

TABLE 2A The Effect on Expenditures for Hospital Services of Using an Additive Rather than a Compounding Method to Determine Hospital Revenue Limits for Fiscal Years 1978–1982 (dollars in billions)[a]

| | CURRENT POLICY | | UNDER ADMINISTRATION'S PROPOSED GROWTH CEILING FORMULA | | | | | |
| | | | Compounding Method | | | Administration's Additive Method As a Percent of Base Year | | |
Fiscal Year	Rate of Growth (in %)	Expenditures for Hospital Services[b]	Rate of Growth (in %)	Expenditures for Hospital Services	Savings Due to Growth Ceiling	Rate of Growth (in %)	Expenditures for Hospital Services	Savings Due to Growth Ceiling
			Medicare Hospital Expenditures for Inpatient Services					
1978	17.3	16.7	6.3	15.2	1.6	6.3	15.2	1.6
1979	16.1	19.4	11.2	16.9	2.5	10.2	16.7	2.7
1980	16.1	22.5	9.5	18.5	4.1	7.8	18.0	4.5
1981	16.2	26.2	9.0	20.1	6.1	6.8	19.2	6.9
1982	16.6	30.5	8.9	21.9	8.6	6.3	20.5	10.1
1978 to 1982	16.4	115.3	9.0	92.5	22.8	7.5	89.5	25.8
			Hospital Expenditures for Inpatient Services by All Payers					
1978	15.2	55.8	8.2	52.4	3.4	8.2	52.2	3.4
1979	14.1	63.7	11.2	58.3	5.4	10.2	57.7	6.0
1980	14.1	72.7	9.5	63.9	8.9	7.8	62.3	10.5
1981	14.2	83.1	9.0	69.6	13.5	6.8	66.5	16.6
1982	14.6	95.2	8.9	75.8	19.5	6.3	70.7	24.5
1978 to 1982	14.5	370.6	9.4	320.0	50.6	7.9	309.7	61.0

[a]Congressional Budget Office estimates. Entries do not sum to totals because of rounding. Rates of growth shown are based on a greater number of significant digits than the expenditure levels shown in the table.
[b]The current policy expenditure estimates have been refined slightly from those published in the paper.

The Administration's approach increases the five-year savings of the Hospital Cost Containment Act from $50 to $61 billion (refer to Table 2A). Medicare expenditures for hospital services would be reduced by $26 billion as opposed to $22 billion under a method that took account of compound growth. The effect of the Administration's approach in fiscal year 1982 is particularly significant. About 40 percent of the savings during the entire five-year period is obtained in the fifth year. The increase in hospital industry revenues from 1981 to 1982 permitted from the anticipated ceiling of 8.9 percent would be only 6.3 under the Administration's procedure. For a hospital that did not increase its ceiling by obtaining an exception, adjusting for volume, or passing through wage increases, the growth in revenues permitted between fiscal years 1981 and 1982 would be 5.0 percent of the hospital's fiscal year 1981 revenues, which is less than the 5.6 percent rate of inflation that CBO estimates will occur in 1982.[17]

[17] The rate of increase of the CPI is projected to be 5.6 percent in 1982. The GNP deflator will increase at a slightly slower rate, 5.4 percent. CBO's estimate of the growth ceiling calculated from the formula for 1982 is 7.0 percent. After adding 1.9 percent to this amount to allow for the effects on hospital expenditures of the exceptions process, the wage pass-through provisions and increases in hospital admissions, total growth in the industry will be about 8.9 percent.

Decision Making at
the Institutional Level

Physician Involvement
in Hospital Decision Making

MICHAEL A. REDISCH*

The focus of government health care policy over the past two decades has subtly changed from earlier commitments to provide health care to all who are in need. While assurance of access to care is, of course, still of great concern, the foremost policy issues of today revolve around ways to constrain future increases in health care costs. The major policy battleground is the hospital sector, where the most serious health care cost increases have occurred.

Governmental concern goes beyond the simple figures that show health expenditures rising from 5.2 percent of Gross National Product in 1960 to 8.6 percent of Gross National Product in fiscal 1976 (see Gibson and Mueller, 1977). A similar rise in relative expenditures in the consumer durable sector would traditionally be interpreted as the result of informed choices made in the economic marketplace by consumers of those products. However, medical care in general and hospital care in particular operate in markets so heavily underwritten by public programs and by private insurance that conventional market signals are weak or nonexistent. In 1975, 92 percent of hospital care was paid for by some form of third-party payer, a fact that tends to obscure the cost impact of hospital care on

*Any views expressed in this paper are those of the author and do not necessarily reflect the official position of the U.S. General Accounting Office.

The authors wishes to thank Jon Gabel for a number of comments that were helpful in the preparation of the paper.

the household budget. Furthermore, the individual seeking care is usually not fully informed of the potential outcomes of that care; instead, he must put his faith and trust in a physician who is allowed to commit the individual to utilize a bundle of scarce health resources. Among them is the physician's own time, and thus a potential conflict of interest is created.

The individual, therefore, typically does not purchase health care through the same mechanism or with the same attitudes as he does other goods and services. The result is governmental concern and intervention as the share of the nation's resources devoted to health care continues to rise.

A number of as yet untested proposals are being offered to combat inflation in the hospital without unduly limiting access to or quality of care. These suggestions include certificate-of-need laws, hospital rate review, various forms of prospective reimbursement, return to the direct wage and price controls of the Economic Stabilization era, or market strategies revolving around the growth of Health Maintenance Organizations.

However, too often in attempts to conceptualize the process by which the hospital sector will react to one or more of these control mechanisms, a central and overriding feature of the U.S. hospital system is omitted. The unique relationship between the hospital and the physician in the production of health care in this country is ignored by many of those attempting to understand or predict the reaction of hospitals to specific government policy. Instead, the hospital is typically viewed as an institution differing from ordinary firms only to the extent that a major portion of hospital care is provided in a not-for-profit setting.

An explanation for the lack of a strong physician figure in most models of hospital behavior can probably be traced to the payment mechanism for health care in the United States. The patient hospitalized here is typically subject to two separate billings; one for "hospital" services and one for "personal physician" services. This dual billing system has led to a conceptually false dichotomy whereby the hospital and physician are often erroneously viewed as independent entities selling services in functionally segmented health markets. Yet from the patient's point of view, "health care" in a hospital setting should be viewed as a single product jointly produced by the combined actions of hospitals and physicians. That patients in fact do take this view is suggested by Yett et al. (1971), who estimate that the demand for hospital care in a state aggregated cross-section is more responsive to changes in a physician surgical fee index than changes in the (more heavily insured) price of a bed day. Davis and Russell (1972) also estimate a demand equation for inpatient care that contains a significantly negative coefficient for the physician fee variable.

This paper will examine the hospital-physician relationship more from a perspective of supply-side response to a set of social and economic incentives than from the perspective of consumer demand for hospital-based health care. It is in the area of modeling supply-side behavior that distortions and erroneous implications can be caused by an improper specification of the role of the physician in determining resource use in the hospital. As Jacobs (1974) has noted, many of the attempts to model hospital behavior either view the hospital as controlled completely by administrators' preferences or lump all decision-making groups into a heterogeneous whole, creating a fictional entity not related to reality. These "organism" models, viewing the "hospital" as the acting body, tend to obscure the way operational decisions are jointly arrived at through the individual actions of patients, trustees, physicians, administrators, and other hospital personnel.

Here we will attempt to delineate more specifically the roles that the physician may play in strategies aimed at controlling cost increases in hospitals. Any effective mechanism for containing the ongoing rapid rises in hospital costs must explicitly take into account the involvement of physicians in hospital decision making. Few administrators like to admit how limited is their control over the operation of their hospitals. They would like to believe that by their efforts alone, order and direction are distilled from anarchy. Yet it is the physician, operating as a separate entity outside the control of the Board of Trustees or the administrator, who directs most of the major resource decisions made in the hospital setting. The physician recommends admission, takes responsibility for ordering diagnostic procedures and therapeutic measures, and determines when the patient is fit to leave the hospital. In addition, it is the physician who typically engages in a lobbying effort with hopes of committing the administrator and trustees to invest in additional bed space, in personnel to help him provide more and better patient care, and in new and expensive technology.

A model of complete physician control, while admittedly an abstraction of reality, is still close enough to be considered a useful tool for analyzing various policy formulations (see Pauly and Redisch, 1973, for a rigorous statement of such a model). The two lines of internal authority in the hospital can lead to inevitable conflict between administrators and physicians. Yet the administrator has little stake in opposing physicians, particularly under a regime of unconstrained cost reimbursement. In fact, the administrator typically finds his own job security most closely tied to his ability to satisfy the demands of the medical staff. Viewed in this light, the administrator's role is simply to provide labor, supplies, and facilities to independent physicians. It is the physician who directs the actual provision of care in the hospital.

Trustees are also organizationally structured to exert external control on physician behavior. In a not-for-profit hospital there are no stockholders or owners of equity capital. The Board of Trustees presumably represents the public interest and bears some form of legal and moral responsibility for all activities, professional and otherwise, that occur within the institution. However, while each member of a typical board is a competent individual in his own field, he is unprepared for participation in the types of issues and decisions involved in the management of the hospital. Ordinarily he has limited knowledge of the medical profession, and his knowledge of the hospital is usually restricted to personal contact as a patient or as a relative of a patient.

A group of laymen without training in medicine thus may find it difficult to fulfill adequately responsibilities related in any way to quality of care, the practice of medicine, or the evaluation of medical staff. Almost all resource-related decisions in the hospital can be classified under one or more of these "medical" rubrics. It is therefore not surprising to see a tendency in most hospitals for the board to abjure direct responsibility and to delegate authority to some internal physician group. This tendency is, of course, actively supported by the American Medical Association, which suggests that "the responsibility of the hospital governing board is to provide the foundation for self-governance by the organized medical staff" (American Medical Association, 1974b:12). Once again de facto physician control over resource-related decisions is not hard to establish.

We will discuss in some detail the physician's role in the hospital cost inflation process and examine the impact of hypothesized physician behavior on the expected relative success of alternative policies for containing hospital costs. First, however, a description of the way inflation has taken place in the hospital will prove helpful.

The hospital cost inflation process will be examined with the patient day (or adjusted patient day, accounting for outpatient department care, American Hospital Association, 1969:466) as the reference unit of output. We feel that a specific illness incident treated as a case is a more meaningful measure of hospital "output" in the social welfare sense than the number of days of varying services devoted to patient care. However, use of the patient day is a more tractable measure and will allow us to explain relationships involving resource use (for example, factor input utilization decisions, a hospital investment function, the operational inflationary mechanism in the hospital environment) as well as or better than the case. This is particularly true since there is yet no precise, generally agreed upon way to measure the economic or medical aspects of "case mix."

The 10 to 20 percent annual increases in per diem hospital costs since 1965 are critically related to changes in the quantities, qualities, and sophistication of the services that are lumped together under the output designation of a patient day. Previous efforts to document the rise in cost per patient day have broken down these cost increases into four basic components: (1) rising wage levels of employees; (2) increased personnel per patient day; (3) rising cost of nonlabor inputs; and (4) increased use of nonlabor inputs per patient day. M. Feldstein (1971a), Davis and Foster (1972), and Waldman (1972) have all independently estimated that rising unit input costs and increased real input use have contributed approximately equal amounts to the rise in per diem costs in the late 1960s and early 1970s.

The American Hospital Association has claimed a recent change

in the proportionate share of hospital cost increases related to rising
unit input costs (Council on Wage and Price Stability, 1976:13). It
estimates that pure factor price increases accounted for over 70
percent of hospital cost increases from January 1974 until June 1975.
This reversal, if true, was due to expanded minimum wage laws and
collective bargaining, increased malpractice insurance premiums,
and higher energy costs. While hospital input prices may temporar-
ily move faster than the general rate of inflation, it is still expected
that increases in real inputs have led and will continue to lead, unless
checked, to the growing share of hospital care in our national
product accounts.

The origin of the rise in the volume of labor and nonlabor inputs
utilized per patient day can be traced in part to the ability of the
physician over time to reduce his own input or operating costs by
transference of functions and costs to the hospital. Examples of this
trend include the obstetrician who relies more and more on nursing
staff and who rushes in at the last minute for the actual delivery, or
the attending physician who utilizes house staff to care for his
patients on Wednesdays and Saturdays. Johnson (1969) notes that
nurses now perform many tasks that until two decades ago were
limited to physicians, for example, the starting of blood transfusions,
introduction of intravenous fluids, and injections. Such transference
will continue into the future as attending physicians are relieved of
suturing and many other responsibilities in surgery, coronary care,
emergency room duties, and dialysis.

If this transference were done in an economically and socially
efficient manner, then society could capture the potential gain
generated by substitution of low-cost hospital inputs for high-cost
physician time. While hospital costs would register increases, these
would be more than compensated for by decreases in aggregate
physician bills to patients. However, this does not appear to have
happened. Instead, aided by the separation of bills for the costs of
joint hospital-and-physician services, the physician has shown a
great willingness to bill as much in his "supervisory" capacity over
hospital inputs as when he performs services directly. Physicians are
thus able to increase output (and incomes) without dramatic increases in fees. As an extreme example, the Medicare program often

finds itself asked to pay under Part A (the hospital side of Title XVIII) its proportionate share of the salary of the resident who performs surgery while simultaneously being asked to cover under Part B (the physician side) the bill submitted by the supervising physician.

The physician's growing financial stake in the direction of resources other than his own labor may be seen by examining data from 1955 to 1971. Over this period physician incomes rose by around 7.2 percent per year while physician fees (as measured by the Consumer Price Index) rose by only 4.4 percent per year. Physician practice hours per week and practice weeks per year fell slightly (see Leveson and Rogers, 1976). The maintenance of this high rate of income growth under these conditions was accomplished by increasing physician productivity through dramatic increases in the nonphysician resource intensity of medical care.

Even if the physician did not continue to bill in part for services transferred to the hospital, the trend toward a greater and greater role for hospital inputs has still led to major inefficiencies in the production of health care. The physician and his patient are usually not even cognizant of the costs of basic hospital services. The hospital will typically tend to prorate the costs of all inputs (except those used to produce ancillary services) over all users of those inputs, through the use of room rates or daily service charges, which cover more than 50 percent of daily patient expense in most hospitals. Thus the utilization of increasing amounts of basic services by an individual patient will have a negligible impact on that patient's bill, since these costs are spread over all patients in the hospital. As the medical staff increases in size, each physician will tend to become less and less aware of the effects of his actions on others, since there are large numbers of patients of other physicians who share in the costs of these basic services. Unfortunately, the cumulative effect of this myopic behavior results in the rapid escalation of basic hospital services and of the hospital's room and board charge. The basic service increase is reflected in the time trend of the semiprivate room charge component of the Consumer Price Index, which almost tripled from 1965 to 1975.

The situation is exacerbated by the extent of insurance for

hospital services. Even when the hospital directly bills the patient for use of specific services, the physician is aware that the major burden of that bill will be borne not by the patient but by some third-party payer. To the extent that hospital care is more heavily insured than ambulatory physician care, the physician is likely to suggest a hospital stay for a patient who could be treated as well (and more efficiently) on an ambulatory basis. The practice of admitting patients into the hospital for an overnight stay to run a series of what are essentially diagnostic tests is the classic example of such behavior. But this specific practice has begun to die out as insurors have taken steps both to cover these tests when performed on an ambulatory patient and to reject payments for inpatient admissions whose sole justification is diagnostic testing.

Thus there appear to be three forces at work that mutually tend to reinforce the physician's incentive to utilize hospital services in an economically inefficient manner. The separation of physician and hospital bills for jointly produced health care, the proration of basic hospital service costs over all patients, and the pervasiveness of insurance for hospital services all make the apparent cost to the physician of additional hospital service very small relative to the true social costs of the inputs used to produce that service. Major incentives are created for the physician to oversubstitute hospital inputs for his own labor and to order the production of only marginally beneficial health and hotel services in the hospital.

At the same time, the physician seems reluctant to utilize health care inputs when he himself must bear the full costs and directorial burden of those inputs. For example, Reinhardt (1972) estimates that physicians could profitably employ in their offices more than twice as many physicians' assistants as they now do. Rather than take the risk and the added responsibility of a larger staff to supervise, physicians have chosen to pass up this potentially profitable option. Yet they seem to show no such compunction when it comes to ordering for their patients increasing amounts of hospital inputs, for which they bear no direct financial or managerial burden.

While the number of inputs used to produce basic hospital room and board services have increased over time, the really dramatic increases in hospital resource intensity seem to be largely related to increases in the availability and utilization levels of a set of diagnos-

TABLE 1   **Growth in Selected Hospital Series[a]**

	1968	1969	1970	1971	Percent Change 1968-1971
Operating cost	$55.51	$60.89	$69.60	$78.75	41.8
Operating room visits	.05456	.05071	.05223	.05373	-1.5
Pathology tests	.06327	.11652	.11504	.10914	72.5
Nuclear medicine procs.	.00252	.00705	.00690	.00965	282.9
Pharmacy line items	.35610	.79150	.91918	1.0449	193.4
In- & outpatient lab tests	2.2046	2.2964	2.5393	2.8588	29.7
In- & outpatient radiology procs.	.31753	.31604	.33519	.36378	14.6
Therapeutic radiology procs.	.00685	.01394	.01577	.01894	176.5
Blood bank units	.03759	.05881	.05333	.06333	68.5

[a]All figures are reported in whole units normalized on adjusted patient days. Thus in 1968 operating cost per adjusted patient day in the sample was $55.51 and the average number of pathology tests per adjusted patient day was .06327.

Sources: The data were provided by the Health Services Research Center (the Center) of Northwestern University and the American Hospital Association (AHA). They were obtained by the Center from the Hospital Administrative Services (HAS) Division of the AHA. Data are submitted to HAS on a monthly basis by several thousand voluntarily participating hospitals. These hospitals may then compare their performance in providing services with that of similarly situated institutions.

No payment for services is based on the completed HAS forms, and the data are not audited. HAS puts the raw monthly data onto a computer tape and runs some simple statistical checks that are meant to eliminate "order of magnitude" errors. The Center obtained a tape of this monthly data file for close to four hundred hospitals. The tape was than "annualized" on a calendar year basis for the years 1967 to 1971. Hospitals reporting less than nine months of data were eliminated from the sample, and it was assumed that hospitals reporting between nine and eleven months of data would have reported "average" figures (based on months they did report) for the missing months. In addition, statistical checks were performed to eliminate obviously erroneous outliers. There still appear to be some order-of-magnitude errors in the data, and certain hospitals and unreliable variables will have to be removed in later empirical work.

All identifying hospital characteristics (geographic area, teaching status, affiliations, services offered other than those reported on the HAS forms, etc.) were removed by either HAS or the Center. The data were then made available to the author.

It was quickly decided that the data for 1967 were too fragmented and erratic to be of much use. (HAS was just starting up and many hospitals were unfamiliar with the forms.) Also, those hospitals that did not appear in all years (1968 to 1971) were eliminated from the sample. The original sample consisted of 348 hospitals in 1968, 370 in 1969, 379 in 1970, and 375 in 1971. After removing those hospitals that did not appear in one or more years, we were left with a sample of 285 hospitals. These were fairly evenly spaced out over all hospital bed-size groups. The average bed size in the final sample varied slightly from year to year about an aggregate mean of 249 beds.

tic and therapeutic medical services provided in a hospital setting under the direction and control of physicians. The increases can be seen quite clearly in Table 1. Over a period of time (1968 through 1971) in which the number of operating room visits per adjusted patient day actually declined slightly in these sample hospitals, we can see explosive growth in the utilization levels per adjusted patient day of seven medical services (pathology tests, nuclear medicine procedures, pharmacy line items, inpatient and outpatient laboratory tests, inpatient and outpatient radiology procedures, therapeuradiology procedures, and blood bank units). There is no break in the general pattern when hospitals are grouped into separate bed-size classes. In a separate paper by the author (Redisch, 1974), hedonic cost indices are estimated that suggest that the growth of these seven medical services accounts for more than one-third of the increase in cost per adjusted patient day in the sample hospitals. Since approximately one-half of the per diem cost rise is related to rises in unit costs of basic inputs, these estimates imply that two-thirds of the increase in real inputs per adjusted patient day in the sample hospitals were related to increases in the per diem use of these seven medical services.

Much of this increase can be traced to the growth of highly specialized treatment centers within hospitals. Coronary care units, intensive care units for adults and for newborns, burn units, and so on, contribute to a highly structured form of patient care. (The ratio of private, not-for-profit hospitals reporting intensive care units jumped from 11 percent in 1960 to more than 70 percent today.) There may be a tendency to establish routines in patient monitoring in these units. Patterns of diagnostic ancillary service use can develop that may bear little relation to the needs of the individual patient (see Griner and Liptzen, 1971).

Growth in ancillary service use has also been encouraged by new hospital technology, such as multiple channel autoanalyzers, that lowers unit costs of individual tests when operating at a high volume. However, these scale economies may soon be dissipated through a "Xerox effect" (in many business offices, the surge in volume after the introduction of duplicating machines may more than make up for the drop in unit costs). Physicians who once ordered a small number of lab tests to confirm their original clinical diagnosis now order a full range of ten or twenty tests to "see what comes up." This somewhat spurious demand for laboratory tests can then be used to justify the purchase of still more automated lab equipment.

Moreover, rapid growth in ancillary service use is stimulated by a major new force in the practice of medicine. The rising number of dissatisfied patients who choose to sue their physicians and hospitals for malpractice, the decreasing reluctance of physicians to testify against one another in the contest of such suits, and the growing propensity of the courts to award large sums of money to patients who are successful in pursuing these suits have all contributed to an increasing tendency for physicians and hospitals to practice "defensive medicine."

This ancillary service growth, contributing such a large share to the rise in per diem hospital costs, is under the direct control of the physician. Furthermore, it is not at all clear that this intensive use of a fairly common set of hospital services has positively contributed to the overall level of the "quality" of hospital care. Berki, for example (1972:31), notes that it is not known whether the more intensive use of laboratory procedures corresponds in fact to increases in the quality of care or to medically unjustified overuse of convenient, income-generating services. Ofttimes what may emerge from haphazard diagnostic testing is one or two false positives that lead to further testing or to inappropriate treatment. For example, Schimmel (1964) notes that 20 percent of the patients in Yale's Intensive Care Unit suffered complications from diagnostic tests, drugs, and various therapeutic measures.

Until now we have talked about hospital cost inflation primarily in terms of increases in costs per adjusted patient day. Yet government policy should be directed not just at these "unit" or daily costs, but at the aggregate level of hospital expenditures, as reflected in per capita hospital costs. Per capita costs are determined by the product of per diem costs and the number of patient days per capita. And the latter is determined by the per capita hospital admission rate and by the average length of stay for hospital care. Thus far we have examined the influence of the physician on per diem costs. We must now consider his degree of control over the admission decision and the discharge (or length of stay) decision.

Work by Wennberg et al. (1975), concerning several Maine communities at a single point in time, suggests that the admission decision is the most important explanation of variations in per capita hospital costs and expenditures. They find that average length of stay or cost per admission is less important than per capita admissions in explaining those variations. Physicians' uncertainty about the need for service or the value of alternative therapies is the likely cause of large observed differences in age- and sex-adjusted per capita hospital admission rates across what would be considered fairly homogeneous communities. Wennberg and his associates conclude that "the resource implications of differences in management within hospitals are less important than decisions to manage patients at the ambulatory or the institutional level of care" (Wennberg et al., 1975:305).

While growth in per diem costs plays a larger role than growth in per capita admissions in explaining increases in per capita hospital costs over time, it *is* true that the admission decision is a central one in initiating the hospital cost inflation process. The decision seems dominated by a group of socioeconomic incentives aimed at both the patient and the physician, and by the varying perceptions of individual physicians as to what constitutes medical need.

Perceptions of medical need do vary among physicians. In England, medical care is not rationed by the price mechanism and physicians face identical economic incentives across all of their patients. In a study of over three thousand normal deliveries in the Oxford Record Linkage Study area in 1962, M. Feldstein (1968) found that the most important single factor influencing any woman's expected hospital stay during delivery was the standard practice of the obstetrician in charge of the case. This was found to be more important in determining length of stay than the age of the woman, the number of previous children, her social class, or other characteristics.

Physicians have a great deal of discretion in deciding whether the "medical needs" of the patient include admission to a hospital. Their determination of this need may be influenced by a number of social and economic forces not directly related to the medical condition of the patient. For example, Rafferty (1971) has observed that in two Indiana hospitals increases in the general incidence of illness in the community, resulting in increases in the rate of bed occupancy, made physicians reluctant to hospitalize patients for less severe illnesses or for minor elective procedures. Similarly, Davis and Russell (1972) found that rises in occupancy rates lead to treatment of marginal patients in the outpatient department. When beds are relatively scarce, they are saved by physicians for the seriously ill.

The resource decisions that physicians implicitly make in response to perceived social needs do not have to be minor ones. Titmuss (1950) notes that in 1939 almost half the patients in English hospitals (some 140,000 individuals) were discharged in anticipation of war casualties, at a time when there were 200,000 people on hospital waiting lists. Major changes in the way health care is delivered can be accomplished if they are considered part of desirable public policy with a degree of universal public acceptance.

While it is clear that "medical need" is the major determinant of health care utilization, we have shown that various social forces and differences in the medical perceptions of individual physicians also influence the decision to utilize hospital services. In addition, economic incentives to the patient and to the physician produce nontrivial changes in the level and mix of care. Bishop (1973:29) notes that the simplification of an extended care facility (ECF) transfer form and, more important, an agreement by a third-party payer to cover physician services in the ECF led to net savings by the insuror and the ending of a hospital expansion plan.

New York City provides another example of how physicians' personal economic incentives can affect their behavior in a way that is particularly relevant for future health care policy decisions. In the late 1950s, Group Health Insurance (GHI) and the Health Insurance Plan of Greater New York (HIP) both provided a wide range of health services at a marginal out-of-pocket cost of approximately zero to similar sets of subscribers in New York City. GHI paid participating physicians a fee for each service performed, while HIP contracted with groups of physicians who agreed to provide care to HIP enrollees in return for payment on an annual capitation basis. The rates for nonsurgical, nonobstetrical physician visits were similar for each plan, but GHI enrollees had an average of 7.18 hospitalized surgical procedures per hundred persons per year, while the rate for HIP enrollees was only 4.18 (Monsma, 1970:151). It may be that "too many" appendectomies, hysterectomies, and tonsillectomies were performed by GHI surgeons, or it may be that "too few" were performed by HIP surgeons. The only statement that emerges with any clarity is that the financial incentive to the physician somehow seems to have heavy impact on definitions of "medical need" when elective surgery is considered.

The impact of personal economic incentives to the physician can be further viewed in the study by Gaus et al. (1976), which compared various aspects of HMO performance with those of the nonprepaid, fee-for-service system for the Medicaid population. It was found that Medicaid beneficiaries enrolled in two medical foundations exhibited no statistically significant differences in hospital use when compared with a matched sample of Medicaid beneficiaries utilizing the fee-for-service system. The foundations accepted capitation payment for their Medicaid enrollees but reimbursed affiliated physicians on a fee-for-service basis. In contrast, Medicaid beneficiaries enrolled in a group of HMOs with non-fee-for-service physicians were observed to have 356 days of hospital care per 1,000 persons per year. This was a remarkable 62 percent lower than the 934 days per 1,000 persons per year measured for the fee-for-service Medicaid control group.

The authors conclude that the fact that foundations show no major differences in hospital use, despite the financial incentives at the organization level to do so, indicates that the financial incentive of capitation payment to the HMO organization may by itself not have significant impact on the hospitalization practices of affiliated physicians. The major cost impact of HMOs appears to lie not simply in having an organization (the HMO) take the risk for total care of the beneficiary. Instead, it lies in having the physician limit his incentives to hospitalize patients by removing him from the fee-for-service setting, by separating to some extent resource control from the medical staff, and by reconstituting medical practice within the context of a salaried, multispecialty group.

These conclusions are partially confirmed at a wider level by Bunker (1970), who observes a much lower rate of surgical procedures per 1,000 persons in England than in the United States. Similarly, Adelstein (1973) shows that the per capita number of x-ray exams is much higher in this country than in other countries.

Surgery and radiology in England are performed by salaried specialists working full time as hospital staff members, while surgery and radiology in the United States are typically performed by independent physicians faced with the perverse incentives of a fee-for-service reimbursement system.

This documentation of the pervasive influence of physicians in determining resource allocations within the hospital implies that control measures to hold down the rate of inflation of hospital costs, if aimed solely at the hospital, will be disappointing. Certificates of need, rate review, or alternative forms of prospective reimbursement all *do* provide the administrator with an added rationale for confronting and standing up to the physician staff. Yet the benefits to the administrator of siding with the staff are usually so high that true confrontations are exceedingly unusual.

Most hospital administrators see themselves in competition with other hospitals for physicians, not for patients, since it is only through a physician that an individual may be admitted to a hospital. As long as there are other hospitals that will admit him to practice, a physician is not totally dependent on a particular hospital for his livelihood. But a hospital that cannot retain a satisfied medical staff will soon find its occupancy rate falling, its per diem costs rising, and its ability to function as a health care institution seriously impaired. Furthermore, if cost guidelines are given to a hospital on a per diem basis, many administrators may find themselves in the seemingly paradoxical situation of allowing certain marginal equipment and personnel decisions or capital projects to attract or keep physician staff so that the occupancy rate will be high enough to move the hospital within the per diem cost constraints.

It is not surprising that administrators will put off as long as possible the inclusion of medical staff into any negative budgetary decisions that must be made. Most physicians practicing in a group of Western Pennsylvania hospitals that were being reimbursed on a prospective basis by the local Blue Cross organization were not even aware of this fact (see Applied Management Sciences, 1975). Cost containment was considered an administrative issue, not a medical one.

If hospital budgetary controls are made so tight that they cannot be met by simply eliminating any administrative slack in the hospital, then affiliated physicians will have to become more directly involved in the hospital's budgetary process. However, even when the administrator is forced to confront his medical staff on cost issues, he is at a disadvantage. Physicians can argue persuasively and with a unique degree of authority about medical need and quality of care. It is difficult for the lay administrator to pick and choose among these arguments and make resource decisions that hurt one physician group but not another. Even when these negative decisions are chosen, they are most likely to be based on the degree of power of the various physician specialty groups within the hospital, rather than on criteria based on some nebulous concept of social efficiency norms. There has been a paucity of sophisticated evaluation relating medical care inputs to health outcomes, even for expensive pieces of equipment. Without such evaluation, hospital administrators have little with which to judge competently or counter physician arguments concerning quality of care.

A more effective control mechanism might make an impact on the physician directly, rather than through the administrator. Yet the costs of policing physicians through direct regulation on a case-by-case basis can be excessive. Medical cases are highly differentiated goods. No two patients are ever exactly the same, even if they exhibit the same general set of symptoms. If the decision to hospitalize were based solely on medical reasoning, the physician would be hospitalizing a disease rather than a person with a disease.

The current method of applying case-by-case regulation is through a form of professional peer review structured around local Professional Standards Review Organizations. Yet peer review in this form may prove more effective as a quality control measure than as a cost control device. Historically, peer review in the health care sector seems to have been oriented toward preventing abuse of patients and not toward preventing abuse of resources. Skeptics have claimed that this orientation will continue, and that hospital costs will rise as PSRO-mandated "resource ceilings" quickly become "quality floors."

A more effective form of case-by-case peer review may be simply to have third-party payers provide full funding on a prospective basis for a second opinion by an "impartial" board-certified surgeon whenever a physician feels that nonemergency surgery is indicated. One study in this area, with a one- to four-year follow-up of cases, showed that "in the voluntary programs, one out of four screened patients, and in the mandatory programs, one out of seven and a half screened patients, appear to be permanently 'deferred' from surgery" (McCarthy and Kamons, 1976:7).

However, peer review in any form should not be expected to play a dominant role in strategies aimed at containing health care costs. The history of peer review in fields other than health has been marginal at best, because of an unwillingness or lack of power to impose meaningful controls. The inability of peer review to function effectively as a cost control device in fee-for-service health care settings gains credence from empirical studies of fee-for-service group practices in California. Physicians in these practices share costs but either bill patients directly or share in the net receipts according to a weighting scheme based on volume of the individual physician's patients. Costs have been observed to be as high as or higher than those in similarly situated solo practices (Newhouse, 1973).

The potential economies of sharing paramedical personnel and office equipment have been dissipated by physician behavior. With a large number (N) of physicians in practice together, each physician knows that by prescribing extensive use of the groups' resources he bears the burden of only $1/N$th of the costs but gains a proportionately greater share of the revenues. Even though physicians have a direct economic stake in the actions of their colleagues, peer group pressures in this ambulatory setting have not been effective cost control devices as physician staff size becomes unwieldy.

And the future may be less bright. Noll (1972) has shown that the regulatory process in areas other than health care has quickly degenerated into a system of peer control. This occurs when the only groups competent to evaluate the regulated firms are themselves current or former members of the industry.

Direct government intervention through the regulatory or rate-review process also does not appear to be the panacea that will bring hospital cost inflation in line with price rises in the rest of the economy. Work by Salkever and Bice (1976) and by Hellinger (1976) in evaluating the early impact of certificate-of-need legislation, and the study by Gaus and Hellinger (1976) of prospective reimbursement systems show that even in those few cases where these regulatory devices evoke a statistically discernible effect in the desired direction, the magnitude of this effect, while large in dollar terms, is quite small relative to cost increases in the hospital sector.

The "co-option" of the regulatory process in health care seems to have already begun in some areas. For example, the Center for the Analysis of Public Issues (1974) makes charges relating to health care regulation in New Jersey. On a more inferential level, Cromwell et al. (1975:121) note that only one out of forty-one certificate-of-need applications was denied to hospitals in the Greater Boston area in 1973.

There is thus a real danger that health care regulation will be proposed and supported by members of the industry as a mechanism for supplanting whatever competitive elements remain with a legal, enforceable cartel. This view would allow for state hospital associations to petition their legislatures to put them under the protective umbrella of a state-mandated prospective reimbursement system that is meant to *guarantee* an "adequate" cash flow to each hospital. This view would also encompass the use of comprehensive health planning by local hospital groups as a vehicle for keeping Health Maintenance Organizations from encroaching on their territory.

Even if direct hospital regulation turns out to be a moderate success, its role will have to be strengthened by some basic structural changes in the way physicians are educated and reimbursed. Today the typical physician, acting in the interests of himself and his immediate patients, puts little weight on the larger issues of economic efficiency and social benefit. This attitude has been reinforced by the strong technological imperative instilled in physicians during their medical training programs (and is tacitly encouraged by the present cost-based system for financing hospital care).

The professional training of physicians has traditionally not emphasized the concept of the physician as a manager of health care resources confronted with complex issues of cost and efficiency. Instead, the physician emerges from his training period with a perception of the hospital as a rent-free workshop, a place where he feels justified in pressing administrators and trustees to add those medical care inputs that allow for full, modern treatment of patients while simultaneously enhancing the physician's income and prestige.

Individual physician and patient issues, not social issues, dominate the training process and are carried over into the medical practice. For example, physicians who specialize in treating patients with a given disease will not agree to the exclusion of facilities at hospital A, where they hold staff appointments, unless they are granted staff privileges at hospital B, where the planning agency would like to concentrate all facilities for diagnosis and treatment. The physician not only has a financial interest involved; there is also the matter of the preservation and employment of professional skills.

At times this type of behavior is costly not only to society but to the individual patient as well. The only one to gain is the physician. Rosenthal (1966:109) quotes, as a not so extreme example, the President's Commission on Heart, Cancer, and Stroke to show that in the early 1960s 30 percent of the 777 hospitals equipped to do closed-heart surgery had no such cases in the year under study, and 87 percent of the 548 hospitals that did have cases performed fewer than one operation per week. Furthermore, 77 percent of the hospitals equipped to do open-heart surgery averaged less than one operation per week, and 41 percent averaged less than one a month. Little of this sporadic surgery was of an emergency nature, and the mortality rate of both procedures when done infrequently was far higher than in institutions with a full work load.

This phenomenon is, of course, closely linked to the explosive growth in the opportunities for application of new and high-cost technology in health care. Recent innovations in medical care have been characterized by an emphasis upon complex diagnostic and therapeutic techniques usually requiring hospitalization and the physician-controlled application of complicated, expensive equipment. Examples include cancer radiation therapy and chemotherapy, renal dialysis, organ transplants, open-heart surgery, brain and body scanners, and intensive care units for burn, trauma, and heart patients. The overall cumulative effect of health care technology in this country, in combination with hospital-oriented, cost-based health insurance, has been to shift the focus of the health system from office-based, primary care medical practice toward hospital-based, specialist care medical practice.

Furthermore, this shift in focus is made more acute by the interaction of technological applications in health care and the current orientation of medical training programs. The new high-cost hospital technology necessitates specialization and fosters a narrow professionalism among new physicians. That is, for reasons relating to income, prestige, and the way that modern medicine is practiced, new physicians are drawn toward the practice of specialized medicine within an urban, institutionalized setting. This trend in turn creates ever greater demands from physicians to induce hospitals to adopt still more technology. Thus the cycle is completed and starts anew. And thus delivery of health care has shifted from general practitioners toward high-priced specialists operating in expensive settings. From 1963 to 1973 the overall number of physicians in the United States increased by 32.5 percent. There was a 53.5 percent increase in medical specialists, a 29.8 percent increase in surgical specialists, a 50.3 percent increase in all other specialists, and a 26.5 percent *decline* in the number of general practitioners (American Medical Association, 1967 and 1974b).

The massive movement toward specialization has helped fuel the hospital cost inflation process through the specialist-technology relationship described earlier. M. Feldstein (1971b:871), using a pooled cross-sectional time series for individual states for the period 1958–1967, estimates that the addition of one or more specialists in a state in that time interval would cause hospital costs to increase by $39,000 per year. Conversely, general practitioners were shown to be a substitute for hospital care. Feldstein estimates that the introduction of an additional GP into a state would cause hospital costs to decrease by $39,000 per year. Thus the true costs of producing ever-increasing numbers of specialists must include these induced hospital costs as well as any added educational costs (in part underwritten by public funds) and higher physician fees associated with specialization. These additional costs should be taken into account in any decisions impacting on the extent of public funding for the production (that is, education) of hospital-oriented physicians.

The greatest potential in utilizing the physician to contain hospital costs, however, may lie in the movement, whenever possible, away from fee-for-service as the method of reimbursing physicians and away from a system in which individual physicians control hospital inputs without bearing any responsibility for them. Such a movement, if feasible at all, would probably have to take place in piecemeal, incremental fashion. Capitation or salaried service may marginally increase in popularity, but it seems clear that, even with a major restructuring of the health care system through national health financing legislation, these two methods of reimbursing physicians will for some time appear only as options to physicians who desire alternatives to fee-for-service. Any new system, to be politically feasible, must meet with at least grudging acceptance by physicians. While most physicians see the hospital as an adjunct to their practice and an extension of their office, a vocal minority visualizes the hospital as a threat to the private practice of medicine. The AMA and individual physicians have fought long and hard to maintain de facto control of resource decisions in hospitals to keep this fear from becoming a reality. The AMA (1974b:20) suggests that "a physician should not bargain or enter into a contract whereby any hospital, corporation, or lay body may offer for sale or sell for a fee the physician's professional services." The only exceptions to this stated AMA principle are salaried "educational" staff appointments. The AMA's position has been that hospitals are "exploiting" salaried physicians by making shadow profits on their activities to support other departments (American Medical Association, 1959).

However, physician groups can no longer severely punish individual physicians who are induced to defect from traditional fee-for-service reimbursement. The courts have ruled that hospitals may not deny staff privileges to a physician simply because he is a member of a group practice or is not a member of the local county medical society.

The amount of money society can afford to spend to induce defections may prove to be quite large. From July 1975 to June 1976 hospital costs increased by $7.2 billion (Gibson and Mueller, 1977). This represents 27 percent of the total cost of physician services in that period, or around $23,000 per U.S. physician, and a much higher figure when divided only by fee-for-service physicians.

We have suggested that a large part of these annual hospital cost increases is related to the growing intensity of care caused partly by the method by which physicians are reimbursed and partly by the way they are free from responsibility for hospital inputs. Movement away from the perverse incentives of fee-for-service, in combination with the separation to some extent of resource control from the medical staff, could produce the dramatic drops in per capita hospital utilization similar to the ones associated with HMOs. It is these anticipated savings that society could decide to use to encourage defections from fee-for-service practice.

Adoption of a European-style health care system, with hospitals primarily the domain of salaried specialists, and with general practitioners operating independently in office-based settings, might be a step in this direction. Many physicians are already practicing in hospitals on a straight salary, such as interns and residents (who comprise more than 20 percent of active physicians in many states), full-time salaried chiefs of staff, and other physicians serving educational functions. Still other physicians could be induced to practice on a salaried basis if the salary were high enough. (While many physicians are ideologically opposed to anything but fee-for-service reimbursement, others are concerned not about ideology but about levels of income and hours of work today and in the future.)

However, adoption of a European-style system for the United States would present many problems. The level of physician salaries and of payment responsibilities would have to be determined. State laws against the corporate practice of medicine would have to be redesigned (they are currently being rewritten in many states to allow for the functioning of HMOs). A way would have to be found to gradually allow new staff privileges only to salaried specialists. And more important, while this system removes many of the perverse incentives individual physicians face with respect to the utilization of hospital resources, it does nothing by itself to provide incentives to the hospital to contain costs.

A more practical approach that should be viewed as a movement in this general direction would be to push for salaried status for three specific hospital-based physicians. Anesthesiologists, pathologists, and radiologists often control small fiefdoms within the hospital. They practice under reimbursement methods that are financially very favorable to them (fee-for-service or some percentage of their departments' gross or net revenues). It is suggested that these reimbursement methods contribute simultaneously to their high average income level and to rising levels of hospital costs resulting from the inordinate growth of their departments' services.

There are, of course, other alternatives to full-scale fee-for-service in addition to the European model. New concepts deserve encouragement, such as variants of the reimbursement plan being developed by the Blue Shield organization in Wisconsin. Individuals or groups of primary care physicians can elect capitation for a number of their patients. That is, they agree to provide a basic set of primary care services "on demand" in return for a fixed monthly fee. (The monthly fee and the set of primary care services can vary from physician to physician.) A pool is set up to pay for referrals to specialists and for hospitalization costs of patients. If the pool is not depleted by year end, the remainder is distributed back to the participating physicians.

Other new methods might be tried that attempt to make the physician responsible for the level of hospital costs. Monetary disbursements could be made to all physicians in an area where hospital costs are below projections, and also for residents or other full-time staff in a specific hospital. While this might create some incentives for the physician peer review process to focus in on some financial criteria, there would be many complications inherent in determining both a projected level of costs and a disbursement method. When variants of this reimbursement method have been tried (as in medical foundations), the evidence appears to show that fee-for-service incentives to the individual physician are stronger than peer group pressure (see Gaus et al., 1975).

The major physician-related impetus to cost containment in hospitals may come from the growth and encouragement of nonfoundation-type HMOs. It has already been suggested that these HMOs keep hospital costs in check not by the organization as an entity going at risk to provide medical care, but from the actions of staff physicians who are removed from fee-for-service reimbursement, who practice in multispecialty groups, and who do not operate with complete autonomy in regard to resource control. Encouragement of HMOs could take many forms. For example, a major insurance plan with deductibles for hospital and physician care and a 20 percent copayment provision for physician services (such as Medicare) could offer to drop all deductibles and co-insurance payments for beneficiaries who joined HMOs that agreed to provide care at a cost to the program of 80 percent of the average beneficiary cost in the area.

In the end it must be remembered that the search for a single panacea to contain hospital and other health care costs is likely to be a futile one. There are major forces at work in the health care arena. They are related to the interaction of physician incentives, patient passivity (induced in part by high levels of insurance), new technology, and cost-related hospital reimbursement. These forces are not unique to the American health care system. Costs of hospital care and other forms of health care can be observed to be rising rapidly in many societies operating under a wide range of regulatory activity and financing arrangements. The lesson to be learned is that there does not appear to be a single, simple solution to the health care cost crisis. Instead, the problem is one that will have to be solved (or at least partially alleviated) through a number of small, discrete steps. Utilizing the physician as a lever to help contain hospital costs is one of those steps.

References

Adelstein, S.
  1973   "The risk-benefit ratio in nuclear medicine." Hospital Practice 8
          (January).
American Hospital Association
  1969   Hospitals, Journal of the American Hospital Association (August,
          Guide Issue).
American Medical Association
  1959   "AMA/Acts on hospital-physician relations." Hospitals, Journal
          of the American Hospital Association (December): 17–19.
  1967   Distribution of Physicians in the U.S., 1963. Chicago: AMA
          Managerial Services Division.

1974a Distribution of Physicians in the U.S., 1973. Chicago: AMA Center for Health Services Research and Development.
1974b Physician-Hospital Relations. Chicago, Ill.

Applied Management Sciences
1975 Analysis of Prospective Reimbursement Systems: Western Pennsylvania. Prepared for the Office of Research and Statistics, Social Security Administration, U.S. DHEW, under Contract No. HEW-OS-74-226.

Berki, S.E.
1972 Hospital Economics. Lexington, Mass.: Lexington Books, D.C. Heath & Co.

Bishop, C.
1973 Public Regulation of Hospitals: Summary of a Conference. Health Care Policy Discussion Paper No. 4, Harvard Center for Community Health and Medical Care (March).

Bunker, J.
1970 "Surgical manpower: A comparison of operations and surgeons in the United States and in England and Wales." The New England Journal of Medicine 282 (January): 135–143.

Center for the Analysis of Public Issues
1974 Bureaucratic Malpractice. Princeton, N.J.

Council on Wage and Price Stability
1976 The Problem of Rising Health Care Costs. Staff Report, Washington, D.C. (April).

Cromwell, J., P.B. Ginsburg, D. Hamilton, and M. Sumner
1975 Incentives and Decisions Underlying Hospitals' Adoption and Utilization of Major Capital Equipment. Prepared by Abt Associates, Inc., for National Center for Health Services Research and Development. Contract No. (HSM) 110-73-513 (September).

Davis, K., and R. Foster
1972 Community Hospitals: Inflation in the Pre-Medicare Period. Social Security Administration, Research Report No. 41. Washington, D.C.: Government Printing Office.

Davis, K., and L.B. Russell
1972 "The substitution of hospital outpatient care for inpatient care." Review of Economics and Statistics 54 (May): 109–120.

Feldstein, M.S.
1968 Economic Analysis for Health Service Efficiency. Amsterdam: North-Holland Publishing Company.
1971a The Rising Cost of Hospital Care. Washington, D.C.: Information Resources Press.

1971b "Hospital cost inflation: A study of nonprofit price dynamics." American Economic Review 61 (December): 853–872.

Gaus, C.R., B.S. Cooper, and C.G. Hirschman
1975 "Contrasts in HMO and fee-for-service performance." Social Security Bulletin 39 (May): 3–14.

Gaus, C.R., and F.J. Hellinger
1976 Results of Hospital Prospective Reimbursement in the United States. Paper presented to the International Conference on Policies for the Containment of Health Care Costs and Expenditures. Fogarty International Center (June).

Gibson, R.M., and M.S. Mueller
1977 "National health expenditures, fiscal year 1976." Social Security Bulletin 40 (April): 3–22.

Griner, P., and B. Liptzen
1971 "Use of the laboratory in a teaching hospital: Implications for patient care, education, and hospital costs." Annals of Internal Medicine 75 (August).

Hellinger, F.J.
1976 "The effect of certificate-of-need legislation on hospital investment." Inquiry 13 (June): 187–193.

Jacobs, P.
1974 "A survey of economic models of hospitals." Inquiry 11 (June): 83–97.

Johnson, E.
1969 "Physician productivity and the hospital: A hospital administrator's view." Inquiry 6 (September): 59–69.

Leveson, I., and E. Rogers
1976 "Hospital cost inflation and physician payment." American Journal of Economics and Sociology 35 (April): 161–174.

McCarthy, E., and A. Kamons
1976 Voluntary and Mandatory Presurgical Screening Programs: An Analysis of Their Implications. Presented at American Federation for Clinical Research, Atlantic City (May 2).

Monsma, G.
1970 "Marginal revenue and the demand for physicians' services." In H.E. Klarman, ed., Empirical Studies in Health Economics. Baltimore: John Hopkins Press.

Newhouse, J.P.
1973 "The economics of group practice." Journal of Human Resources (Winter): 37–56.

Noll, R.C.
1971   Reforming Regulation. Washington, D.C.: The Brookings Institution.

Pauly, M., and M.A. Redisch
1973   "The not-for-profit hospital as a physicians' cooperative." American Economic Review 63 (March): 87–99.

Rafferty, J.
1971   "Patterns of hospital use: An analysis of short-run variations." Journal of Political Economy 79 (January–February): 154–165.

Redisch, M.A.
1974   Hospital Inflationary Mechanisms. Presented at Western Economic Association Meetings, Las Vegas, Nev. (June).

Reinhardt, U.
1972   "A production function for physician services." Review of Economics and Statistics 54 (February): 55–66.

Rosenthal, G.
1966   "The public pays the bill." Atlantic 218 (July): 107–110.

Salkever, D.S., and T.W. Bice
1976   The Impact of Certificate-of-Need Controls on Hospital Investment, Costs, and Utilization. Final report to the National Center for Health Services Research, DHEW, Contract No. HRA-106-74-57 (August).

Schimmel, E.
1964   "The hazards of hospitalization." Annals of Internal Medicine 60 (January): 100–116.

Titmuss, R.
1950   Problems of Social Policy. London: HMS Office and Longmans, Green.

Waldman, S.
1972   The Effect of Changing Technology on Hospital Costs. Research and Statistics Note No. 4, DHEW Publication No. (SSA) 72-11701 (February 28).

Wennberg, J., A. Gitteljohn, and N. Shapiro
1975   "Health care delivery in Maine III: Evaluating the level of hospital performance." Journal of the Maine Medical Association 66 (November).

Yett, D., L. Drabek, M. Intriligator, and L. Kimball
1971   A Macroeconomic Model for Regional Health Planning. Presented at the 46th Annual Conference of the Western Economic Association (August).

Hospital Cost Containment

and the Administrator

WILLIAM ZUBKOFF

Introduction

The purpose of this article is to discuss cost containment from the viewpoint of a local hospital administrator, specifically, an administrator at a moderate-size, private, nonprofit, community hospital in an urban setting. Because of the position, the local administrator cannot be limited to an in-depth view of a single issue, but by necessity is exposed to the entire spectrum of issues and programs involving cost-containment measures. It should be recognized that the local administrator's reactions to the issue of cost containment may be based on personal experiences. Yet any discussion of cost containment that excludes this subjective element would be lacking in depth.

It is well to ask, "What is the definition of cost containment to a hospital administrator?" Is it to limit costs by discouraging or slowing down applied research into selected areas that may be desirable for long-range benefits but not essential to immediate patient care requirements? Is it to decrease costs by better management of medical services? Is it to limit costs of ancillary services that are desirable but not essential to the eventual recovery of the patient? Is it possibly to decrease costs at the local level by calculated risks in lessening both care and services to the patient? Is it to sponsor and practice the delivery of health care to selected medical conditions rather than responding to demand medical care?

Is it to cause personnel pay to drift downward to a point where the minimum federal wage law is the principal concern?

Perhaps the issue of cost containment involves all of these questions plus many more concerns. Of primary importance is the issue of whether cost containment is feasible only through programs directed by high echelons and imposed upon the local level to combat inflation, or whether substantial savings can be realized through local level managerial improvements. Answers to these questions are contingent upon the cost-containment problems revealed by the market in which hospital care trades, and can only be arrived at by a down-to-earth view of the various factors with which a hospital administrator must deal.

The Marketplace

To sell any product there must be an anxious or at least willing consumer to purchase it. Practically no consumer, however, desires to purchase "cheaper" medical care. At the most, when neither the consumers nor their family members are acutely ill, they are willing to participate in objective discussions about hospital bills being too high. When consumers or their family members require hospitalization, however, these same consumers will shop for the most expensive hospital that they and their insurance can afford, often *more* expensive than they can afford. There appears to be no limit to how much money could be spent on medical care based solely on demand.

In one hospital service area, a questionnaire was distributed to 200 consumers (100 recent hospital dischargees and 100 randomly selected consumers in the community) to test their willingness to allow certain changes in the interest of reducing hospital costs and their bills. The questions involved both personal services and medical care. The respondents overwhelmingly rejected such things as black-and-white televisions instead of color sets, one telephone for two patients, less attractive hospitals, and elimination of routine screening tests unless ordered by the attending physician. No attempt is made to generalize from this very small and limited sample, but the responses seem to support the contention that the most inclusive and expensive services are desired by the consumer, as well as to indicate that not many people would be content with fewer amenities, let alone less medical care.

A hospital administrator, therefore, has little incentive to create a product for which there is no market. Savings that might be realized through managerial improvements must be presented in such a way as to ensure that no question exists concerning the possible compromise of the quality of services. If costs were actually reduced, the local administrator, concerned about varying significantly from the cost per patient day of neighboring hospitals, might attempt to hide the savings in ancillary services or perhaps use the money for other expenditures, rather than passing the savings on to consumers in the form of lower room and board charges. The motivation, obviously, is the belief by the administrator that the public equates higher cost with better quality of medical services.

Despite this gloomy picture of the marketplace, the local administrator will still feel that containing costs is the proper thing to do, and will want to examine various aspects of hospital administration in terms of their cost-containment potential.

Local Tools

Are tools to "contain costs" actually within the grasp of an individual hospital administrator? Let us answer this question in terms of:

Salaries—No. The local administrator has little or no control over the salary structure. The geographic area and the immediate community dictate the salary marketplace in which the hospital must compete.

Supplies—No. Supplies, particularly the ten highest dollar value items, such as films, parenteral solutions, and pharmaceuticals, are priced almost on a national basis.

Selection of Supplies—Partially. Selection of supplies may effect minor cost reductions through an active Therapeutics Committee supported by a firm and effective hospital formulary program.

Utilities—Minimally. Utilities may be subject to a 5-to-10 percent reduction through a program available from qualified engineering consultants that mechanically eliminates or reduces wasted energy. These savings, however, are projected and require a current outlay of investment. The potential savings in other utilities (such as telephone long-distance controls) are so small when compared with the "bad feelings" they engender that action is generally not worthwhile.

Equipment and Bonded Indebtedness—Minimally. Equipment expenditures and, in particular, changes in families or systems of equipment do offer significant savings, especially when the usual increase in personnel costs associated with the new equipment is considered. To a large extent, the administrator is at the mercy of the medical staff. A knowledgeable, respected, and firm director of professional services, assisted by an effective Equipment Committee, is necessary to keep these costs reasonably low, consistent with current advances in the delivery of medical care. This area of expenditure cannot be controlled by the administrator alone. The same holds true for any other capital expenditures resulting in bonded indebtedness.

Manpower Requirements—Yes. It is in this area, almost wholly within the administrator's authority, that the greatest control over costs can be exerted. While the administrator does not control salaries, there is almost no limit to the ability to perform any given task with fewer man hours. This is accomplished through good personnel selection procedures, proper motivation of employees, and effective utilization of all manpower resources. For instance, in a hypothetical $5,000,000 annual operating budget, here are some "nuts and bolts" types of savings that the local administrator could consider and accomplish:

	Savings per annum
1. Reduce the number of security guards or eliminate completely (often for parking with little effect upon security)	$35,000
2. Keep personnel manpower and procedures to a minimum (for example, unnecessary physical examinations)	$15,000

3. Keep Public Relations Office to a minimum $20,000
4. Eliminate desk position of executive housekeeper by having a working executive housekeeper $10,000
5. Eliminate formal, staffed mail room $15,000
6. Eliminate formal, staffed reproduction room $10,000
7. Eliminate formal, staffed message center and messenger service $30,000
8. Keep to a minimum middle management executives and secretarial staff $40,000
9. Avoid unnecessary and expensive position of chief engineer and supportive clerical help $30,000
10. Use night administrators to provide many coverages (admitting, security, etc.) $20,000
11. Avoid establishing an in-house patient transport service (function to be performed by each department) $20,000
12. Reduce postage expense and personnel expense by providing simple box pick-up system (to disseminate information to attending staff, etc.) $5,000
                                             $250,000

This list is only an illustration of the types of activities in which potential savings exist. The specific activities in which savings can be realized are dependent upon the individual hospital's organization, priorities, and administration. This example is intended to show the relative ease with which $250,000 can be saved in an operating budget of only $5,000,000 by cost-conscious administration. The emphasis is on savings realized through reduced or more efficient utilization of man hours. Since payroll expenditures account for the majority of total U.S. hospital expenditures (57.5 percent in 1974; see American Hospital Association, 1975: Table 11, p. xiv), this approach would seem to provide the greatest potential for savings.

Local Government Planning—Minimally. Sporadically, the administrator participates in or at least provides opinions to local governmental planning agencies (sometimes by invitation and sometimes because of vested interest). These opinions, however, rarely seem to have any real effect on planning decisions that may be translated into savings.

Federal and State Programs—Minimally. The local administrator is frequently asked by state and federal authorities to complete questionnaires and surveys, and occasionally is asked for other opinions and input. Somehow, however, administrators often feel that all this material feeds into one vast wastebasket, and that governmental officials expediting the laws and regulations will pay no heed. In the case of the newly established PSROs, for instance, the administrator may see little possibility of fiscal savings or quality improvement, only increased administrative costs. A 150-bed hospital might need at least three additional employees at a per annum cost of $27,000 just to handle the PSRO paperwork.

Hospital Size and Cost

There appears to be a great deal of controversy concerning the relationship between hospital size and cost. The issue of the realization of economies of scale in hospital operations is far from resolved. According to Berki (1972:115):

The answer from the literature is clear: the exact general form of the function is unimportant but whatever its exact shape and depending on the methodologies and definitions used, economies of scale exist, may exist, may not exist, or do not exist but in any case according to theory they ought to exist.

Various estimates of optimal hospital size have ranged from a low of 160 beds (Cohen, 1967) to a high of 905 beds (Feldstein, 1968). Carr and Feldstein (1967) reported a U-shaped curve for all hospitals with a minimum at between 250 and 350 beds, a rise to about 600 beds, and no change thereafter. Regardless of the controversy concerning hospital size and cost, there appears to be some agreement that a U-shaped curve exists. Donabedian (1973:285) mentions the "increasing difficulties in management and coordination, as well as decreases in personnel morale and productivity" that occur as hospital size increases. Additionally, according to Donabedian (1973:287), studies of the relationship of hospital size and cost are often "concerned only with the internal economies or diseconomies. If external costs were to be added, the optimal size of the service-producing unit would be smaller than that indicated by considering internal costs alone." Feldstein (1968:56) states that "hospital 'distribution costs' per case, including social as well as money costs, increase with the size of the catchment area served." Consideration of these various factors would tend to indicate a lower optimal hospital size (in terms of minimum cost per patient day) than has been reported in many studies.

Since costs for the same procedure are generally accepted to be higher at the largest and most complex hospitals, it should be equally accepted that delivery of services should be so designed as to provide for them at the least costly competent level. Consumers, however, are convinced that "big is better" and "costlier is better." The consequence of this belief is the major problem in the delivery of medical services. For example, this belief seriously undermines any attempt at developing voluntary referral networks. Hospitals should continuously and routinely redistribute patients according to the individual hospital's respective capabilities. Such redistribution should permit concurrent financial exchanges among hospitals to encourage this program and to ensure that the transferring hospital does not suffer financially—a system somewhat similar to blood exchange programs.

No hospital must feel ashamed, hurt, or hesitant to tell a patient that at this time Hospital B would be more appropriate given the patient's specific medical needs. Each hospital should be recognized both within the hospital field and throughout the community for those areas of care in which it specializes and excels. Newspapers and neighborhood activities responsible for citizen participation and input should be actively used for dissemination of such information. Concurrently, the "medical center syndrome," that "big is better," must be deemphasized. No one facility should ever feel or subtly advertise that it is so complete that seldom if ever does it have to transfer patients to other medical facilities in the area. Nor should it imply that the others are "lesser" facilities with "lesser" competence. These combined, across-the-board actions will teach the public that the inability to provide a specific service for a specific medical need in no way is a barometer of the overall effectiveness of a hospital. In fact, it should be stressed that specialization and moderate size frequently enhance the quality of services rendered each patient. In this regard, appropriate changes in consumers' thinking and actions probably offer the best returns on investment—if it is possible to accomplish this herculean task.

The issue of centralization is also affected by the belief that "big is better." The path to bigness is traveled the first time one accepts the theory that centralization saves money. As a solution to problems of organizational coordination in large hospitals, Starkweather (1970:35) proposes reorganization into "mini-hospitals" of approximately 100 beds, hoping to reduce "the organization barriers and operating inflexibilities which are characteristic of large hospitals." Starkweather states "that it is worth decreased efficiency in some components to obtain greater overall efficiency—a type of efficiency which recognizes patient service rather than hospital operation as the fundamental criterion" (p. 44).

Hospital Cost and Quality

It is first necessary to develop a rough definition of what is meant by the term "quality." A measurement of quality index should encompass more than just technical competence. Overall quality includes the issues of access, continuity of care, and consideration of social and psychological factors that affect health.

Many studies that have purported to examine quality have really measured technical competence. Presently, the highest technical competence is associated with the largest, most complex, and most costly facilities. This need not, however, be the case since high technical competence is related to the amount of care provided by specialists rather than to the size of medical care facilities.

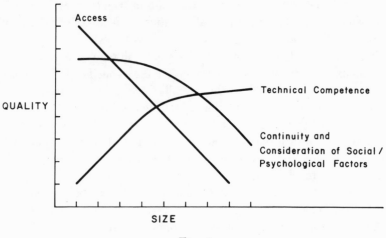

SIZE

Fig. 1

A broader definition of quality would encompass more than just technical competence, and the relationship between quality and size might be like that in Fig. 1. All of these curves represent only hypothesized relationships between the variables and would probably vary greatly based on the severity of the diagnosis (case mix). For example, in extremely complex cases, technical competence may take precedence over all other aspects of quality whereas, in the usual or routine cases, technical competence may be of lesser importance than continuity, access, or consideration of social-psychological factors. For the majority of routine cases, I would contend that Fig. 1, when weighted appropriately, would reduce as in Fig. 2.

Concerning the relationship between cost and size of medical care facilities, as already discussed, there appears to be some agreement that a U-shaped curve exists, with cost first decreasing with increasing size as economies are realized, and then increasing as diseconomies and management and coordination problems develop (Fig. 3).

Consideration of size as a proxy measure for cost might be of

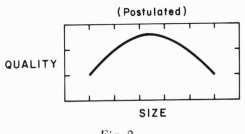

Fig. 2

value since high cost could either be caused by too small or too large a facility.

1. High cost —low quality (lacks adequate ancillary or
   (small facility) support services)
2. High cost —low quality (ignores all aspects of qual-
   (large facility) ity except technical competence. Actually provides high technical competence in spite of organization rather than because of it.)
3. Lower relative cost—high quality (technical competence
   (moderate-size through use of specialists
   facility) combined with possibility of increased access, continuity, and consideration of social-psychological factors.)

If Figs. 2 and 3 accurately reflect reality, then the optimal size of a medical care facility could be the same for maximum quality as well as for minimum cost (although this sounds somewhat outrageous). The relationship between cost and quality (for usual or routine diagnoses) could therefore be that illustrated in Fig. 4, with the lower cost facilities (moderate size) providing the highest quality, and the higher cost facilities (either small or large) providing the lowest quality (but for different reasons).

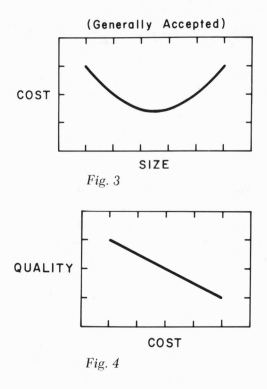

(Generally Accepted)

COST

SIZE

Fig. 3

QUALITY

COST

Fig. 4

Government's Role

To facilitate appropriate financial management by the local administrator, the government needs to clarify for the public what services will or will not be provided and paid for by various governmental levels. The murky atmosphere surrounding services authorized by each level of government pervades the fiscal and planning functioning of nonprofit community hospitals. It may be well to say that medical services are a "right," but some responsible agency must list for the public all potential medical services and then identify those that are or are not to be provided. Similarly, clarity of the legal contracts for medical services between local governments and providers is a basic requirement for common knowledge among consumers.

It is well for a community planning mechanism to promote

sharing among hospitals of expensive supporting services and avoid unnecessary duplication of hospital facilities and/or services. But this policy is a delusion or at least is limited in its usefulness if the transferring hospital must plead, wait, and lose prestige when it desires to transfer a patient to a receiving hospital for specialized services.

It is well for a community planning mechanism to promote accessibility of services to all consumers without regard to age, sex, race, ethnic background, or ability to pay. Yet the planning mechanism belies its goal if at the same time by the distribution of its funding resources, it directly or indirectly creates deliverers of medical services limited only to ghettos. Efforts should be made to eliminate the ambiguity of a hospital's role in what is grossly labeled "indigent care." Theoretically, this concept rests upon a definition of poverty, but this definition presently is vague and uncorroborated. Such vagueness makes a mockery of the planning attempts by hospital administration.

County, municipal, and other governments that collect millage and disburse funds for hospital medical services should be required to perform on a businesslike basis with local community hospitals. In an area where governmental facilities to exist, other nongovernmental hospitals still are frequently nudged or almost required to provide nonreimbursable services to the same people for whom the governmental agency has collected and disbursed tax money to the governmental hospitals.

The multiplicity of cost-sharing programs on the federal, state, and local levels has a tendency to cloud the fiscal picture and is prohibitive to sound fiscal planning and practices at the hospital level. For example, although a federal law may espouse "reasonable cost reimbursement," the funding on the state level may seriously alter the reimbursing formula. Complex sharing programs, therefore, should be eliminated or at least clarified.

Planning the Wrong Way

There is a feeling that all planning is good and economical. Nothing could be further from the truth. It often appears that learning from experience is slight and that a tendency exists to change radically entire systems rather than to build block upon block in a nondramatic but probably more productive manner.

The experiences in the inpatient field indicated that constructing more beds whenever "beds were full" was a mistake; this policy has resulted in the current oversupply of beds. Hindsight appears to indicate that instead of building more beds, a wiser course of action would have been to concentrate on management by improving the utilization of facilities. However, the prevailing philosophy was the more beds in the facility, the more prestigious the hospital. Achievement of a certain number of beds would magically transform a hospital into a medical center theoretically ready for conducting research. In this chase for a magic wand, we championed "big is better" and "the greater the concentration of specialties and specialists, the better." These mottos are perhaps the major issue today in government itself—although signs now point to both decentralization and lessening of all aspects of "bigness."

Disregarding this history and the future trend of inpatient services, planning, for example, is taking the same wrong route in providing emergency services. Planning typically designates three categories of emergency facilities: (a) regional emergency centers; (b) comprehensive emergency service; and (c) emergency standby and referral service. While the planning reads smoothly and perhaps has no ulterior motive, it clearly would have you believe that (a) is best, (b) is next best, and (c) is all right if you have to "live with it." Again, big is better (and usually the most costly). The envisioned economies of scale that never materialized in the inpatient service may very well never materialize in emergency services. The ineffectiveness and managerial shortcomings associated with huge medical complexes, however, can be relied on to materialize very quickly.

Of major importance is the likelihood that the indoctrinated consumer will once again conclude that big is better and will tend to go to the largest, most expensive location rather than to the nearest emergency facility that could probably well handle 95 percent of the emergency room demand and could certainly handle the emergency aspects of the other 5 percent—life saving, stabilization, and transfer of patient in perhaps 1 or 2 percent of the cases.

Thus the capable, less expensive facility is continually belittled, discouraged, or phased out in favor of the more expensive, bedlam type of centralized emergency service. The financial consequences of centralizing emergency room services may have far-reaching effects on all hospitals, since emergency room admissions represent a sizable portion of total hospital admissions.

The present course in emergency medical services development will reinforce the current dilemma of inaccessible, overly expensive medical centers, which in many urban areas are now in the process of decentralization, if this is at all possible. The discouraging error in inpatient services is in the process of being repeated for emergency care, to create a product we cannot afford in order theoretically to take better care of about 1 to 2 percent of emergency consumers. Obviously, this is not cost containment but an irresponsible act by the provider, whose attitude is the consumer and the national economy be damned.

The issue of emergency services is an example of the planning-without-regard-to-cost attitude that infests many echelons in the field of medical services. Today's medical care system overprovides; it encourages needless and sometimes inferior services at more expense. We talk economy, we sponsor economy, we fool ourselves into thinking that we plan economy, yet we actually promote and practice increased spending whether we can afford it or not.

All proposed programs, while still a gleam in the eye of the originator, particularly government, should have a potential cost figure attached. Also, this figure should not include deduction of the envisioned savings in dollars, since more frequently than not the savings are imaginary or not truly recapturable in dollars. If cost containment is to be the number one priority, then all proposals must first be evaluated as to whether or not the economy can afford them and only second as to whether or not the product is worth the cost or how it compares in priority with other programs.

Licensure and Other Bosses

The need for reexamination of the personnel licensure system
has been a controversy for many years. In 1971, the DHEW report
Licensing and Related Health Personnel Credentialing pointed out
that "The concept of expanding institutional licensure to include the
regulation of health personnel beyond the traditional facility licensure has important potential as a supplement or alternative to
existing forms of individual licensure" (p. 77). The various claims for
moratoriums on licensure and for reexamination of the personnel
licensure system, however, appear to have resulted in little action
and less success in curtailing the proliferation of groups seeking
individual licensure, with resultant rigidity and increased costs for
the hospital.

Licensure should be a tool for enhancing quality consistent with
the practicalities of its fiscal implications. Licensure should not be
enacted primarily because of vested interest-group pressure but
should be reserved for situations where other controls are not
sufficient and where the number of potential abuses warrants the
expensive and usually disagreeable financial outgrowths resulting
from licensure.

A similar situation exists concerning inspectors and accrediting
agencies whose "standards" are frequently established by self-
centered pressure groups without due regard to implementation
cost or actual need. These inspectors or accrediting agencies impose
a multitude of staffing and procedure standards upon providers who
by law or prestige require their approval.

Licensure, staffing prerequisites, employee industrial standards,
frequency of repetitive fire drills, and duties that may and may not
be performed by specified personnel all cost money and should not
be mandated by law or higher echelons but should be made the
responsibility of the individual hospital whose performance will be
evaluated on an institutional basis.

Pursuit of the Costly Impractical

Funds are frequently squandered on impractical, nonproductive
programs, or, even worse, on "hanging on" programs that no one is

willing to eliminate; for example, the variety of utilization review programs that have been a "paper farce" since the enactment of Medicare. These will soon be replaced by a probably equally unproductive paper mill, the PSRO. Traditional utilitization review has primarily focused on length-of-stay controls in an attempt to reduce total inpatient days. Whatever savings could be realized from this approach have already been made. In short-term, acute care, general hospitals, having a sizable portion of admissions of three days or less, controls that attempt to shave down slightly the average length of stay will be ineffective.

Only an effective admission certification approach would significantly reduce inpatient days. However, as long as it is financially advantageous to hospitalize patients, admission certification programs will continue to be a paper farce. Basically, the only way to reduce hospital admissions is for the government to assign qualified personnel to each hospital on a twenty-four-hour, seven-day-a-week basis, who have the authority to say "yes" or "no" to every admission. Once the patient is admitted, no amount of concurrent or retrospective utilization review by local level peer groups or PSROs will reduce inpatient days significantly over a sustained period. I am not, of course, proposing such drastic or unrealistic action, but I do stress that only such an authoritarian weapon would be effective in reducing inpatient days on a population basis.

Given the present concern for "cost containment," my point is merely this: to stop spending the hospital's money for those impractical programs and concentrate instead on practical measures that are direct and simple. One could properly ask me or any local hospital administrator, "What sort of practical programs do you propose?" To which I, and undoubtedly others, would reply, "That's your job. I comply with and make judgments on the programs you design." By "you," I mean any level of authority above me. While this reply may seem to be avoiding the question, it is not. The local administrator's responsibility is not to prescribe laterally or upward. The hospital administrator is not yet convinced that "cost containment" is a pressing problem that must now be solved. It has not yet reached the top of the administrator's stack of papers; at the top is still the attempt to satisfy the daily desires of each patient, the patient's family, and the attending staff. This ordering of priority, however, does not prevent the daily attempt to manage effectively, economically, and with a clear fix on reimbursement.

Expectations from Cost-Containment Measures

From a local administrator's point of view, the expectations from various cost-containment measures are limited. Increasing costs per patient day may very well be inherent in hospitals with increasing personnel salaries. Anderson and Neuhauser (1969) compared health systems as varied as those in the United States, England, and Sweden and concluded that "hospitals in all three countries are experiencing the same dramatic increases in expenditures." The authors further expressed the belief that "these rising expenditures should be regarded as inherent in progressive health care systems rather than the result of the loosely organized nature of the systems themselves" (p. 50).

In the long run, simple and direct controls are needed over duplication of services, incentives are needed to establish functioning referral networks, and, most important, significant adjustments are needed in public attitudes or values concerning medical care delivery systems. Given the poor history of regulatory attempts, the potential success of recent measures such as the new health planning legislation (P.L. 93-641), rate-review commissions, or token efforts at the development of hospital consortiums is quite debatable. Of crucial importance is the realization of the incompatibility of additional programs with cost control measures. More responsible program proposals with realistic consideration of the financial implications are needed, which may, in turn, result in some refinement of the rather crude attempts at conducting cost-benefit analyses of various proposals.

Local level administrators are not convinced that cost containment is as serious an issue as the rhetoric it engenders might indicate. Nevertheless, in the short run, moderate savings can be realized by the individual hospital through a variety of managerial improvements, primarily focusing on the reduced or more efficient utilization of man hours outlined previously.

Aftermath of Cost Containment

Oddly enough, the eventual problem in this area may not be how to contain costs. Equally or maybe more important and more difficult may be what to do with the "cost-containment savings." Should the savings be returned to the consumer in the form of reduced charges? Should the savings be set aside for future capital expenditures or to support special community projects? Whether the individual, the institution, or the government provides the principal motivation, the question of why, what, and for whom am I saving is most essential and presents a more complex problem than the process of saving.

References

American Hospital Association
  1975   Hospital Statistics, Table 11, p. xiv.
Anderson, O.W., and D. Neuhauser
  1969   "Rising costs are inherent in modern health care systems."
          Hospitals, Journal of the American Hospital Association 43
          (February): 50–52.
Berki, S.E.
  1972   Hospital Economics. Lexington, Mass.: Lexington Books, D.C.
          Heath & Co.
Carr, W.J., and P.J. Feldstein
  1967   "The relationship of cost to hospital size." Inquiry 4 (June):
          45–65.
Cohen, H.A.
  1967   "Variations in cost among hospitals of different sizes." Southern
          Economic Journal 33 (January): 355–366.
Donabedian, A.
  1973   Aspects of Medical Care Administration. Cambridge, Mass.:
          Harvard University Press.

Feldstein, M.S.
   1968   "Effects of scale on hospital costs," in Economic Analysis for Health Service Efficiency. Amsterdam: North-Holland Publishing Company.
Starkweather, D.B.
   1970   "The rationale for decentralization in large hospitals." Hospital Administration (Spring): 27–45.
U.S. Department of Health, Education, and Welfare
   1971   Report on Licensure and Related Health Personnel Credentialing. DHEW Publication No. (HSM) 72-11. Washington, D.C.: Government Printing Office.

Medical Technology

and Hospital Costs

JUDITH L. WAGNER
AND MICHAEL ZUBKOFF

Introduction

Medical technology, particularly the kind found in hospitals, has undergone a curious shift in public acceptability over the past five years. Those who influence and shape national health policy have shown increasing alarm over the way in which new technologies are developed and introduced into the health care system. With few exceptions, the present concern is with the proliferation of new technologies in hospitals.[1] New equipment, procedures, or systems appear to be introduced by hospital decision makers often without knowledge of or concern for their relative effectiveness or efficiency. Technology purportedly follows its own imperative, eluding effective control by regulatory or financing agencies (Rabkin and Melin, 1976). Most important, new hospital technologies have allegedly raised health care costs, and herein lies the major source of

[1] The exceptions are important. Some observers have noted the low development or implementation of technologies for use in primary care that would allow the substitution of low-cost for high-cost manpower (see White, Murnaghan, and Gaus, 1972). Barriers to development and diffusion of technologies that would be very useful to the handicapped have been noted in a recent report by the National Research Council (1976).

alarm. Clifton Gaus of the Social Security Administration recently stated:

> The long-term cumulative effect of adopting new health care technologies is a major cause of the large yearly increases in national health expenditures and in total Medicare and Medicaid benefit levels [Gaus, 1975:12-13].

Technology has clearly acquired a bad name; increasingly, policies to assess, evaluate, or control the introduction of new technologies on the federal and state levels have been suggested as cost-containment strategies (see, for example, Russell, 1976; Rabkin and Melin, 1976; Gaus and Cooper, 1976; Weiner, 1976). Debates over the nation's ability to continue to pay for new technologies as it has in the past have flourished (DeBakey and Hiatt, 1976).

The obvious question arises as to why technology, and particularly hospital technology, has been singled out at this time as a particular problem of hospital behavior. The answer lies in the convergence of three lines of criticism of the health care system.

First, recent studies decomposing hospital cost inflation into its constituent parts have provided some circumstantial evidence linking technology to increased hospital costs. In 1972, Waldman estimated that increases in real inputs accounted for 50 percent of the annual changes in per diem hospital costs between 1951 and 1970. Similar findings by Worthington (1975) and, most recently, Feldstein and Taylor (1977) have demonstrated the changing nature of the hospital product. Feldstein and Taylor found that about 75 percent of the rise in hospital costs relative to the general economy can be attributed to increases in labor and nonlabor inputs per patient day. Although there is no one-to-one correspondence between the increasing level of intensity of care (as measured by increasing inputs) and the rate of technological change, a clear implication of these studies is that the introduction of new technologies is responsible for much of the trend.

The second factor leading to the assault on hospital technology is the mounting evidence that many health services, indeed perhaps *all* medical care, have made little difference in health outcomes. Nonmedical factors appear to have been more important in reducing mortality and morbidity rates over the past fifty years than has medical care. The works of Cochrane (1972) and McKeown (1976) have raised considerable doubt about the efficacy of many medical procedures. It has become increasingly clear that clinical research is not organized to provide definitive information on the effectiveness of existing or new medical procedures. In the absence of hard scientific proof, several observers have suggested that we should avoid heavy investments in technologies that enhance the delivery of dubious services (see, for example, White, Murnaghan, and Gaus, 1972; Banta and McNeil, 1977). Arguments for redistribution of health dollars to areas of health promotion and prevention are based on an acceptance of this thesis (Lalonde, 1972).

A third source of concern lies in the disappointing record of programs designed to control hospital capital expenditures. State certificate-of-need laws and state programs for approval of large capital expenditures under Section 1122 of the 1972 Social Security Amendments have been in existence long enough for some evidence to be accumulated about their effectiveness in controlling the proliferation of expensive pieces of capital equipment. The record has been dismal. Not only have health planning agencies proved to be unprepared to make appropriate judgments about new technologies, but certificate of need appears to have shifted the composition of capital spending from investments in new beds to investment in sophisticated equipment (Salkever and Bice, 1976). Capital equipment expenditures should not be unequivocally equated with adoption of new technologies, but the lack of effective control over this aspect of hospital expenditure has raised the question whether any control over decisions of hospitals to adopt new and expensive technologies exists.

The convergence of these three separate types of evidence has created an environment of cynicism about the value of new technologies to the delivery of health care. If health care services make so little difference to the community's health level, then investments in an increasing level of sophistication embodied in new technology become especially suspect. As the major repository of the visible symbols of sophisticated technology, the hospital is a natural target for criticism. Sensitive to this emerging anti-technology trend, the authors of DHEW's 1976 *Forward Plan for Health* defended technology's contribution to the well-being of the nation:

During the past 30 years, national investment in biomedical and behavioral research has been enormously productive and has revolutionized clinical care. It is true that it is not yet possible to prevent many of our most frequent and costly illnesses, but that is not because such "high technology" (in Lewis Thomas' concept) is not a goal of research; rather, it is that research progress has not yet permitted the kind of definitive interventions that antibiotics brought for many infectious diseases. . . . Nevertheless, 30 years and billions of dollars of public funds have been invested in this progress against disease, and the public believes it has a right to the benefits of its investment whether such benefits are "half way" or not [pp. 93–94].

Because the issue of technology is so visible at present and the policies that have been suggested to deal with problems of technology are so varied and in some cases extreme,[2] it is important to differentiate among the kinds of "technology problems" that have been identified. As the previous discussion indicates, inferences about the improper use of technology by the health care system have been drawn from very different kinds of evidence, including the volume of inputs devoted to the production of hospital services and the level of capital expenditures undertaken by hospitals. For the most part, critics have not distinguished among the particular problems that they address. Confusion stems partially from the broad scope of hardware and software activities that are often thought of as technology. According to the definition offered by the U.S. Congressional Office of Technology Assessment (OTA), medical technologies include techniques, drugs, procedures, or systems combining these elements, used in the practice of medical care (U.S. Congress, OTA, 1976a). The very comprehensiveness of this definition blurs some of the critical policy problems currently under consideration. More important, however, is a general failure to

---

[2]See, for example, Bogue and Wolfe (1976), calling for the establishment of a moratorium on the purchase of CAT scanners.

distinguish between problems associated with the improper use of existing technologies and the process by which new technologies are developed, introduced, and diffused into the medical care system. Often, the two problems are lumped together, as in a recent article by Banta and McNeil (1977), focusing on problems associated with new and existing diagnostic technologies. Policy recommendations often involve combined strategies to control both the use of existing capabilities and the introduction of new technology. As a result, exactly which problems specific policies address and how these policies will affect different aspects of the "technology problem" are often unclear.

For the purpose of this chapter, the technology problem can be divided into two subproblems, each with its own policy implications. The first is the problem of the way in which the health care system allocates resources to and uses existing technologies. The second is the problem of technical change involving the introduction of new equipment, systems, or procedures into the health care system. Each of these problems must be defined separately, although it is obvious that the way in which existing technologies are used has immense impact on the direction and speed of technical change in the health care system.

Problems Involving Existing Technology

If we accept the OTA definition of medical technology, the problem of existing technology becomes synonymous with the more general problems of resource allocation and use of health care services. And if, as Perrow has claimed (1965), the hospital itself is the technological instrument of the medical profession, then all problems of utilization of hospital services and allocation of resources to hospitals are inherently problems of the inappropriate use of existing technologies. Most frequently, critics of "existing technology" focus on particular elements of hospital behavior or resources that are "technological" by nature, such as equipment (U.S. Congress, OTA, 1976b), capital-intensive facilities (Russell and Burke, 1975), diagnostic tests (Rushmer, 1976; and Banta and McNeil, 1977), or surgical procedures (Orloff, 1976). These particular elements are identified as sources of abuse of existing technology because they represent the "sophisticated" element of medical care. The tendency of the health care system to bias the allocation and use of resources toward these more sophisticated elements is often referred to as the "technological imperative" (Rushmer, 1976). To the extent that the tendency to overinvest in and overuse sophisticated services is just part of a larger tendency to overuse health services or to invest too many labor or nonlabor resources in the production of hospital services, the problem is not related to technology itself and should not be singled out as one of technology. The impact of present reimbursement and regulatory policies on hospital resource allocation, particularly on decisions to overinvest in capital assets and overuse services, should be viewed as a problem of cost control and not of technology per se.

However, insofar as decisions to invest in or use certain equipment, procedures, or drugs are made on the basis of their level of technical sophistication, the existence of the "technological imperative" must be accepted. A number of arguments have been put forth to justify the view that technology is a problem in its own right. Changes in medical education have purportedly placed increasing emphasis on objective tests and precise measurement when less technologically advanced methods might still be adequate for diagnosis and treatment (Gellman, 1971). Medical students and residents, trained in the most sophisticated institutions, expect and depend upon the availability of diagnostic and therapeutic assists in the form of instrumentation and facilities. Thus, clinical decision makers may be functionaries of the technological imperative.

Several economists have theorized that patient demand for medical care is, among other things, a function of the perceived quality of care (Feldstein, 1976). Others postulate that the objective of the hospital is to maximize a weighted function of the quality and quantity of the services it produces (Newhouse, 1970). How quality is perceived by patients and hospital decision makers thus has a major influence on the behavior of the health care system with respect to technologically sophisticated procedures and services. Feldstein (1976) hypothesizes that hospital decision makers' perceptions of quality depend on the amount of labor and nonlabor inputs devoted to the production of medical care. However, perceived quality may be correlated as much with the level of sophistication of those inputs as with their absolute amounts.[3] If, too, patients perceive quality in terms of high levels of sophistication in the delivery of services, including the application of many and frequent diagnostic tests, performance of equipment-bound procedures (such as respiratory therapy), and increases in the number and training level of health care personnel, then physicians and hospitals will respond by emphasizing those inputs. Similarly, if an important element of the patient's perception of hospital quality were the efficiency of its billing procedures, then the hospital would invest capital and labor resources to improve these. Thus, to the extent that it does exist, the source of the technological imperative rests largely on the value that patients and hospital decision makers place on technological sophistication for its own sake.

Newhouse (1970) has posited that under a predominantly charge- or cost-based system of third-party payment, the hospital decision maker could conceivably push both quality and quantity to the point where the additional utility to the hospital is zero. If quality is equated with the availability and use of sophisticated services, then this hypothesis implies a level of sophistication much beyond that which would result were marginal utility equated with the marginal cost of these services.

The problem of existing technology can thus be related to three factors: structural changes in the nature of medical education, which stresses dependence on scientific instrumentation; patient demands for technological sophistication as a surrogate for high "quality" care; and the failure of the cost-reimbursement system to constrain hospitals from increasing their investment in expensive and sophisticated technological capabilities. On balance, these factors create powerful incentives for the hospital to invest in the showpieces of technological sophistication, including clinical instrumentation, special care units, specialized facilities for complex procedures (for example, cardiac catheterization and cardiac surgery), and automated clinical laboratory systems.

[3] See for example, Grimes and Moseley (1976), relating hospital characteristics with indices of their performance.

The implications for public policy to deal with these sources of abuse of the existing armamentarium of equipment and procedures available to hospitals and physicians are fairly clear. First, the present reimbursement system as it is currently structured needs a major overhaul. Either detailed regulation of the investment decisions of hospitals and health care facilities must be undertaken, or reimbursement systems must be so structured as to provide different incentives to hospitals and health care facilities. Certificate-of-need programs represent one regulatory approach, but these laws generally fail to require the approval of capital purchases under some threshold level or to apply to all health care settings. Furthermore, the separation of the responsibility for regulation of health care expenditures from the responsibility for paying for the services produced creates an institutional weakness in the certificate-of-need arrangements.

Rate setting on a prospective basis is also a potential solution for the bias toward the use of sophisticated technology, but as Bauer's paper in this book points out, rate setting may not lead to the cost control results that many expect of it. Rate setting does not apply to decisions to use sophisticated services. These decisions remain for the most part the exclusive domain of physicians. Thus, rate setting may keep unit costs low, but it cannot be expected to control the utilization of services effectively. Also, hospital rate setting would not alter the internal bias within the hospital decision-making structure toward technologically advanced services. Because the hospital administrator views quality as related to sophistication, the tendency to invest in these services will still remain.

Ellwood (1975) has suggested that a system of competing prepaid group practices would provide the incentives to health care providers to make resource allocation decisions in the light of the relative cost effectiveness of each decision. With appropriate information on measures of performance of such prepaid plans, patients could trade off quality against cost in a fashion that would approach a more conventional market decision.

A second policy implication arising from the tendency to equate technological sophistication with quality of care is the need for a reexamination of the efficacy of medical practices, particularly those involving the use of expensive equipment, facilities, or personnel. Furthermore, the results of this reexamination must be transmitted or communicated to physicians and patients so that a more informed set of demands can be made for quality. Indeed, the results could also be used to control utilization of sophisticated services.

The organization of such deliberate and ongoing research into efficacy requires the delegation of a new set of responsibilities to some federal agency or the establishment of an agency to perform this role. At present, no federal health agency has the specific charge of evaluating the efficacy of existing medical practices.

The third policy implication argues for changes in methods of medical education, including incorporation into the educational process the information on efficacy produced through research efforts. Some critics of the medical education system have noted that medical schools do not provide any training in statistical decision theory to enable medical students to evaluate the relative information content of diagnostic tests (Schwartz, 1976). Of course, if the reimbursement system were altered so that hospitals and physicians had to choose among alternative uses of limited economic resources and if appropriate information on efficacy were produced by a research organization, medical education would be likely to reflect the new incentives and knowledge.

The Problem of Technical Change

Technical change refers to the complex and not well understood process by which new capability is developed and brought into use. New technical capability in health care refers to the ability to produce new products or services that did not previously exist or to produce existing products or services in a new way, with greater reliability or less cost. Because the nature of the hospital product is so poorly defined, these two kinds of capability are often difficult to distinguish from one another. For example, was gastric freezing a new service, or was it a "better" way to perform an old service—the treatment of ulcers? The most important distinction for policy purposes is between changes that at least theoretically enhance the quality of care and changes that lower the cost of providing care. Gastric freezing was clearly intended to fall into the former category.

Technical change implies that the new capability has resulted from scientific progress, not from changes in the hospital's economic environment. For example, if the hospital reorganizes previously scattered services into a separate respiratory therapy unit for economic reasons, it has not introduced a new technology, as some would claim (see, for example, Russell, 1976), but has merely adjusted methods of providing services. However, the introduction of intermittent positive pressure breathing (IPPB) as a new service clearly represents the adoption of a new technical capability, as would the replacement of existing laboratory methods with new automated laboratory equipment.

Technical change is a dynamic process that involves several identifiable but somewhat overlapping phases. The process has been classified in a number of ways (U.S. Congress, OTA, 1976a), but it can be summarized in terms of four major phases: (1) generation of clinically useful knowledge; (2) prototype development; (3) testing; and (4) diffusion. The first phase can be equated with scientific and biomedical research, or in some cases with technological development outside of health care. The development phase may occur as part of the first or may involve a significant time lap (President's Biomedical Research Panel, 1976a). Testing in the clinical environment is likely to be concurrent with development activities to some extent. Diffusion represents the final phase in which a technology is adopted for nonexperimental use by individual or organizational decision makers.

The dependence of diffusion of new technology on the outcome of scientific and biomedical research has complicated the policy problems associated with the process. Two major strains of criticism appear to be in direct conflict with each other. The first is that the process of technological change has raised health care costs too high; the second is that the pitfalls in each step of the process of technical change render it extremely delicate and in need of assists at critical points, particularly in the research and development phase. The first criticism implies that too much technology is emerging from the process; the second that too little results.

The result of this schism is a spate of policy recommendations that on their face appear contradictory. Those whose focus and experience lie in the early phases of the process are extremely sensitive to the obstacles that must be overcome to reach the testing and diffusion phases and the high mortality rate of ideas and inventions along the way (see, for example, Anderson, 1976). Among the obstacles cited are biomedical research funding policies that bias the kinds of clinically useful knowledge that develop (RAND Corp., 1976); property rights policies that provide inadequate incentives to developers of new technologies (U.S. Federal Council for Science and Technology, 1975); the small size and disaggregated nature of the potential markets (National Research Council, 1976); inadequate networks for communicating the results of clinically useful research to the health care community (U.S. DHEW, 1977) and the host of regulatory processes required before new technologies can reach their markets (Noll, 1975).

Those whose primary concern is the cost of new technologies cite the failure of those who test new technologies to consider the important concepts of efficacy and effectiveness in a complete or consistent fashion (Hiatt, 1975); the willingness of hospital decision makers to serve as an easy market since they bear no risk if the technology proves to be inadequate or quickly outmoded (Brown, 1972); the apparent bias in the system toward the development of hospital technologies instead of ambulatory or home setting (Hiatt, 1975); and the lack of any responsibility for early assessment of the impact of new technologies on costs or effectiveness (Arnstein, 1976).

The first set of arguments would call for public policy to facilitate the development and diffusion of new technologies and the elimination of bureaucratic and regulatory barriers. The second set would imply the intensification of public efforts to shape and control the process through research funding and regulatory avenues. The recent passage of the medical device amendments, which will require significantly new devices to obtain clearance prior to entry in the market is an interesting example of the conflict. Critics cite the impact that new drug regulation has had on both the rate of introduction of these new technologies and the structure of the drug industry (U.S. Congress, 1973). Supporters point to the need for intervention in a field that poses ever increasing safety and efficacy questions, and to the savings that have resulted from the inability of unsafe or ineffective new drugs to reach the market.

The source of the conflict expressed in this context arises from the paucity of information now available about several critical aspects of the process of technical change. First, the empirical evidence on the impact that new technology has had on medical and social costs and effectiveness is fragmentary and inconclusive. We need to know the extent to which the process has worked inefficiently and whether new technologies have indeed raised costs as so many claim. Some recent research efforts have been devoted to this question. The results of that research are summarized in a subsequent section of this paper.

Second, we know very little about the way in which new medical technologies are developed. We do not even have a clear picture of who the developers are and what environments produce what kinds of technologies. The impact of government funding of biomedical research on the development of different kinds of technology is also unclear. The settings for development of different kinds of technology unquestionably vary. Considering the many different procedures, techniques, equipment, and systems that have come into being in the past ten years, it is reasonable to assume that the patterns of development among these will be highly varied. Research and development can occur in universities, hospitals, medical schools, large or small research and development laboratories, manufacturing firms, and even in physicians' offices; frequently, the process involves a combination of these settings. Although it is easy to theorize about the motivations of various kinds of participants in the development process, there is very little evidence to support a model to explain the determinants of technology development. The background studies commissioned by the President's Biomedical Research Panel (1976b) made a start in this direction, but they did not focus on the different kinds of developers and the differences among them. A frequently described model is the "advocacy" theory (Anderson, 1976). The individual scientist, engineer, or clinician has a strong personal faith in the value of his idea and mothers it through the paths of development. The success of a technology at least to the prototype state is said to be a function of the degree of advocacy it engenders as well as its usefulness. But we know so little about who actually does research and development and how they interact, that it is virtually impossible to diagnose failures in the development process.

Third, the evidence on how hospital decision makers adopt new medical technologies is scattered among several research disciplines with different approaches; consequently, the results are somewhat equivocal. It is important to identify not only the early adopters of new technologies and the time and spatial patterns of diffusion, but also how these factors differ among different classes of medical technologies. Unfortunately, the research has not looked directly at these questions; rather, individual studies have focused on a single technology or a specific type of hospital behavior, such as capital equipment purchases. Nevertheless, some tentative conclusions can be drawn from this literature. Indeed, there appears to be more systematic analysis of the process of medical technology diffusion than of any other important policy-related question in the area. The major findings of the literature on this question are summarized in a subsequent section.

The Economic Costs of New Technology

A number of studies have attempted to estimate the economic impacts of new technology. These studies measure different concepts of cost, including hospital costs, total costs of medical care, and net social costs. They also vary in the operational definition of technological change. These variations render objective comparison difficult; nevertheless, the results do provide some insight into the relation between technology and health care costs.

In a study of the impact of new technology on the cost of hospital care, Davis (1974) used data from approximately 200 non-profit hospitals for the period 1962 to 1968. Using time as a proxy for technological change, Davis found that when demand and supply variables had been taken into account, hospital expenses per admission rise about 2 percent annually. The time trend variable is an imperfect proxy since it also includes effects due to gradual changes that influence demand, including changing attitudes about hospital care, improved methods of ambulatory care, or other changes in behavior over time that are not accounted for by explicit variables in her model. Davis suggests that the time estimate provides an upper limit for an estimate of the effect of technological change on hospital costs, but the other influences represented by the time variable could have had a negative effect, leading to an understatement of technology's effect on hospital costs.

Several researchers have studied the impact of technical change on total medical care costs. Mushkin et al. (1976) analyzed the total impact of biomedical research on health expenditures from 1930 to 1975. Using a time residual as a proxy for biomedical advances, they found that this factor was responsible for an annual reduction in total health expenditures of 0.5 percent. This result compared favorably with a twenty-year study by Fuchs (1972), which found that technology and biomedical change had a positive residual effect on total health care expenditures in the amount of 0.6 percent annually. The difference in these studies may be attributable to differences in the study periods (Fuchs' study compared the years 1947 to 1967) and to other effects included in the studies. These longitudinal studies include the effects on medical care costs of the significant advances in the treatment of communicable diseases during the period under study. They also include the net effect of shifting disease patterns of the population. Thus, the relatively favorable outcome with respect to the role of technology and biomedical research over the entire study period obscures some of the changes in the health of Americans. The pattern of cost changes in the recent past may not be consistent with long-run trends.

Scitovsky and McCall (1975) have analyzed the changes in cost of medical care associated with selected illnesses. Between 1964 and 1971, the net increase in the average cost of treatment of an episode of illness was calculated for eight conditions: otitis media; forearm fractures; appendicitis; maternity care; cancer of the breast; pneumonia; duodenal ulcer; and myocardial infarction. In almost every instance, there were cost-raising and cost-saving changes in treatment. However, Scitovsky and McCall noted that "the costs of treatment of conditions requiring hospitalization rose at a considerably faster rate than those of conditions treated on an ambulatory basis" (p. 15). Cost-raising sources were found to include shifts to more expensive drugs, an increase in the number of laboratory tests per case, and an increase in the number of miscellaneous inpatient and outpatient services. However, the most dramatic cost increases occurred in the treatment of myocardial infarction; these changes were traced principally to the increasing use of intensive care units. Thus, we see that sources of medical cost increases reflect an epidemiological shift from diseases requiring outpatient to those requiring inpatient care, and a shift of setting of care within the hospital from less specialized services to more specialized units. Unfortunately, the analysis does not permit any comparison of cost-increasing conditions with cost-decreasing conditions because of the selected nature of the conditions considered. Combined with Mushkin's results, these findings show that the ultimate impact of technological change on medical care costs is not clearly cost-increasing. A more selective approach to analysis is required. Cooper (1976) has observed that the important policy issues lie not in the total impact of technological change across all diagnoses and settings of care but in the misallocation of resources in whatever settings they occur. However, if the overall effect of the introduction of technology does not clearly lead to inordinate increases in the cost of medical care, then the impact of an elaborate system to control the introduction of new technologies may not be worth the administrative costs involved.

Although the application of benefit-cost analysis to health programs has a long history (see Klarman, 1974), only one study has attempted to measure the "social" costs of a broad class of technological developments. This study, by Orloff (1976), estimated the net contribution to medical and nonmedical social costs of research in surgery over the study period. Using the life-cycle earnings approach to valuation of changes in morbidity and mortality, this study found that the most significant research contributions had resulted in a net saving of $2.8 billion for the year 1970. The study suffers from the bias of dealing only with selected surgical advances, but there was some attempt to consider the leading advances in the period under study as identified by a panel of surgeons. It is possible that the surgical advances not considered would have shown systematic increases in hospitalization and total social costs.

Although the studies described here represent significant advances in the economics of technological change in medical care, they fall short of providing policy guidance. New technologies appear to be raising hospital costs, but it is not altogether clear that these increases are not offset by savings in other sectors of the health care delivery system or by nonmedical benefits to society.

A major problem with these analyses is the lack of a normative base for comparison. The real question is not how much total health care costs increased or decreased, but how far that change differed from what would be possible under an ideal system of technical change, that is, a system in which development and adoption decisions were made with full information and with the maximization of social benefits as the objective.

The Diffusion of New Hospital Technologies

In order to devise good policies to control the introduction of new technologies, it is necessary to know a great deal about how they find their way into hospitals and into the practice of medicine. What factors determine whether and when a hospital adopts a new technology? How do these factors differ among classes of hospital technologies? What are the characteristics of early adopters and of late adopters? How do they differ? What determines the speed with which new technologies are introduced? And, most important, how does the process diverge from patterns of diffusion that would occur in an ideal situation?

The literature offers answers to some of these questions but leaves the central question of the ultimate effectiveness of the diffusion process unanswered. What we do know must be synthesized from several independent bodies of research, representing different disciplines. Economists have studied the economic characteristics of the adopting unit and the new technology; sociologists have studied the attributes of organizations and individuals determining their propensity to adopt new technologies; political scientists have considered the political environment in which change takes place.

Definitional problems pose significant barriers to comparison of research studies. Not only do operational definitions vary because of constraints on data available to various researchers, but there are also basic conceptual differences in various approaches. In order to avoid confusion, we must define some terms commonly used in this literature. First, the adoption of a new technology refers to a decision by an adopting unit (defined as an individual or organization) to make use of the technology's capability. Adoption is often confused with utilization of a new technology. For many hospital technologies, adoption is synonymous with the purchase or lease of equipment, construction of a facility, or decision to offer a new service. When, however, the adopting unit is likely to be the physician (as is the case with new drugs or surgical procedures not requiring extraordinary equipment), then adoption cannot be easily distinguished from the first use of the technology. Because so many hospital technologies require a decision to make capital expenditures, the determination of whether and when a hospital has adopted a new technology is often based on the time of the commitment of capital resources.

Diffusion refers to the pattern of adoption decisions over time and sometimes space. The diffusion process is often expressed as the number of units adopting a new technology as a function of the time or distance from its first availability on the market. Diffusion studies often differentiate early adopters from late adopters and attempt to characterize them. The time path of adoption of new medical technologies may be either too fast or too slow depending on the real social value of the change.

Many studies focus on the determinants of "innovation" by individuals or organizations. Innovation is defined as the first use of a product or program by a given adoption unit.[4] The adoption of a new technology is, then, one kind of innovation possible within the hospital. Innovations can include program or organizational changes

[4]See Mohr (1969) for a discussion of alternative definitions of innovation.

as well. Much of the literature on innovation in health care organizations has involved the study of these nontechnological innovations. Using these studies to make inferences about the determinants of technological innovations may be dangerous, as the external validity of such studies across innovation types has not been demonstrated in the literature.

Economic studies of technological diffusion outside of health care have provided empirical support for the hypothesis that the rate of innovation is a function of the profitability of the innovation and the resources required for adoption relative to the size of the firms in the industry (see Mansfield, 1961, 1968). To apply these findings to technological innovation in health care, it would be necessary to redefine "profitability" to be more consistent with the objectives of hospitals. In fact, it is the generalization of this concept that most studies of the diffusion of medical technologies address. Substitutes for profitability must be found to explain differences in the way that particular technologies are adopted by hospitals. As discussed above, these substitutes are most often postulated to be some combination of quantity and quality of services provided by the hospital, where quality may be perceived in different ways by hospital decision makers. Economic studies of diffusion of hospital technologies relate adoption of specific technologies to variables believed to be related to these objectives and to the resources available to the hospital.

In a recent study of nuclear medicine facilities, Rapoport (1976) used statewide data to regress the speed of diffusion over different time periods against a number of factors, including the ratio of the state's population in urban centers, state income, availability of physicians, hospital size, percent of hospitals affiliated with medical schools, and the variation in size among hospitals. Depending on the time period under study, these variables explained between 50 and 75 percent of the total variation in diffusion rates across states. The most interesting result was the strong negative relationship between the medical school affiliation variable and the diffusion rate in all time periods. Rapoport offers the explanation that in areas with many affiliated hospitals, which acquired nuclear medicine early, the nonaffiliated groups may not have considered themselves capable of competing in this arena and thus did not adopt this new technology as rapidly as hospitals in states with few such medical school affiliations. Thus, regionalization of this service may have occurred by default.

Cromwell et al. (1975) have studied the relationship between the existence of particular high technology facilities in a state and a number of explanatory variables. Their results show that the diffusion of equipment-intensive hospital services such as intensive care units, open heart surgery, x-ray therapy, cobalt therapy, radium therapy, diagnostic radioisotope, and therapeutic radioisotope services is significantly and positively related to per capita income, age, total per capita number of physicians in the state, the ratio of specialists to total physicians, and for certain facilities, the existence of a certificate-of-need law.

Studies of innovation in health care organizations have related adoption of innovations to factors such as organizational size, wealth, or access to resources; organizational structure; the nature of the environment facing the organization; and attributes or attitudes of individual decision makers within the organization. In a study of respiratory therapy technologies, Gordon et al. (1974) showed that innovation in hospitals is a function of several structural characteristics of the organization, including the degree of decentralization of decision making, the visibility of consequences of medical care within the organization, and the complexity of the medical staff resources of the hospital. This study looked only at respiratory therapy services which were judged by an expert panel to be elements of "good" medical care. Whether these factors would remain important as determinants of adoption of technologies of questionable efficacy is uncertain; the study also failed to include any technologies requiring substantial capital resources.

Resource availability has surfaced as the leading determinant of innovation in health departments and other public health agencies (see Gordon and Fisher, 1975). Studies of innovations in these agencies have concentrated on program changes rather than on the adoption of new medical technologies; therefore, their external validity for the adoption of medical technology in hospitals is suspect. However, evidence from the economics literature tends to support this finding. In a study of capital expenditure decisions by hospitals, Ginsburg (1972) showed that the availability of capital funds and hospital size were important determinants of the overall level of capital investment, whereas composition of investment depended on demand factors. In a more recent study of capital equipment expenditure decisions by fifteen hospitals, in the greater Boston area, Cromwell et al. (1975) found that larger hospitals spend proportionately more on capital equipment than smaller hospitals, but the relationship between capital expenditures and the availability of financial resources was found to be insignificant.

Taken together, these studies show that hospitals are likely to adopt new technologies when they are large, complex, and wealthy institutions. Medical centers and teaching hospitals can be expected to be the early adopters of new technologies, although there is no information on how well these early adopters differentiate between "good" and "bad" technologies.

The diffusion literature has provided virtually no information on the channels of communication responsible for the dissemination of information on new technologies. What role early adopters such as medical schools play compared with suppliers in communicating information on new technologies has not been studied. Nor have researchers studied at what stage in the process of diffusion new technologies become standards of medical practice, virtually guaranteeing their ultimate penetration of the health care system. The impact of the emergence of health planning and concepts of regionalization on different patterns has also not been assessed.

If, as one might expect, medical centers offering a full array of services and training are the early adopters of new medical technologies, followed by the rest of the hospitals, then it would be useful to focus policy development on these units. The impact of recent experimental reimbursement policies on adoption decisions may be perverse. Many hospital prospective reimbursement systems group hospitals according to certain characteristics for the purposes of rate setting. Often these include teaching status, bed size, case mix, or "service intensity." By so doing, these formulas are likely to compare the costs of early adopters with one another and thus ensure the continued resource availability to future adoption of new technologies by these hospitals. As other groups of hospitals respond to the new standards of medical practice developed in these centers, their costs get pulled upward as well.

Conclusion

The one clear implication of this discussion is that there are major gaps in what we know about the real impact of hospital technologies, new or existing, on social costs and benefits. We do not fully understand the nature of the development process, nor do we know how sensitive that process is to changes in the health care delivery or financing system.

This lack of knowledge does reveal that there needs to be increasing federal attention paid to the generation of valid information on the efficacy of medical procedures, particularly those involving the use of new and existing "sophisticated" services (that is, capital-intensive, equipment-oriented, requiring a high level of staff capabilities). That such information is not currently generated is reflected in our inability to determine the extent to which the hospital industry makes appropriate adoption decisions. We do not even know to what extent we are wasting our health care dollars on relatively ineffective but technically sophisticated services.

In the long run, the problem facing policy makers will be where on the trade-off curve between health care costs and benefits we should be and how to ration the availability of expensive technologies whose benefits are clear. To date, we have shown that the health care system as it works today cannot ration such technologies effectively (witness the renal dialysis program). Up to now we may have wasted resources, but we have been able to offer the benefits of new technologies to an ever wider class of beneficiaries. In the future, we may not be able to do so.

Refernces

Anderson, N.
  1976 "Critical steps in the development of new health technology."
         Paper prepared for the Conference on Health Care Technology

and Quality of Care, Boston University, November 19-20, 1976. Boston: Boston University, Program on Public Policy for Quality Health Care.

Arnstein, S.
1976   Statement by Sherry Arnstein, Senior Fellow, Intramural Research Section, National Center for Health Services Research, U.S. DHEW, at the Conference on Health Care Technology and Quality of Care, Boston University, November 19-20, 1976. Boston: Boston University Program on Public Policy for Quality Health Care.

Banta, H.D., and B.J. McNeil
1977   "The costs of medical diagnosis: The case of the CT scanner." Photocopy. Washington, D.C., Office of Technology Assessment.

Bogue, T., and S.M. Wolfe
1976   "CAT scanners: Is fancier technology worth a billion dollars of health consumers' money?" Washington, D.C.: Health Research Group.

Brown, R.E.
1972   "Managing the mushrooming growth of America's hospital system." In Regulating the Hospital, a report of the 1972 National Forum on Hospital and Health Affairs. Durham, N.C.: Department of Health Administration of Duke University.

Cochrane, A.L.
1972   Effectiveness and Efficiency: Random Reflections on Health Services. London: The Nuffield Provincial Hospitals Trust.

Cooper, B.
1976   Statement by Barbara Cooper, Office of Research and Statistics, Social Security Administration, at the Conference on Health Care Technology and Quality of Care, Boston University, November 19-20, 1976. Boston: Boston University Program on Public Policy for Quality Health Care.

Cromwell, J., et al.
1975   Incentives and Decisions Underlying Hospitals; Adoption and Utilization of Major Capital Equipment. Cambridge, Mass.: Abt Associates.

Davis, K.
1974   "The role of technology, demand and labor markets in the determination of hospital costs." In Mark Perlman, ed., The Economics of Health and Medical Care. New York: John Wiley & Sons.

DeBakey, M.E., and H.W. Hiatt
1976   "Medical technology: How much is enough?" In Proceedings of the National Leadership Conference on America's Health Policy. Washington, D.C.: National Journal.

Ellwood, P.M., Jr.
1975   "Alternatives to regulation: Improving the market." In Institute of Medicine, Controls on Health Care. Washington, D.C.: National Academy of Sciences.

Feldstein, M.S.
1976   Quality Change and the Demand for Hospital Care. Discussion Paper No. 475, Harvard Institute of Economic Research, Cambridge, Mass.

Feldstein, M.S., and A. Taylor
1977   "The rapid rise of hospital costs." Discussion Paper No. 531, Harvard Institute of Economic Research, Cambridge, Mass.

Fuchs, V.
1972   Essays on the Economics of Health and Medical Care. New York: Columbia University Press.

Gaus, C.R.
1975   "What goes into technology must come out in costs." Excerpt from testimony of the Social Security Administration before the President's Biomedical Research Panel, September 29, 1975, in The National Leadership Conference on America's Health Policy. Washington, D.C.: National Journal.

Gaus, C.R., and B.S. Cooper
1976   "Technology and Medicare: Alternatives for change." Paper prepared for the Conference on Health Care Technology and Quality of Care, Boston University, November 19-20, 1976. Boston: Boston University, Program on Public Policy for Quality Health Care.

Gellman, D.D.
1971   "The price of progress: Technology and the cost of medical care." Canadian Medical Association Journal 104 (March 6): 401-406.

Ginsburg, P.B.
1972   "Resource allocation in the hospital industry: The role of capital financing." Social Security Bulletin 35 (August): 20-30.

Gordon, G., and G.L. Fisher, eds.
1975   The Diffusion of Medical Technology. Cambridge, Mass.: Ballinger Publishing Co.

Gordon, G., et al.
1974   "Organizational structure, environmental diversity and hospital adoption of medical innovations." In A.D. Kaluzny, J.T. Gentry, and J.E. Veney, eds., Innovations in Health Care Organizations: An Issue in Organizational Change. Chapel Hill, N.C.: School of Public Health, University of North Carolina.

Grimes, R.M., and S.K. Moseley
1976   "An approach to an index of hospital performance." Health Services Research 11 (Fall): 294.

Hiatt, H.H.
1975   "Protecting the medical 'commons'—who has the responsibility?" The New England Journal of Medicine 293 (July): 235–241.

Klarman, H.E.
1974   "Application of cost-benefit analysis to health systems technology." In Morris F. Collen, ed., Technology and Health Care Systems in the 1980's. DHEW Publication No. HRA-74-3016. Rockville, Md.: National Center for Health Services Research and Development.

Lalonde, M.
1972   A New Perspective on the Health of Canadians: A Working Document. Ottawa: Government of Canada.

McKeown, T.
1976   The Role of Medicine. London: The Nuffield Provincial Hospitals Trust.

Mansfield, E.
1961   "Technical change and the rate of imitation." Econometrica 29 (October): 741–766.

1968   Industrial Research and Technological Innovation: An Econometric Analysis. New York: W.W. Norton & Co., Inc.

Mohr, L.B.
1969   "Determinants of innovation in organizations." American Political Science Review 63 (March): 111–126.

Mushkin, S.J., L.C. Paringer, and M.M. Chen
1976   "Returns to biomedical research 1900–1975: An initial assessment of impacts on health expenditures." Photocopy. Washington, D.C.: Georgetown University, Public Services Laboratory.

National Research Council
1976   Science and Technology in the Service of the Physically Handicapped. National Research Council, Assembly of Life Sciences, Division of Medical Sciences, Committee on National Needs for

the Rehabilitation of the Physically Handicapped. Washington, D.C.: National Academy of Sciences.

Newhouse, J.P.
1970   "Toward a theory of nonprofit institutions: An Economic Model of a hospital." American Economic Review 60 (March): 64–74.

Noll, R.G.
1975   "The consequences of public utility regulation of hospitals." In Institute of Medicine, Controls on Health Care. Washington, D.C.: National Academy of Sciences.

Orloff, M.J.
1976   "Contributions of research in surgical technology to health care." Paper prepared for the Conference on Health Care Technology and Quality of Care, Boston University, November 19–20, 1976. Boston: Boston University, Program on Public Policy for Quality Health Care.

Perrow, C.
1965   "Hospitals: Technology, structure, and goals." In J.G. March, ed., Handbook of Organizations. Chicago: Rand McNally.

President's Biomedical Research Panel
1976a   Report of the President's Biomedical Research Panel, Appendix B: Approaches to Policy Development for Biomedical Research: Strategy for Budgeting and Movement from Invention to Clinical Application. DHEW Publication No. (OS) 76-502. Washington, D.C.: Government Printing Office.
1976b   Report of the President's Biomedical Research Panel, Supplement 1: Analysis of Selected Biomedical Research Programs: Case Histories. DHEW Publication No. (OS) 76-506. Washington, D.C.: Government Printing Office.

Rabkin, M.T., and C.N. Melin
1976   "The impact of technology upon the cost and quality of hospital care, and a proposal for control of new and expensive technology." Background paper prepared for the Conference on Health Care Technology and Quality of Care, Boston University, November 19–20, 1976. Boston: Boston University, Program on Public Policy for Quality Health Care.

RAND Corporation
1976   "Policy Analysis for Federal biomedical research." In President's Biomedical Research Panel, Appendix B: Approaches to Policy Development for Biomedical Research: Strategy for Budgeting and Movement from Invention to Clinical Application. Washington, D.C.: Government Printing Office.

Rapoport, J.
1976   "Diffusion of technological innovation in hospitals: A case study
        of nuclear medicine." Photocopy. South Hadley, Mass.: Mount
        Holyoke College.
Rushmer, R.F.
1976   "The technological imperative." Editorial, American Journal of
        Roentgenology 127 (August): 356–357.
Russell, L.B.
1976   "Making rational decisions about medical technology." Paper
        presented at the National Commission on the Cost of Medical
        Care, November 23, 1976, Chicago, Ill. Photocopy. Washington,
        D.C.: L.B. Russell.
Russell, L.B., and C.S. Burke
1975   Technological Diffusion in the Hospital Sector. Washington,
        D.C.: National Planning Association.
Salkever, D.S., and T.W. Bice
1976   "The impact of certificate-of-need controls on hospital invest-
        ment." Milbank Memorial Fund Quarterly/Health and Society
        54 (Spring): 185–214.
Schwartz, William
1976   Statement by William Schwartz, Vannevar Bush University
        Professor, Tufts University School of Medicine, at the Confer-
        ence on Health Care Technology and Quality of Care, Boston
        University, November 19–20, 1976. Boston: Boston University,
        Program on Public Policy for Quality Health Care.
Scitovsky, A.A., and N. McCall
1975   Changes in the Costs of Treatment of Selected Illnesses
        1951–1964–1971. San Francisco: Health Policy Program, Univer-
        sity of California School of Medicine.
U.S. Congress
1973   Senate, Select Committee on Small Business, Subcommittee on
        Monopoly, Present Status of Competition in the Pharmaceutical
        Industry: Hearings. 93d Congress, 1st Session, February 5–8 and
        March 14, 1972. Washington, D.C.: Government Printing Office.
U.S. Congress, Office of Technology Assessment
1976a   Development of Medical Technology: Opportunities for Assess-
        ment. Washington, D.C.: Government Printing Office.
1976b   The Computerized Tomography (CT or CAT) Scanner and Its
        Implications for Health Policy. Draft. Washington, D.C.

U.S. Department of Health, Education, and Welfare
  1976   Public Health Service, Forward Plan for Health: FT 1978-82.
          DHEW Publication No. (OS) 76-50046. Washington, D.C.:
          Government Printing Office.
  1977   National Institute of Health, "The responsibilities of NIH at the
          Health Research/Health Care interface." Draft. Bethesda, Md.:
          National Institute of Health.
U.S. Federal Council for Science and Technology
  1975   Executive Subcommittee of the Committee on Government
          Patent Policy, University Patent Policy Ad Hoc Subcommittee,
          Report. Photocopy.
Waldman, S.
  1972   The Effect of Changing Technology on Hospital Costs. Research
          and Statistics Note No. 4, DHEW Publication No. (SSA) 72-
          11701 (February 28).
Weiner, S.M.
  1976   "State regulation and health technology." Paper prepared for the
          Conference on Health Care Technology and Quality of Care,
          Boston University, November 19-20, 1976. Boston: Boston Uni-
          versity, Program on Public Policy for Quality Health Care.
White, K.L., J.H. Murnaghan, and C.R. Gaus
  1972   "Technology and health care." The New England Journal of
          Medicine 287 (December): 1223-1227.
Worthington, N.L.
  1975   "Expenditures for hospital care and physicians' services: Factors
          affecting annual changes." Social Security Bulletin 38 (Novem-
          ber): 3-15.

Federal, State,
and Local Experiences

Impact of the Economic Stabilization Program on Hospitals: An Analysis with Aggregate Data

PAUL B. GINSBURG

Introduction

In August 1971 the federal government froze all wages and prices for a period of three months and then controlled increases in them with varying degrees of earnestness through April 1974. Special regulations were developed for health care providers because of unique characteristics of that industry. These special regulations allowed the controls program for the health industry to evolve toward one with goals different from those of the rest of the controls program.

At the time the initial controls on the health industry were drawn up, rate regulation was a radical departure from federal thinking on policies to deal with health care cost inflation. Measures such as utilization review and planning were more frequently mentioned than controls, particularly so considering the prevailing philosophy of the Nixon Administration. Nevertheless, early debates on the design of wage and price controls for health care focused on issues that are still debated today.

In the ensuing years, controls on hospital rates and reimbursement have become more central to policies to reduce inflation in the health care sector. A significant number of states are now involved in rate setting or prospective reimbursement, a particularly varied form of price control applied to hospital reimbursement from third-party payers.[1] Further, many plans for national health insurance propose reimbursing hospitals for services on a prospective rather than on a cost basis.[2] Finally, whenever new wage and price controls are discussed, health care is considered a prime candidate for programs of selective controls.

The purpose of this study is to assess the impact of the Economic Stabilization Program (ESP) on key hospital variables. Hospital costs rather than prices are the major concern. Fat profit margins have never been alleged to be a cause of rising hospital prices by those who have studied hospital inflation (Feldstein, 1971a, 1971b; Salkever, 1972; Davis, 1974; and others). Comparing precontrols profit margins of 2–3 percent of revenues with annual per diem price increases of almost 15 percent rules this out immediately. Thus if controls only reduced price increases without reducing cost increases, their short-run effects would only be transfers from the hospital to patients or their insurers.

Hospital costs depend on factor prices, productivity, and the nature of hospital output. This last factor makes the hospital industry difficult to control and to study. Each year a hospital day or stay involves the use of more inputs and delivery of more services to patients. While some equate this increase in intensity of care with an increase in quality, economists in particular have expressed doubts as to whether all of them are worthy of their price. According to Feldstein (1971a), increases in inputs per day accounted for one-half of recent increases in hospital costs. Thus, intensity is one of the major sources of potential inflation reduction, but even though intensity decreases reflect productivity gains, we lack a consensus as to whether this is a desirable outcome of a controls program.

[1] See Dowling (1974) for a review of the range of types of prospective reimbursement plans and where they are in use.

[2] See Waldman (1974), and American Enterprise Institute (1974) for discussions of current proposals.

ESP Controls and Their Environment[3]

Hospital wage and price controls were initiated at a time when hospital inflation was more rapid than the rate of increase in consumer prices in general, but had already begun to decline from the extreme rates experienced after the initiation of Medicare. Table 1 shows the behavior of a number of time series over the period covered by this study (1963–1973). The period is broken down into a pre-Medicare period (second quarter 1963 to second quarter 1966), a post-Medicare period (to second quarter 1969), a precontrols period (second quarter 1969 to second quarter 1971), and a controls period (to second quarter 1973). The time series examined include revenues and expenditures per unit of output (patient days and admissions for revenues, adjusted patient days, and adjusted admissions for expenditures), input use per unit of output, hospital wage rates, and hospital nonlabor input prices. Both real and nominal values are reported.

The expenditure and revenue series move closely together, although they are sensitive to the unit of output used in the denominator. These series show a sharp rise after Medicare, and then a decline for the 1969–1971 period. For expenditures, there was some further decline during ESP, but the additional decline was quite small, especially in real terms. During 1971–1973, revenues diverged somewhat from expenditures, presumably reflecting ESP pressures. The time series for real expenditures shows clearly that the major retrenchment from Medicare inflation rates occurred *before* the initiation of controls. This adds to the difficulty of assessing the impact of ESP on hospital costs.

The series on input use per unit of output (derivation described below) reflects a pattern similar to expenditures. Rates of change in input use increased during the Medicare period and declined thereafter. However, this decline only shows up in inputs per adjusted admission because of a substantial drop in mean stay. During the controls period, increases in input use *accelerated* to reach rates that were the highest of all of the periods examined.

[3]See Ginsburg (1976) for an extensive description and evaluation of the regulations.

TABLE 1   Annual Rates of Increase,
Selected Hospital Time Series
(percentages)

Series	Period			
	1963 II–1966 II	1966 II–1969 II	1969 II–1971 II	1971 II–1973 II
A. Nominal Terms				
Expenditures per adjusted admission	8.4	16.7	10.0	8.2
Expenditures per adjusted patient day	8.6	14.0	12.2	10.2
Inpatient revenue per admission	8.7	16.7	10.2	7.3
Inpatient revenue per patient day	8.9	14.1	12.6	9.3
Inputs per adjusted admission	3.4	6.8	2.7	9.9
Inputs per adjusted patient day	3.6	4.3	4.9	12.0
Wages	4.9	9.5	7.2	6.6
Nonlabor input prices	1.8	3.7	3.1	5.1
B. Real Terms				
Expenditures per adjusted admission	6.3	12.2	4.6	3.7
Expenditures per adjusted patient day	6.5	9.6	6.6	5.6
Inpatient revenue per admission	6.6	12.2	4.8	2.9
Inpatient revenue per patient day	6.8	9.7	7.0	4.8
Inputs per adjusted admission	3.4	6.8	2.7	9.9
Inputs per adjusted patient day	3.6	4.3	4.9	12.0
Wages	2.9	5.2	1.9	2.2
Nonlabor input prices	-0.1	-0.3	-2.0	0.7

Sources: National Hospital Panel Survey; Altman and Eichenholz (1974; nonlabor input prices).

Wage rates (obtained by dividing payroll expense by full-time equivalent employees) followed the pattern of expenditures. Their rate of increase accelerated during the Medicare period and then declined afterward. There was little difference in wage increases between the ESP period and the two years before. Indeed, there was a slight increase in real wage increases. Finally, the nonlabor input price index (described below) followed a pattern not very different from the Consumer Price Index, as shown by the series in real terms.[4]

In summary, we see that behavior of these key series during the ESP period did not depart radically from the experience of the preceding two years, especially when one focuses on real as opposed to nominal values. This interpretation does not appear to be consistent with some other accounts of hospital behavior during the period (such as the report of the Council on Wage and Price Stability, 1976), which describe dramatic declines in rates of hospital *price* increases during the ESP period.

There are three explanations for this discrepancy. First, the council's analysis is in nominal terms. Since the rate of increase in the Consumer Price Index was lower during the 1971–1973 period than in the 1969–1971 period (4.4 percent as opposed to 5.2 percent per annum), nominal series will overstate any deceleration in rates of increase. This phenomenon is clear from Table 1. Second, the council's analysis focuses on prices, not on costs. There does appear to have been a squeezing of hospital profit margins during the ESP period. However, since nobody has ever pointed to hospital profits as a cause of rapid rates of price inflation in the industry, and the intent of ESP in the hospital industry was to reduce *cost* inflation, use of a price series is misleading.

The most serious problem however, is the use of charge data (from the Consumer Price Index) instead of data on revenue per unit of output. With the extensive use of third-party cost reimbursement, charges are paid only by a minority of patients. Thus a series on charges is an imperfect indicator of revenues. This was the case for the ESP period. From 1971 (second quarter) to 1973 (second quarter), semiprivate room charges increased at an annual rate of 5.8 percent, while inpatient revenues per inpatient day increased at a 9.3 percent annual rate. The fact that hospital charges were much easier to monitor than revenues from reimbursement of costs probably accounts for this large discrepancy.

---

[4]See page 310 for a description of the derivation of the input measure and of the nonlabor input price index.

In regard to the regulations themselves, hospital wages and prices were initially frozen along with those in the rest of the economy. While wages probably did not change during this initial period, it is likely that only posted prices such as the daily service charge were frozen by the price controls. The concept of controlling the price of a day of hospital care had not been addressed by the early regulations, so increases in input or service intensity probably continued during the freeze period.

As a result of DHEW pleas for separate regulations for health providers, the Committee on the Health Services Industry, composed of provider representatives and "consumers," was appointed to advise the Price Commission on regulating health care providers. The committee recommended for institutional providers (hospitals and nursing homes) a series of controls on service charges. The 6 percent limit recommended was obtained by taking one-half of the then current rate of increase in hospital daily service charges. Consistent with the rest of the controls program, all price increases had to be cost justified, and an institution's profit margin could not exceed that from a base period. In addition, there were limitations on cost increases that could be used for justification of price increases. The limitations were 5.5 percent for wages (consistent with the intent though not necessarily the reality of wage controls), 2.5 percent for nonlabor costs (the goal of the general price controls), and a fudge factor (to enable a 6 percent price increase to be justified) of 1.7 percent for new technology. These suggested regulations clearly were not designed to influence service intensity, since the prices of services rather than days were being regulated. They could be characterized as backups for wage controls and controls on profit margins with some incentives for productivity improvements.

While these recommendations were essentially accepted by the Price Commission, a key change altered their concept drastically and left them poorly defined for many months. Noting that hospital revenue would not be controlled under these recommendations because most patients were financed by third-party payers that reimbursed the hospital for its costs, the Price Commission, in a preamble to its regulations, defined payments from reimbursers to be prices. Limitations were applied to *revenue increases due to price* instead of to increases in charges. As a result, a method to separate revenue changes corresponding with changes in volume from those due to price increases was needed. Many months went by, however, before the extent of ambiguities in the regulations was perceived. The period from August 1971 through September 1972, at which point a special form (S-52) was published for institutional health care providers, must be characterized as one of substantial confusion with regard to the price controls. While it could be said that hospitals knew that productivity gains would pay off in permitting them greater potential freedom from the price controls, incentives to alter mean stay, service intensity, or other variables were not clear.[5]

The methodology finally put forth to adjust for volume was a strange and hastily compromised creation with substantial internal inconsistencies. Hospitals had a choice of adjusting for volume through detailed service data or through use of a formula. The formula was initially a weighted average of admissions and outpatient visits with an adjustment for intensity increases (per admission) based on recent national trends in input intensity. Ultimately, patient days joined admissions in the denominator of the formula (presumably to avoid incentives to alter length of stay). Thus, one of the alternative volume adjustments did not control intensity in any way while the other limited *each* hospital's intensity to a continuation of past *industry-wide* trends. Thus the issue of whether to regulate intensity was avoided. In practice, because of limitations of many hospital data systems and ambiguity as to how to adjust for volume by service data, most hospitals used the formula. Intensity was thus in fact regulated.

An exceptions procedure was established along with the regulations. State advisory boards were authorized to advise whether the requested exception was in the interest of the community in which the hospital operated. Exceptions decisions tended to allow price

[5] Research through American Hospital Association bulletins informing hospitals of ESP regulations shows no attempt on the part of the AHA to anticipate the resolution of the ambiguities. Consequently it is difficult to determine how hospitals interpreted the rules before publication of Form S-52.

increases necessary to avoid a negative cash flow but rarely allowed them on other grounds. Once a hospital fell into the negative cash flow situation, it was essentially free from the controls. The exceptions process became an extension of the formula, but with an opportunity for negative subjective input from the state advisory boards.[6]

The regulations were enforced by the Internal Revenue Service. While voluntary compliance was thought to be high, undoubtedly some hospitals accidentally violated the regulations. The ambiguities prevented the IRS from detecting violations. The most effective enforcement was performed by Medicare, which refused to pay more than 109 percent of the previous year's per diem unless an exception had been granted by the Price Commission.[7]

A brief assessment of hospital regulations can be made at this point. From an administrative view, the long-term persistence of ambiguities and frequent changes in important details of the regulations (such as the base period from which to calculate increases) must have diminished their effectiveness. From an economic point of view, the cost-justification requirements were the worst aspects. No incentives were placed on hospitals with price increases below 6 percent. Any gains in efficiency could not be used to increase profit margins. In fact, fears of current cost and price levels becoming a base for the future actually provided an incentive to increase costs. Separate limitations on labor and nonlabor cost increases were counterproductive. They interfered with intrahospital resource allocation and gave irrational incentives to shift input mix. Cost justification may have been a legacy from regulating hospitals within

[6] Cost of Living Council survey data showed a tendency for boards in the Northeast to deny or reduce many requests while those in the South and West approved most. Denial rates appeared to be related to the extent of state activity in health planning and regulation.

[7] Medicare used patient days as a volume adjustment for administrative feasibility. The 109 percent was derived from the 6 percent price ceiling and the portion of intensity increase trends not already allowed for in the 1.7 percent new technology allowance. This 109 percent per diem limit was inconsistent with Price Commission regulations because of the latter's use of admissions as well as patient days in its volume adjustment.

the context of the economy-wide controls which used such rules, but it diminished the potential efficacy of the hospital program. The formula to separate volume and price changes was crude. Possibly its major drawback was its treatment of average costs as constant. Economic studies (Lave and Lave, 1970; P. Feldstein, 1961) have shown marginal costs to be substantially less than average costs in the short run. Another was the arbitrariness with which price limits were set. Theoretical work (Ginsburg, 1975) has shown the importance for resource allocation of the level of the regulated price as it determines the service intensity and output levels. However, without agreement as to the validity of influencing these variables, it is difficult to set an appropriate level of the controlled price.[8]

Theory

Using a simple model of the nonprofit hospital, one can obtain hypotheses concerning the effects of *price* controls on a number of hospital variables. Since this has been done elsewhere (Ginsburg, 1975), only a summary is given here. The hospital is assumed to maximize an objective function of quantity, intensity, and a variable that I call "managerial slack." The last includes the cost of inputs above the minimum necessary to produce a given output-intensity combination and payments to labor in excess of opportunity costs.[9] The hospital is constrained by the necessity of breaking even in the long run. Quantity demanded is a function of price, intensity, and exogenous variables. Costs are a function of output, intensity, and exogenous variables.

To examine the effects of regulation, we assume price to be exogenous, and with comparative static analysis, obtain the effects of a change in the regulated price on the endogenous variables in

[8] In the design of Phase IV, which was aborted by the expiration of legislative authority for controls, an attempt was made to set the price ceiling rationally. However, with regard to intensity, continuation of previous trends was aimed at.
[9] This variable would include "philanthropic wages" discussed by M. Feldstein (1971a).

question. With some modest assumptions,[10] a fall in the regulated price should reduce quantity and intensity. The effect on slack is ambiguous, however, because of opposite income and substitution effects.[11]

While formal theory predicts the effects of pure price controls, it does not do as well in predicting the effects of ESP. The principal reason for this is that the wage controls associated with the program should have qualitative effects generally opposite to those of price controls.[12] For this reason, no attempt is made to include the details of ESP regulations in an expanded formal model. Instead, the incentives of the regulations and short-run adjustment considerations are discussed informally.

Wage Controls

While wage controls should affect variables such as intensity, output, and slack in a direction opposite to that of price controls, is there any evidence that one effect should be stronger than the other? It appears that the price controls should be stronger. This is because the containment of prices required for the average hospital was greater than the potential savings from wage limitations. Since the 2.5 percent limitation on nonlabor expenses was unrealistic, and the 1.7 percent allowance for new technology not usable by many

---

[10] The assumptions are: (a) an increase in intensity does not lower the quantity demanded; (b) the response of quantity demanded to intensity is not reduced by higher prices; (c) marginal costs do not fall with output; (d) intensity is not an inferior good. In an environment where the marginal patient's demand is not sensitive to price (from third-party coverage), assumptions (b) and (c) are automatically fulfilled.

[11] When the regulated price falls, slack becomes cheaper relative to quantity and intensity. Thus the substitution effect works to increase slack, while the income effect works to decrease it (assuming that it is not an inferior good).

[12] To an extent, ESP was designed so that wage and price controls offset each other to minimize distortions in resource allocation. However, in the health area, distortions were sought by some in order to offset previous distortions from factors such as the subsidy effect of health insurance. An exception to these offsetting tendencies is that both wages and prices are hypothesized to decline.

hospitals,[13] one would expect that the net impact of wage and price controls would be similar to that of a price control program.

The particular form of wage controls used should induce changes in the skill mix of labor. "Low-wage" labor was exempted from wage controls, and any wage increases in excess of 5.5 percent paid to low-wage labor could be passed through in the form of higher prices. Since most hospitals expected ESP to be short-lived, it is not clear to what extent relative wages changed. However, to the extent that they did, an incentive to move to a higher skill mix existed.

Changes in the mix between labor and nonlabor inputs are more difficult to predict. Prices on nonlabor inputs were controlled through the general economy-wide controls. If controls on hospital labor prices were more effective than those on the prices of nonlabor inputs, a tendency to substitute labor would exist. However, if hospitals face a positively sloped supply curve for labor, excess demand for labor would develop, and the opposite would occur. Dynamic considerations discussed below are likely to be far more powerful, however, particularly considering the short duration of controls and expectations that they would be temporary.

Admissions and Mean Stay

The model summarized above referred to "output" without defining it operationally. While the ultimate output of the hospital is the improvement of patients' health status attributable to hospital services, measurement problems prevent its use in regulation or empirical analysis. Instead, we deal with admissions and patient days (related by mean stay). Although patient days have been used more commonly as an output measure, economists have preferred admissions, since they are closer to the "true" output of health

---

[13] New technology was defined as "new equipment and new services directly related to health care, to the extent they are not charged directly to persons benefiting directly from that equipment or those services . . ." (Federal Register, 1972). Thus, increases in ancillary services (lab tests, x-rays) charged to patients could not be included under this category, even if the service was new.

improvement. The models referred to can be modified to include mean stay and admissions as output variables. However, this does not take us very far because (a) the literature on hospital behavior does not indicate what aspects of output should be in the objective function; (b) length-of-stay decisions have a heavy physician input—the model would have to be expanded to include physicians' behavior in shifting demand functions via their role as advisers to patients; and (c) the offsetting effects of wage and price controls add substantial uncertainty to signed results.

Instead of a formal approach, we examine the formulas used to determine price ceilings. Since the distinction between average costs and marginal costs was not recognized,[*] and studies show that in the short run the difference is substantial (P. Feldstein, 1961; Lave and Lave, 1970), there was a powerful incentive to increase both admissions and mean stay. Since the formula was based on an average per admission limit and a per patient day limit, and costs per day are higher during the earlier days of a stay, no obvious incentive is obtained to alter length of stay, given the number of patient days. However, since there was a strong incentive to increase the number of patient days, one would expect length of stay to be increased.[14]

Case Mix

Rafferty (1971) has shown that hospitals (via their medical staffs) are capable of altering case mix over time. ESP regulations introduced a number of incentives to alter case mix. Possibly the most important was one to shift diagnostic mix toward less costly types. If a hospital's costs increase by 9 percent, but only 6 percent can be passed along in higher prices, a means of avoiding a loss is to emphasize lower cost case types. A more subtle readjustment might

[*]But see the paper by Lipscomb, Raskin, and Eichenholz, below.—ED. NOTE.
[14]Thirteen months elapsed from the time controls began before the formula was announced. Research through bulletins issued by the American Hospital Association to its members during this period revealed no advice or hints as to what was the likely denominator in the formula. As per diem was used in the Medicare program for purposes of preliminary reimbursement, anticipations of the formula might have leaned in this direction.

involve shifting to a less profitable case mix. In a model of case-mix optimization,[15] those case types that are most desirable to the hospital at the margin are least profitable at the margin. If the margin of net revenue is forced down by 3 percent as above, the hospital may shift case mix toward the less profitable. If the profit margin must fall, the hospital might as well switch to more preferred case types.

Of least empirical importance is the fact that demand elasticities vary by case type. If price controls are effective, case mix could shift as patients respond to the reduction in real price. However, the magnitude of any price declines should be small enough so that this effect is not particularly important.

Expectations and Dynamic Adjustment

Thus far adjustment costs have not been considered. Since it is less costly to vary labor inputs than to vary fixed inputs, the former are varied more extensively when output levels are changed. Expectations as to whether output changes are temporary or permanent will influence the type of adjustment. The more temporary the adjustment, the more variation in labor relative to nonlabor inputs can be expected. It is clear the hospitals expected the controls to be short-lived. Consequently, if output increased as a result of ESP, there should be a shift toward labor intensity, while if output fell, the shift in factor proportions should be in the other direction.

---

[15] Assume that the hospital maximizes the objective function

$$U = U(x_1, x_2 \ldots x_n)$$

where x_i is the number of cases of type i, and is constrained by

$$R_1(x_1) + R_2(x_2) \ldots R_n(x_n) - C(x_1, x_2, \ldots x_n) = 0.$$

Then, first order conditions are

$$U_i + \lambda(R_i - C_i) = 0 \qquad i = 1, \ldots n.$$

Taking any two case types, $i \neq j$, we have

$$\frac{U_i}{U_j} = \frac{R_i - C_i}{R_j - C_j},$$

or, the ratio of the marginal utilities is equal to the ratio of the marginal net losses.

Within labor, similar changes should occur. It is more costly to train skilled workers, so one would expect short-run adjustments to involve more variation in unskilled employment than in skilled. Thus if output increases, the skill mix should decline, and if output declines, relatively more skilled workers will be used. Since data on wages are usually not adjusted for skill mix, such effects make monitoring wage trends difficult.

A final dynamic consideration is the impact of controls on hospital profits. In the long run, there should be no change, as breaking even is a constraint. However, as the ability to adjust in the short run is limited, and complete adjustment to temporary controls is irrational, one should expect a decline in profits because of controls.

Summarizing this section, if price controls were more powerful than wage controls, a formal approach would predict a reduction in service intensity and output, with an ambiguous effect on slack. Also, prices and wages should be reduced. A number of additional factors were examined which do not fit easily into a formal model. Admissions and mean stay should increase because in the short run, marginal costs are less than average costs. If output should fall as a result of controls, there will be a movement toward a higher skill mix of labor, and a reduction of labor relative to nonlabor inputs. The details of wage regulations also should induce an upgrading of labor skills employed. Finally, changes in case mix are induced.

Specification and Data

Both the AHA and the Cost of Living Council have issued periodic "back of the envelope" assessments on the effects of this program.[16] Looking for changes in trends from the precontrols period to the period covered by controls can be highly misleading because (a) other factors affecting the variables in question are not held constant and (b) the statistical significance of changes in trends is usually not assessed. In order to avoid these problems, a complete model of a hospital is estimated.

[16] For example, see statements by both parties in U.S. Congress (1974).

Two alternative approaches were available to estimate an empirical model of hospital behavior. One could estimate a series of structural equations, and then calculate a reduced form in order to assess the total impact of controls. On the other hand, one can estimate reduced form equations (where each endogenous variable is regressed on all of the exogenous variables) directly.[17] Direct estimation of reduced form equations was considered to be most useful for the task at hand.[18]

The choice of data for this study was dictated by special requirements of the task. A large number of observations both before and during the period covered by controls were needed to obtain statistically significant results on the effects of controls. The AHA's National Hospital Panel Survey (NHPS) was chosen because of its frequency of appearance (monthly) and its rapidity of collection and processing. The NHPS consists of a stratified sample of approximately 1,000 community hospitals. Information similar to that in the Annual Survey is obtained on capacity, utilization, personnel, and finances. Data on individual hospitals were not available for the precontrols period. Inflations of the sample to

---

[17] Feldstein (1971b) has estimated a particularly simple structural hospital model with state data. Davis has estimated a structural model (1972) and reduced form models (1973, 1974).

[18] The reasoning behind this judgment is based upon the unusual kind of structural shift associated with the imposition of controls on this industry. In moving from a model of an unregulated hospital to one where price is regulated, we do not see shifts in demand, cost, or production functions. The change in the structure occurs in the nonstochastic optimizing conditions. This rules out the usual approach of estimating structural equations over two periods and entering shift variables. Since shifts are in the nonstochastic equations, the only method for executing a structural approach would be to estimate a structural model for the precontrols period and use the calculated reduced form to forecast values of the endogenous variables for the controls period. Comparison of predicted with actual values would assess the impact of controls. However, solving for the reduced form would be a problem here since the marginal conditions involve marginal utility. (Davis, 1972, avoids this by assuming profit maximization; Feldstein, 1971b, assumes desired output to be exogenous.) Further, as a result of nonlinearities in the functional form of the cost or production function (necessary for realism), the equations are too complex to solve exactly. Only a numerical solution can be obtained, making it impossible to calculate a confidence interval for forecasts.

aggregates (by census division and by bed-size class—but not both) were available and were used instead.

Most of the analysis was performed on a pooling of data on nine census divisions for forty-four quarters (1963–1973).[19] The regional cross-section was preferred to one of bed-size groups to permit more variation in exogenous variables. Also, all of the hospitals in an area comprise a more meaningful aggregate than those hospitals in a certain size class. However, the bed-size cross-section was used to estimate equations where service intensity or productivity variables were endogenous, since only this file could be merged with data on these variables from Hospital Administrative Services (HAS).[20] Unfortunately, the lack of cross-sectional variation in exogenous variables caused such instability in estimated coefficients due to multicollinearity among the various time series that meaningful results could not be obtained from this file. The major drawbacks of this situation are the inability to treat productivity as a separate endogenous variable, and the necessity of using input intensity rather than service intensity as a proxy for quality of care. Productivity change and service intensity are both encompassed by the input intensity variable.

The variables used in the reduced form estimation (classified as endogenous or exogenous) are as follows:

Endogenous
    ADM   Admissions
    DAYS   Inpatient days

---

[19] Monthly observations were aggregated to quarterly because data from other sources tended to be available with less frequency.

[20] HAS is a service to enable hospital administrators to compare productivity and service indicators from their institutions with those from others. While a great deal of information is provided which is not available from other sources, a number of difficulties in using the information for research are encountered. First, the sample of participants is self-selected. Second, individual observations tend to be closely guarded, and published aggregates are medians rather than means or totals. Finally, the form in which the data are published changes frequently, making it impossible to use a time series over more than a few years. Published data aggregated by region had more consistency problems than those by bed-size group, so the latter were merged with the NHPS bed-size file. The resulting file consisted of six bed-size classes and twenty quarters (1969–1973).

OPV	Outpatient visits
INP	Index of input use
π	Net revenue (profits)
IR	Inpatient revenue
OR	Outpatient revenue
MS	Average length of stay
AA	Adjusted admissions
SURG	Surgical procedures
EXP	Costs
WGE	Hospital wage rate
FTE	Full-time equivalent personnel
NL	Nonlabor inputs

Exogenous

INS	Proportion of community hospital expenditures financed by third-party payments
INS-M	Proportion of medical and surgical expenditures financed by third-party payments
CPI	Consumer Price Index
INC	Per capita disposable income
POP	Population
PDENS	Population per square mile
UE	Percentage of those eligible for unemployment compensation receiving it
TIME	Time trend
BEDS	Beds in community
MD	Physicians in office-based practice/capita
GP	Proportion of such physicians that are general practitioners
DEM	Index of age, sex, and race of the population
PHP	Physician price index
MFW	Manufacturing wage
NLP	Nonlabor input price index
PRP	Percentage of hospitals organized for profit
SL	Percentage of hospitals owned by state or local governments
TCH	Percentage of hospitals with medical school affiliation

AVSIZE   Average bed size of hospitals in an area
CR   Proportion of community hospital expenditures fi-
           nanced by reimbursement of costs.
ESP   Dummy variable for Economic Stabilization Pro-
           gram

Some explanation about the variables used is in order. INP is a Laspeyres index of labor and nonlabor inputs. The measure of labor inputs is FTE, while nonlabor inputs (NL) are obtained by dividing nonpayroll expenses (supplies, explicit capital costs) by NLP, an index of hospital nonlabor input prices developed by Altman and Eichenholz (1974). Both FTE and NL are divided by their 1963 values, and are weighted by the proportion of 1963 expenses classified as payroll and nonpayroll respectively.

Adjusted patient days (APD) and adjusted admissions (AA) are composites of inpatient days or admissions and outpatient visits. They are defined as:

$$APD = DAYS \left(1 + \frac{OR}{IR} \right)$$

$$AA = ADM \left(1 + \frac{OR}{IR} \right)$$

Among the exogenous variables, INS, INS-M, INC, POP, PDENS, DEM, and UE are demand variables. INS is obtained by summing hospital benefits from Blue Cross plans, commercial insurers, Medicare, and Medicaid and dividing by total expenditures in community hospitals.[21] The variable tends to be too large since some hospital benefits go to providers other than community hospitals. INS-M is constructed in the same way. Medical-surgical benefits are summed in the numerator, and the denominator is physician expenditures. CR is similar to INS, except for the omission from the numerator of Blue Cross benefits in charge reimbursement plans and commercial insurance benefits. BEDS, MD, and GP are added as demand variables as well, following others such as

[21] Data on Blue Cross and commercial insurance are obtained from annual editions of *Source Book of Health Insurance Data*, published by the Health Insurance Institute. Data on Medicare are from the *Social Security Bulletin*. Data on Medicaid are obtained from various publications of the Medical Services Administration, DHEW. The Annual Grade Issues of the American Hospital Association are the source.

Feldstein (1971b). PHP is seen as a demand variable reflecting the price of a substitute (or complement—the literature is not clear on this).

The variables TCH and AVSIZE reflect output mix (and possibly scale economies). The dummy for the Medicare program (MED) reflects a structural shift in demand (aside from the insurance aspect) reflecting relatively greater demand by the elderly and a consequent shift in the age distribution of the hospital population. MFW is an exogenous variable in a supply of labor function. NLP reflects a cost identity variable. The ownership variables (SL, PRP) could reflect differences in the hospital objective function. Finally, TIME reflects technological change in the production of hospital care, including secular increases in service intensity not associated with demand shifts.

Estimation

As noted above, direct estimation of reduced form equation is the most practical way of assessing the impact of controls on the hospital variables of interest. The model to be estimated is:

$$G^1_{jt} = \beta^1_{0j} + \sum_i \beta^1_i Z_{ijt} + \mu^1_{jt}$$

$$\cdot \qquad \cdot \qquad \cdot \qquad \cdot$$
$$\cdot \qquad \cdot \qquad \cdot \qquad \cdot$$
$$\cdot \qquad \cdot \qquad \cdot \qquad \cdot$$

$$G^n_{jt} = \beta^n_{0j} + \sum_i \beta^n_i Z_{ijt} + \mu^n_{jt}$$

In this system, $G^1 \ldots G^n$ are the endogenous variables, Z_i ($i = 1 \ldots k$) are the exogenous variables, j denotes the cross-sectional unit, and t refers to the time period. A logarithmic functional form is used, and a different constant is estimated for each cross-sectional unit.[22]

[22] The regional dummies (which are statistically significant) are added to prevent potential specification bias from omission of variables correlated with included independent variables (see Johnson and Lyon, 1973). Certain exogenous variables, such as PDENS, which did not vary over time in these data, could not be included along with the regional dummies because they would have caused the intercorrelation matrix to be singular. Dummies are preferred to these variables, since the latter essentially constrain the regional constants to be in proportion to the values of the variables, but regional dummies do not add this undesirable constraint.

Some assumptions of the general linear regression model are not fulfilled. Probably the most important violation is autoregressive disturbances. Durbin-Watson statistics showed significant positive autocorrelation to exist in most of the equations (that for profit margins was an exception). Assuming a first order autoregressive relationship, estimates of ρ were obtained from ordinary least squares (OLS) estimates. For each equation, a Cochrane-Orcutt transformation was performed, and then the equation was reestimated with OLS.[23] Kmenta (1971) has shown that this technique is asymptotically equivalent to Aitken's generalized least squares (GLS). The former is computationally simpler, but one time-series observation is lost. The homoscedasticity assumption of the general linear regression model is not a problem. Efficiency of estimation can be improved by taking into account the lack of independence of disturbances over the cross-section through Aitken's GLS. Unfortunately, an appropriate computational program was not available, so this was not pursued.

Results

Table 2 contains the results of a basic reduced form model, estimated by OLS after autoregressive transformations. Alongside is a model that is identical except that mean stay is included as an exogenous variable instead of an endogenous one.[24]

[23] To ease computational difficulties, the estimate of ρ for each equation was rounded to either 0, .35, .50, or .65. The value used for each equation is indicated in Table 2.
[24] The exogenous variables used in these models are listed in Table 2. Hospital bed capacity is treated as exogenous here, although the regression spans eleven years. This is due to the lack of success by economists in explaining bed construction. Ginsburg (1972) was only able to explain 14 percent of variation in bed construction over a five-year period on cross-sectional data. Lave and Lave (1974) have argued that beds should be viewed as exogenous because government subsidies are a major determinant of construction. It is unlikely that ESP affected bed stock because of the brevity of the program. Whether or not beds per capita was included as an exogenous variable had little effect on ESP coefficients in regressions, however.

Cost and price variables are in nominal terms. The CPI is entered as an exogenous variable. Those variables that would enter structural equations in real terms (e.g., INC, PHP) are maintained in that form in the reduced form model.

TABLE 2   Regression Coefficients on ESP Dummy:
Log-Linear Reduced Form Equations

Dependent Variable	$\hat{p}$	Basic Model β	t	MS Exogenous β	t
WGE	.65	-.068	-2.7	-.074	-2.9
FTE/NL	.65	-.041	-2.7	-.042	-2.7
ADM	.35	.004	0.9	-.005	-1.7
MS	.5	-.011	-3.0	—	
PD	.35	-.007	-2.2	-.005	-1.7
OPV	.65	.011	0.8	.011	0.8
INP/AA	.35	-.010	-1.9	.001	0.1
INP/APD	.35	.001	0.1	.001	0.1
EXP/AA	.35	-.007	-1.6	.001	0.3
EXP/APD	.35	.004	0.9	.001	0.3
IR/ADM	.35	-.008	-1.8	-.002	-0.5
IR/PD	.5	-.001	-0.2	-.005	-1.1
OR/OPV	.5	-.014	-0.8	-.020	-1.1
π	0	-.046	-1.2	-.053	-1.3
SURG	.35	.013	2.3	.013	2.3

Exogenous variables: INS, INS-M, CR, TIME, BEDS/CAP, CAP, MD, GP, UE, NLP, MFW, PHP, CPI, INC, MED, PRP, SL, TCH, SURG, QUARTERLY DUMMIES, REGIONAL DUMMIES.

Looking at results with the basic model, coefficients on the ESP dummy for all of the variables in per unit of output terms differ according to whether admissions or patient days are used in the denominator. When admissions are used in the denominator, costs, inputs, and prices tend to decline (though by small amounts), while when patients days are the unit, there are no significant changes. It is apparent that a decline in mean stay attributed to the controls by the model is responsible for this divergence.

Since hospital length of stay is generally considered to be too long on the average, cost savings per admission accomplished through reductions in mean stay would be considered a real accomplishment of controls. However, there are reasons to believe that the decline in mean stay econometrically attributed to ESP resulted from other factors. The discussion of the incentives from the ESP regulations showed that mean stay should have increased rather than declined; the strongest incentive was to reduce average costs by filling empty beds, and increasing mean stay is a way of achieving this. One of the factors accounting for the decline in mean stay might have been utilization review. The period in question was one of more general use of utilization review committees in hospitals. In addition, availability of beds in extended care facilities increased. Since a major exogenous shift in mean stay may have occurred, an alternative model treating mean stay as exogenous was also estimated.[25]

An important result seen in both models is a substantial reduction in wage increases attributed to controls. It is estimated that wages (or more accurately payroll per full-time equivalent employee) were 7 percent lower at the end of 1973 than they would have been in the absence of controls. This is a substantial reduction but is not surprising to those familiar with the program, since compliance with the limitations on wage increases was apparently quite high. The result is a strong one, as a number of *downward* biases are seen. Since the period was characterized by a decline in the rate of growth of hospital output and personnel, there may have been a shift in skill mix toward a more highly skilled labor force. This is because in those institutions where layoffs occurred, one would expect a preponderance to be in the unskilled category, where there is little investment in on-the-job training. An additional tendency to alter skill mix arose from the exemption of low-wage employees from the controls. If hospitals moved to a work force of a higher skill mix during this period, then the reduction in wage is attributed to the controls.

In regard to input intensity, no significant impacts of ESP are shown, with the exception of the model where mean stay is endogenous. Here, inputs per adjusted admission decline while inputs per adjusted patient day are unchanged. Since occupancy rates declined during the period, and reduced occupancy might lead to an increase in input use per unit of output, one could argue that factors not captured by the model were forcing occupancy rates down, and that the effects of this on input use were offsetting the effects of ESP. A crude test of this hypothesis involves adding the occupancy rate as an exogenous variable in the manner in which mean stay was added. However, when this is done, the results on the effect of ESP on input use are unchanged.

---

[25] Technically, mean stay is added to the exogenous variables to avoid specification bias from the omission of those factors influencing mean stay which are positively correlated with the ESP dummy.

The results on expenditures parallel those on input use. If the decline in length of stay is seen as exogenous, then no significant effects are seen. This result is somewhat perplexing, however. Since wages were reduced by controls, and input intensity was unaffected, expenditures should have been shown to be reduced. This inconsistency may be due to deficiencies in some of the price indices used, notably the nonlabor input price index, but a completely satisfactory explanation is not yet at hand. The inconsistency does not show up in one of the dynamic models discussed below.

Prices tended to parallel expenditures, but small negative effects for controls appeared. However, these effects were not statistically significant. A 2 percent reduction in the prices of outpatient services was seen, but the *t* statistic was only -1.1. The difference in impacts on prices and costs does show up in the equation for profits. In the exogenous mean stay model, a 6 percent reduction in the profit margin is seen—an effect almost significant at the 10 percent level.

An interesting change in input proportions occurs. There is a decline in the ratio of labor to nonlabor inputs attributed to controls, although the quantitative magnitude is sensitive to the model used. The much smaller (and marginally significant) impact in the exogenous mean stay model indicates the importance of the apparently exogenous output reduction in explaining this effect. Labor expenses are more variable in the short run. The remainder of the result may be due to the incentive to increase fringe benefits as opposed to money wages. The former were not controlled, and the AHA statistical gatherers include fringes in nonpayroll expenses.

As noted above, there is a decline in mean stay attributed to controls by the model. When mean stay is entered as an exogenous variable, a small negative impact of controls on admissions is shown.

Up to this point, case mix has been treated as exogenous. The only such variable available to this study (the proportion of admissions that were for surgery) was entered as an independent variable in all of the above equations. While it tended to be statistically significant, it did not change the results for the effects of ESP on the endogenous variables. When the surgery variable was used as a dependent variable, a statistically significant 1 percent increase is attributed to controls by either model. Again, it is necessary to ask whether this result is predicted by theory.

It was stated that there were incentives to alter case mix toward the low-cost and low-profit types. To classify surgical cases as to their relative costliness and profitability, the coefficients of the surgery variable in the reduced form equations for costs and profits were examined. In neither was the coefficient significant. Thus, as a whole, surgery cases do not appear to be more costly or more profitable. While the change in case mix could have been along these lines, we have no evidence to support it. As in the case of mean stay, exogenous variables not included in the model must be considered as an explanation. However, utilization review is not a likely explanation, since the results were not altered by inclusion of mean stay (a presumed proxy) as an exogenous variable, and I am not aware of any drastic changes in medical technology occurring at the time that would explain this. Thus, while the mechanism is not clear, ESP could very well have affected surgery rates.

A number of other versions of the basic reduced form models were investigated. In one, wages were included as exogenous in order to concentrate on the effects of price controls only. However, no changes in the results occurred. In another, all variables influenced by the nonhealth segments of ESP (the various price indices and wages) were dropped on the theory that their correlation with ESP could affect the ESP coefficient. However, again no important changes in the results emerged. The assumption of a log-linear time trend was relaxed. A squared term was added, to allow the effect of time on the dependent variable (in log terms) to increase or decrease over time. Alternatively, time was entered logarithmically. The results were not very sensitive to varying time trend assumptions. The time period covered by the ESP dummy was altered to begin with the fourth quarter of 1972, which is when Form S-52 was issued, and a great deal of ambiguity was removed. Again, the basic thrust of the results was continued.

A potentially more important model estimated was a lagged adjustment model. Hospitals may not adjust to changes in exogenous variables immediately because of adjustment costs, expectations, and other factors. Thus some changes in endogenous variables are seen as delayed response to prior changes in exogenous variables. One general form of lagged adjustment is the Koyck distrib-

TABLE 3   Lagged Adjustment Model

Dependent Variable	$\hat{\rho}$	ESP Dummy β	ESP Dummy t	Lagged Dependent β	Lagged Dependent t
WGE	.5	-.25	-2.2	.21	1.6
FTE/NL	.5	.081	0.9	.05	5.3
ADM	0	.000	0.0	-.01	-0.4
MS	0	-.003	-1.5	.71	21.
PD	0	.000	0.2	1.6	74.
OPV	0	.008	0.7	.06	0.7
INP/AA	0	-.005	-1.1	-0.4	-0.9
INP/APD	0	.003	1.0	-.000	-0.3
EXP/AA	0	-.002	-0.4	.48	4.2
EXP/APD	0	.004	1.2	.29	6.8
IR/ADM	0	-.002	-0.5	.004	3.5
IR/PD	0	.005	1.2	-.01	-1.7
OR/OPV	0	-.007	.4	singular	
π	0	-.045	1.1	.03	0.5
SURG	0	.015	3.2	.02	0.9

Exogenous variables: same as Table 2.

uted lag, which is obtained by adding a lagged value of the dependent variable to the independent variables. This specification assumes a uniform adjustment pattern with respect to all of the exogenous variables. While this specification causes bias in small samples, large sample estimation is consistent as long as autocorrelation is absent. Since Durbin-Watson statistics are biased in this context, the Wallis (1967) procedure was used. An instrumental variable is used in place of the lagged dependent variable (in this case, the predicted value of the lagged dependent variable) to estimate the value of ρ. Then a Cochrane-Orcutt transformation is performed, and the lagged dependent variable (as opposed to the instrument) is used in estimation with the transformed data set. Results of these regressions are given in Table 3.[26]

The distributed lag models are plagued by high correlation between the lagged dependent variable and the bulk of the other independent variables. This causes the coefficients on the lagged variable to be unstable, and indeed they are. It is difficult to assess the extent of this multicollinearity's influence on the ESP coefficient. It is reassuring, however, that the signs (if not the magnitudes) of these coefficients are generally consistent with the static models.

[26] In most cases, a Cochrane-Orcutt transformation was not called for by the Wallis procedure.

One exception is that the ESP effect on mean stay is reduced (and not significant at the 10 percent level)—although results still differ according to whether admissions or patient days are used in the denominator. Another exception is that the impact on labor intensity changes from a significant negative to positive but insignificant.

A special case of the distributed lag model avoids some of the econometric problems. If the coefficient on the lagged dependent variable is predetermined, then it can be moved to the left-hand side of the equation. If a coefficient of 1.0 is chosen, this makes the dependent variable a first difference. This implies that hospitals behave entirely marginally—that changes in endogenous variables (but not levels) are based on exogenous variables. Such a model is not particularly realistic, but is useful because of its contrast with static models, where the coefficient on the lagged dependent variables is set equal to zero.[27]

The results of this special case of the distributed lag model are shown in Table 4. No transformations were necessary to eliminate autocorrelation. There are a number of interesting contrasts with the static model. One is that the alleged negative impact of ESP on mean stay disappears (it is positive but not significant here). Another is that inpatient revenue per day is reduced by ESP, although the reduction is less than 1 percent and is significant only at the 10 percent level. Unit costs declined also, but these results are slightly less significant than those for prices. Input use increased, though the results were not significant. In this model, there is no inconsistency between the results for wage rates and input intensity on the one hand, and unit costs on the other.

ESP is seen to reduce labor intensity, here, in contrast to an increase in the static model. A final difference is that the effects of controls on profits and on surgery rates are no longer significant.

The first difference model provides useful corroboration for the static model. The most important results of the latter—the strong

[27]A problem with this model is that no static equilibrium is possible as long as the endogenous variables are equal to zero. Its role, however, is not as a substitute for the other models, but as a type of sensitivity analysis. If the results from the static model are maintained in this overly dynamic one, we can have more confidence in the results.

TABLE 4   **First Difference Dependent Variable Model**

Dependent Variable	β	t
WGE	-.061	-4.3
FTE/NL	.006	2.3
ADM	.002	.7
MS	.003	1.2
PD	.006	1.6
OPV	-.010	-1.1
INP/AA	.007	1.6
INP/APD	.004	1.1
EXP/AA	-.002	-0.5
EXP/APD	-.005	-1.4
IR/ADM	-.003	-0.8
IR/PD	-.006	-1.7
OR/OPV	.010	0.7
π	-.037	-0.7
SURG	.003	0.6

Exogenous variables: same as Table 2. MS is endogenous.

negative effect of controls on wages and the quantitatively (and often statistically) insignificant effect on input use, unit costs, and prices—are maintained. However, many of the previous results not consistent with theory—such as the decline in mean stay, the decrease in labor intensity, and the increase in surgery—are not maintained when a dynamic model is used.

Conclusion

The Economic Stabilization Program was very effective in reducing rates of increase of hospital employees' wages, but not with regard to hospital costs. In neither the static or dynamic models did input intensity decline as a result of controls. In one model, prices declined slightly, but this appeared to result from wage reductions and a possible reduction in profit margins.

It is useful to consider why the program did not have important impacts on costs. First, the influence of the economy-wide controls over the design of health care controls created serious disincentives. Cost justification requirements eliminated all incentives from hospitals not experiencing difficulty in staying under the 6 percent limit. Since base period data for calculating price increases were each institution's own, many hospitals were not limited by the controls.

For example, those hospitals with increasing occupancy rates were seldom constrained, since the formula did not distinguish between average and marginal costs. If hospitals feared that their current performance might become a base for the future, incentives to increase costs may have existed. Finally, those hospitals forced into a negative cash flow position by the limitations had no incentives to cut costs.

A second negative factor was the persistent confusion and ambiguity of the regulations. It is difficult for a hospital to take constructive action when its position vis-à-vis the regulations is in doubt.

A final negative factor was the expectation that controls would be short-lived. Initially, hospitals were skeptical of whether the controls would be seriously enforced. Afterward, a (correct) belief that controls would be temporary was prevalent. Most organizations would not pursue important managerial changes to respond to temporary controls; hospitals are even less likely to do so. During the program, hospital administrators complained that they were not in a position to pursue cost reduction, since so many decisions on the nature of the product and productivity were under the control of the medical staff. Clearly, changing this relationship or organizing the medical staff to contain costs is a long-term project, unlikely to be induced by temporary controls. Thus the nature of hospital organization requires long-term changes to deal constructively with cost containment, and the expectations that controls would not be long term discourages such changes.

Are there any implications for increasingly used prospective reimbursement programs that can be drawn from the ESP experience? Unfortunately, not many. In the area of wages, where ESP appears to have had a most substantial impact, we do not know the roles played by wage versus price controls. Since prospective reimbursement systems tend to have only the latter, the ESP experience cannot be used to predict the wage effects. As to the effects of ESP controls on input use and costs, there are many reasons for not expecting the same to hold true under prospective reimbursement. Inhibitions in design and expectations that the controls would be short-lived have been discussed. Perhaps one of the most basic difficulties in projecting from the ESP experience is one of research design. Since all hospitals were affected, there was no control group. While the statistical techniques used here are adequate to distinguish shifts in the functions from random variation with a degree of confidence, we must always wonder whether some change in technology or other systematic influence roughly coincided with controls, and whether the effects attributed to ESP are really those of some other factor (or whether the absence of effects is the result of an offsetting influence).

References and Acknowledgments

An earlier version of this paper, entitled "Price Controls and Hospital Costs," was presented to a joint American Economic Association–Health Economics Research Organization session at the Allied Social Science Association meetings, San Francisco, December 29, 1974. The author is grateful to the National Center for Health Services Research for financial support (HSM 110-73-467), the American Hospital Association for access to data, to Robert Henry and Terry Halpin for research assistance, and to Lawrence Officer, John Rafferty, and Kenneth Raske for useful discussion.

Altman, S.H., and J. Eichenholz
   1974   "Control of hospital costs under the Economic Stabilization Program." Weekly Compilation of Presidential Documents, Federal Register 39, No. 60 (March 27): 11398-11405, Appendix to Subpart R.
American Enterprise Institute
   1974   National Health Insurance Proposals, Legislative Analysis #13.
Davis, K.
   1972   An Empirical Investigation of Alternative Models of the Hospital Industry. Paper presented to American Economic Association meeting, Toronto.
   1973   "Hospital costs and the Medicare program." Social Security Bulletin 36 (August): 18-36.
   1974   "The role of technology, demand, and labor markets in the determination of hospital cost." In Mark Perlman, ed., The

Economics of Health and Medical Care. New York: John Wiley
& Sons, Inc.

Dowling, W.L.
1974   "Prospective reimbursement of hospitals." Inquiry 11 (September): 163–180.

Federal Register
1972   Code of Federal Regulations, Title 6, Economic Stabilization,
Section 300-18, Institutional Providers of Health Services. Federal Register 37 (April 18): 7622.

Feldstein, M.S.
1971a   The Rising Cost of Hospital Care. Washington, D.C.: Information Resources Press.
1971b   "Hospital cost inflation: A study of nonprofit price dynamics."
American Economic Review 61 (December): 853–972.

Feldstein, P.
1961   An Empirical Investigation of the Marginal Cost of Hospital
Services. Chicago: University of Chicago Press.

Ginsburg, P.B.
1972   "Resource allocation in the hospital industry: The role of capital
financing." Social Security Bulletin 35 (August): 20–30.
1975   Regulating the Non-Profit Firm: Hospital Price and Reimbursement Controls. Mimeographed. Department of Economics,
Michigan State University.
1976   "Inflation and the Economic Stabilization Program." Pp. 31–51 in
Michael Zubkoff, ed., Health: A Victim or Cause of Inflation?
New York: Prodist for Milbank Memorial Fund.

Johnson, K.H., and H.L. Lyon
1973   "Experimental evidence on combining cross-section and time
series information." Review of Economics and Statistics:
465–474.

Kmenta, J.
1971   Elements of Econometrics. New York: Macmillan Publishing
Company, Inc.

Lave, J.R., and L.B. Lave
1970   "Hospital cost functions." American Economic Review 60
(June): 379–395.
1974   The Hospital Construction Act: An Evaluation of the Hill-Burton
Program, 1948–1973. Washington: American Enterprise Institute,
Evaluative Studies 16.

Rafferty, J.
1971 "Patterns of hospital use: An analysis of short-run variations."
Journal of Political Economy 79 (January–February): 154–165.
Rosenthal, G.
1970 "Price elasticity of demand for short-term hospital services." In
H. Klarman, ed., Empirical Studies in Health Economics. Balti-
more: Johns Hopkins Press.
Salkever, D.
1972 "A microeconomic study of hospital cost inflation." Journal of
Political Economy 80 (November): 1144–1166.
U.S. Congress
1974 House of Representatives Committee on Interstate and Foreign
Commerce, Subcommittee on Public Health and Environment,
Hospital Cost Controls. Hearings held December 19, 1973. Serial
No. 93-60. Washington, D.C.
Waldman, S.
1974 National Health Insurance Proposals. Provisions of bills intro-
duced in the 93d Congress as of July 1974. U.S. Department of
Health, Education, and Welfare.
Wallis, K.F.
1967 "Lagged dependent variables and serially correlated errors: A
reappraisal of three-pass least squares." Review of Economics
and Statistics 49: 555–567.

Hospital Rate Setting—
This Way to Salvation?

KATHARINE G. BAUER

Hospital rate setting is a new type of regulatory activity rapidly spreading in the United States. Between 1970 and 1975 the number of rate-setting programs grew from two to twenty-seven. These programs, most of which are administered by Blue Cross plans or state governments, now control the hospital rates or charges to one or more major type of payer in twenty-three states, and affect to some degree more than 25 percent of the nation's acute care hospitals (U.S. DHEW, 1975).

The federal government's involvement in hospital rate setting has up to now been minimal. Both Congress and the executive branch have been moving cautiously, made sensitive, perhaps, by the misfortunes that attended the massive switch to cost-based reimbursement when the Medicare program was introduced in 1966. This time, the federal government is closely scrutinizing experience in the states before adopting new methods of hospital reimbursement for Medicare or in plans for the administration of national health insurance.

Congress has, however, offered positive inducements to the states to develop rate regulation. Both the 1972 Amendments to the Social Security Act and the 1974 National Health Planning and Resources Development Act provide for federal support of new state and regional experiments in hospital rate setting and for the evaluation of results of programs in current operation. As the paper by Fred Hellinger describes, so far there is no conclusive evidence that rate-setting programs constitute an important means of containing hospital costs.

This paper reviews highlights in the state and regional experience as of 1975. After outlining the nature of rate setting and the impetus behind the movement, it examines some of the major issues that implementation has brought to the fore. In particular, we will note the kinds of assumptions on which this new and highly demanding form of regulation was premised, the sometimes contradictory expectations held for it, the strengths and weaknesses of various types of structures for its administration, and certain problems of methodology and information that handicap efforts of rate-setting bodies to accomplish their intended purposes. The final section deals with the kinds of risks and incentives that rate-setting programs introduce to the hospital industry, sometimes by intention, sometimes by inadvertence, and often because of the still limited state of their art.

Case studies of major rate-setting programs conducted or supervised by the author between 1973 and 1975 under contracts with the Social Security Administration provide the material for most of the descriptions and discussions of issues (Bauer and Clark, 1974a, b, c, d; Bauer, 1974a; Arthur D. Little, 1974a, b, c, d, e, f).

The What and Why of Hospital Rate Setting

Controls on the amounts of future reimbursement to which hospitals will be entitled take many forms. "Rate setting," by the purest definition, is only one of these forms. For purposes of convenience, however, we will use the term here in the broadest sense to include any means for determining the financial remuneration of hospitals whereby the amounts to be paid for specified units of service are established by some external authority prior to the period in which the services are to be given.[1]

[1] One could argue persuasively that this definition should be broadened to include the imposition of ceiling limits beyond which hospital price increases would not be reimbursed, such as under the federal wage-price control program, and under the regulations implementing Section 223 of the Social Security Act Amendments of 1972. For purposes of this paper, however, the narrower definition of rate setting has been used, since other sections of the book deal with price limit controls.

The rate-setting programs in operation at the end of 1975 are extraordinarily heterogeneous. They operate under different types of auspices and organizational structures, cover different kinds of payers, use different types of methodologies, and present varied degrees of risks and sometimes conflicting incentives. While they pursue a common goal of trying to contain rates of increase in hospital costs, their specific objectives often differ considerably. Some emphasize controls on new spending for facility and program expansions, some stress improved hospital management, and some simply try to keep hospital cost increases in line with the movement of the general economic indicators. The approaches they use to achieve these objectives range from education, jawboning, and public disclosure to formula-derived rate projections. Their means for resolving conflicts may take the form of negotiation, mediation, and arbitration or of formal hearings, administrative case law precedents, and court decisions.

This diversity among the programs is stressed at the outset to warn the reader against summary statements about rate setting that will inevitably appear in the pages to follow. In fact, as will be seen, there is considerably more commonality in the activities rate-setting agencies *fail* to pursue than in the ones they do pursue. As a major example, no program aims its reimbursement risks and incentives at the physician members of hospital staffs, although all fully recognize that the day-by-day decisions such physicians make in hospitals are by far the most cost-consequential ones. Similarly, no program yet takes into systematic account the considerable differences among hospitals in respect to case mix, patient characteristics, and types of surgical procedures performed, although cost function analyses show these to be highly explanatory factors (Lave and Lave, 1971; Feldstein and Schuttinga, 1975). The most comprehensive study to date, analyzing the experience of all hospitals in two Canadian provinces, showed that diagnostic and age variables together accounted for more than 80 percent of the variation in costs among hospitals (Evans and Walker, 1972).

Finally, although hospitals and rate-setting bodies alike give considerable lip service to the quality issue, no program has tried to use the results of medical audits or other systematic quality of care measures as factors in rate-setting decisions.

Before describing the rate-setting programs in further detail, we will review the reasons behind their development.

The Rationale for Rate Setting as a Cost Control Measure

The current trend toward prospective rate setting rests on the premise that a major reason for the recent rise in hospital costs was the adoption by Medicare and Medicaid of retroactive cost-based reimbursement. By agreeing to reimburse hospitals for the actual "reasonable costs" incurred in providing services to patients, plus a share of depreciation and interest, it is argued, the third-party payers have encouraged these hospitals to spend freely—secure in the knowledge that they will get back whatever dollars they put out.

Former DHEW Secretary Caspar W. Weinberger summed up this position when he told the Subcommittee on Health of the House Ways and Means Committee in hearings on June 12, 1975:

> I ... firmly believe that the faulty design of Medicare and Medicaid is the principal culprit responsible for this super inflation in health care costs. The guaranteed government payment of health care costs is virtually any amount submitted by the provider, and with normal market factors absent in the health care area, inflation was bound to happen, and it did.

The third-party payers adopted one type of defense by the provisions of laws or contracts that excluded certain classes of hospital costs, such as bad debts and research, from the allowable cost-reimbursement obligation. Besides the federal wage-price control program, and the Section 223 ceiling limits on Medicare payments, the next major attempt to contain costs through reimbursement has been the move to rate setting. The advantages seemed obvious: if a hospital could know its payment rate before it rendered its services, it would have the highest possible motivation to see that these services were produced in the most efficient manner, since its solvency would depend on keeping its spending within the limits of its anticipated revenues. The hospital would have positive incentives for efficiency as well, since if it could produce its service more cheaply than the predetermined rate had allowed, it could pocket the difference (P. Feldstein, 1968; Waldman, 1968).

Cost savings through improved hospital efficiency was to be the key: the public statements of theoreticians and program designers alike always stress that cost containment from rate setting will never be at the expense of access or quality.

Thus the rationale for cost containment through rate setting rests on several basic assumptions:

- rising costs are importantly associated with inefficiencies in the delivery of hospital services;
- these inefficiencies can be identified, and are amenable to control by hospital trustees and managers, were they to be so motivated;
- a more public and visible process of rate determination, with external review of institutional practices, can provide such motivation;
- those who establish prospective rates will have the skills and information required to calculate rates that will neither underpay nor overpay each individual hospital for the particular mix and quality of products it provides;
- the point at which these rates are set will be sufficiently exact to motivate each hospital to overcome the particular inefficiencies in its own production process and to avoid future actions leading to new inefficiencies, but without affecting patient access or quality of care.

None of these somewhat heroic assumptions appears to have been based on empirical observation of the experience of existing hospital rate regulation programs, such as the Canadian experience during the 1960s, nor the accomplishments of rate setting in improving production efficiency in other industries, such as railroads and public utilities. On the contrary, the rush to hospital rate setting appears to have been almost entirely reactive. To state legislators with their feet to the fire of hospital cost inflation, moving away from retrospective cost-based reimbursement seemed only logical; problems of implementing an alternative system of prospective reimbursement could be dealt with as they arose.

To be sure, most Blue Cross plans, already sensitive to the complexity of the issues surrounding hospital reimbursement, entered the arena more pragmatically. Rate setting seemed an approach worth trying; they would learn how to do it as they went along. But whoever the sponsor, little or no systematic analysis was made to project the magnitude of the benefits to be expected from rate setting, nor were doubts expressed as to the ability of rate setters first to define the "efficient production" of hospital care, second to measure efficiency in relation to the quality of the product, and finally to fashion incentive and risk structures that would induce behavior changes in the actors responsible for creating the inefficiencies. Nor was the possibility of creating perverse, cost-increasing incentives considered.

The Impetus behind Rate Setting

While many of the forces that moved Blue Cross plans and state governments to adopt hospital rate setting were unique to each locality, some were widely shared. They are important to understand, since they shaped the objectives of the ensuing programs.

In regions where hospital cost rises were the most precipitous, they forced corresponding rises in Blue Cross premiums that the plans feared might price them out of their markets. State insurance commissions joined them in anticipating insolvencies if the trend could not be halted. Similarly, governors and legislators in a number of states began to fear that rising hospital costs in Medicaid and other state programs if continued unchecked would bankrupt state treasuries. Meanwhile, constitutents concerned about their taxes were pressing for controls, while constituents who paid their own hospital bills or were insufficiently protected by indemnity-type hospital insurance were pressing for relief.

Hospitals, too, were early backers of the rate-setting concept; their associations were usually active participants in program design. They saw several types of advantages. First, many hospital leaders believed that most of the rises in operating costs were stemming from a multiplicity of conditions genuinely beyond the power of hospital administrators to control. They believed that the external reviewing authorities would discover these facts for themselves once they began to scrutinize the details of operating costs. In the face of the public's concern and resentment, the arguments that hospitals mounted in their own defense appeared self-serving. Were the same arguments to be presented by independent rate-setting bodies, the credibility of hospitals would be enhanced.

The hospitals perceived a second advantage, namely in cash flow. Cost-based reimbursement is characterized by long-delayed retroactive adjustments by third-party payers that often plunge hospitals into fiscal crises; rate setting would allow hospital managers to predict their revenues for future periods and keep payments current with expenditures.

Most important, however, hospital leadership saw rate setting as a possible answer to the problem of cost shifting by major third-party payers. As over the years each payer tried to define ever more narrowly the particular hospital costs it would consider "allowable," expenses for items such as free care and losses from emergency room and outpatient care were falling between the cracks, becoming no one's responsibility. Hospitals were increasingly having to load such expenses on the bills of self-pay patients. The American Hospital Association's 1969 *Statement on the Financial Requirements of Health Care Institutions and Services,* a policy statement advocating elimination of such inequalities, proposed changes in reimbursement methods so that all legitimate hospital costs would be covered fairly by all payers. In subsequent guidelines (AHA, 1972), the association formally accepted the principle that hospital rates be reviewed and set by independent state hospital commissions.

Thus, although the phenomenon of rising costs clearly sparked the move toward rate setting in the 1970s, we find that the major proponents, Blue Cross plans, insurance commissioners, taxpayers, state governments, and hospitals, often had quite different expectations of what rate-setting programs should accomplish. In summary, these diverse objectives included:

- curbing the rate of increase in the *unit price* of services (per diem, billed charges, etc.) for which hospitals would be reimbursed by some *particular class of payer,* such as Blue Cross, Medicaid, self-pay patients;

- curbing the rate of increase in *overall expenditures for hospitalization,* i.e., unit price times volume of service, for which the taxpaying public and insurance subscribers must eventually foot the bill;
- curbing the *shifts of legitimate hospital costs* from one type of payer to another.

Certain national commissions had even broader expectations, seeing rate setting as one component of a broad armamentarium of measures to bring about system changes that would increase not only the cost effectiveness of hospital care but of total health care expenditures (National Advisory Commission on Health Manpower, 1968).

Unfortunately, the methods employed to accomplish any one of these objectives can well block the attainment of other objectives. For example, the hospital's classic answer to criticism of high unit costs is to stimulate more admissions and increased volumes of services. Yet increased volumes (unless accompanied by bed reductions) can easily translate to higher total expenditures for hospital care. Further, if volume increases are obtained by rendering types of care that patients do not in fact need, or could obtain less expensively on an ambulatory basis, the level of cost effectiveness will decline.

Again, to the extent that any single class of payer is successful in minimizing his own share of hospital cost increase, the tendency to shift costs to other payers is encouraged. Conversely, successful fair share efforts will inevitably augment the reimbursement obligations of those payers from whom costs had previously been shifted.

In short, a basic schizophrenia of purpose confuses the efforts of many programs and introduces fundamental problems in the evaluation of their results. However, before further analyzing these and other types of issues associated with hospital rate regulation, it will be helpful to review the major features of the various rate-setting programs functioning in the United States as of the end of 1975.

An Overview of Current Rate-Setting Programs

Blue Cross plans and state governments administer most rate-setting programs; in three localities hospital associations do so. The University of South Carolina is conducting a rate-setting experiment in sixteen hospitals.

Under special contract provision, twenty-two of the nation's seventy-four Blue Cross plans currently negotiate or establish Blue Cross rates or charges for their member hospitals. These plans, listed in Table 1, unless designated as pilot programs, cover virtually all the hospitals in their region or state. Four Blue Cross plans—Indiana, Kentucky, Missouri and North Carolina—establish charge rates that hospitals voluntarily apply to their self-pay as well as to their Blue Cross patients. The Medicare program, under special waivers, accepts the prospective payment rates set by Blue Cross plans in Western Pennsylvania and Rhode Island as well as by the University of South Carolina program.

Nine states have rate-setting laws. The types of agency that perform the function and the types of payers whose rates they cover are shown in Table 2.[2] It will be seen that four states have independent commissions, with a structure roughly similar to that of Maryland's described in the paper by Harold Cohen; five others administer rate setting through some existing state government agency. The unique private-public structure in New York and Rhode Island will be described later.

The unit of payment chosen for control is usually, but not always, that which had been customary for the payer affected. Although the largest number of programs use hospital charges as the payment unit, the per diem unit is used in programs that control the largest number of hospitals. Payment by the case and capitation have been tried only in small experiments involving a few hospitals (Arthur D. Little, 1974c; Sigmond, 1968).

[2]An attentive reader comparing Tables 1 and 2 will discover that Colorado and Connecticut have separate rate-setting programs, administered both by Blue Cross plans and by state government. The Colorado Blue Cross plan covers only a few hospitals; in Connecticut, the two programs are estimated to control about 65 percent of hospital revenues.

TABLE 1   Blue Cross Plans with Rate-Setting or Review Programs as of January 1976[a]

State or Area within State	Name of Blue Cross Plan	Number Short-term General and Other Special Hospitals Covered	% Plan Area Population Enrolled in Blue Cross
Connecticut	Connecticut Blue Cross	40	51
Indiana	Indiana Blue Cross	115	38
Kentucky	Blue Cross Hospital Plan	107	43
Missouri:			
Kansas City area	Blue Cross of Kansas City	57	34
New York:	(under state regulations & approvals)		
New York City	Blue Cross-Blue Shield of N.Y.C.	185	73
Upstate	7 upstate plans; as consortium	140	59
North Carolina[b]	Blue Cross and Blue Shield of N.C.	133	34
Ohio:			
Cincinnati area	Blue Cross of Southwest Ohio	35	59
Oklahoma	Blue Cross and Blue Shield of Oklahoma	40	24
Rhode Island	(with State Office of Budget) Blue Cross of Rhode Island	15	80
Wisconsin	Associated Hospital Service	149	34
Colorado	Colorado Hospital Service	8 (pilot)	36
Michigan	Michigan Hospital Service	12 (pilot)	58
Ohio:			
Cleveland area	Blue Cross of Northeast Ohio	2 (pilot)	56
Pennsylvania:			
Pittsburgh area	Blue Cross of Western Penn.	17 (pilot)	56
Wilkes-Barre area	Blue Cross of Northeastern Penn.	2 (pilot)	57

[a]Blue Cross plans in Delaware and New Mexico also have rate-review and negotiating provisions in their contracts but are not included here because implementation, so far, has been minimal.
[b]Voluntary compliance.
Sources: Communication with Blue Cross Association, January 30, 1976; *Hospital Statistics*, 1975 edition (1974 data from the American Hospital Association Annual Survey), American Hospital Association, Chicago, 1975; Blue Cross Association Enrollment and Utilization Report, third quarter, 1975.

Enabling statutes specify the types of providers and payers whose rates are to be regulated. In most states, the rates of nursing homes as well as those of hospitals are covered. Table 2 shows that the share of total hospital revenues affected by state rate-setting bodies varies considerably; only in Arizona and Rhode Island is the proportion clearly commanding. The absence of control on a

TABLE 2   Hospital Rate-Setting Activities of State Governments as of December 1975

Name of State	Type of State Agency	Number of Hospitals Covered	Type of Payer Rates Currently Regulated	Estimated Share of Hospital Revenue Affected
Arizona[a]	Dept. of Health Services	75	Charges to self-pay patients Blue Cross	85
Colorado	Dept. of Social Services	89	Medicaid	8
Connecticut	Independent commission	40	Charges to self-pay patients	30
Maryland	Independent commission	54	Blue Cross Charges to self-pay patients	55
Massachusetts[b]	Independent commission (full-time commissioners)	133	Medicaid; Charges to self-pay patients & others	45
New Jersey	Dept. of Health with concurrence of Dept. of Insurance	104	Blue Cross Medicaid	55
New York	Dept. of Health with concurrence of Dept. of Insurance; recommendation from Blue Cross plans	320	Medicaid Blue Cross	55
Rhode Island	State Budget Director with R.I. Blue Cross	15	Blue Cross Medicare Medicaid	90
Washington	Independent commission	119	Charges to self-pay patients Workmen's Compensation	50–55

[a]Hospital rate review is mandatory under Arizona law, but compliance is voluntary. (To date there has been almost 100 percent compliance.)
[b]The Massachusetts Rate Setting Commission has approval power over the terms of Blue Cross contracts; since the current contract incorporates controls on charges consonant with the state's charge control law for self-pay patients, the 45 percent figure understates the commission's overall leverage.
Sources: Telephone interviews with state agencies, December 1975; January 1976; *Hospital Statistics*, 1975 edition, American Hospital Association.

hospital's total revenue allows it to make up for an unusually tight rate from one payer by inflating charges to others. The University of South Carolina's sixteen-hospital experiment is the only place where the rates set cover 100 percent of the payers.

In a later section we will review some of the principal cost-containment targets and the mechanisms these programs have developed for reviewing hospital costs and budgets and for projecting rates. First, however, we will discuss certain questions of structure and organization that affect their administrative feasibility and limit or strengthen their power.

Who Sets the Rates?

Successful implementation of a hospital review and rate-setting system requires that there be a sound legal or contractual mandate, an effective organizational base, adequate resources of budget and staff, power to enforce decisions, and a feasible and appropriate rate-setting and appeals process. In most of these matters the issue of who sets the rates is crucial.

Issues Surrounding Rate Setting by State Governments

The clear legal authority given by state legislatures to regulate hospital rates, together with the statement of purpose that usually prefaces such laws, obviously provides a far stronger framework for regulation than do the voluntary contractual arrangements of the Blue Cross plans. The message is clear to all parties that action must and will be taken, and that it will continue over time.

The place within the structure of state government where the rate-setting responsibilities are placed is important, although it will not be discussed at length, since what may be most appropriate depends heavily on the particular history of organizational relationships within each state. Hospital associations prefer the independent commission model. They object on principle to having any one of the major third-party payers, such as a state department administering Medicaid, given the responsibility for setting rates, claiming that for a major purchaser of service to determine the price at which it buys that service constitutes a clear conflict of interest (AHA, 1972).

The case for rate-setting commissions is also made on grounds of independence from the direct political interference to which regular agencies of state government are usually exposed. Such independence, of course, also complicates the process of public accountability unless there is an accompanying public disclosure law.

In states with large numbers of hospitals, rate-setting responsibilities appear to demand full-time, well-paid commissioners; so far only the Massachusetts law provides them. The composition of commission membership is obviously important to both its acceptance and its effectiveness. Systematic analysis of what constitutes desirable numbers, types, and proportions of consumer and provider representation has yet to be made.

The commission structure predisposes toward certain problems in the rate-setting and appeal process. John Dunlop, the former Secretary of Labor, commenting on regulation in other types of industries, recently cited two of these (Dunlop, 1975). First, the traditional regulatory approach discourages the posture of negotiation; the rule-making and adjudicatory procedures prescribed in administrative practice laws militate against the development of mutual accommodation among conflicting interests. Second, the regulatory process

. . . involves legal game-playing between the regulatees and the regulators; the tax law is a classic example, but it is typical of regulatory programs in general. The regulatory agency promulgates a regulation; the regulatees challenge it in court; if they lose, their lawyers may seek another round for administrative or judicial challenge.

Meanwhile time passes—the regulatory lag. And legal services become one more factor in hospital costs. The stakes in legal battles are high, particularly during the first few years of a new regulatory commission's life, since the case precedents that are set will set the limits on its future activities. It is not improbable to suppose that more time and skills may be devoted to beating the system in the courts than are devoted to improving efficiency in the hospitals.

Placement of the rate-setting function within an established state agency may provide more flexibility. If that agency also has concurrent responsibilities for other regulatory functions affecting hospitals, such as licensing, inspections, planning, and certificate of need, such placement should minimize duplications of hospital reporting requirements and avoid regulations written at cross purposes. Most important, a centralizing of regulatory functions should force the agency to formulate some coherent overall health policy and regulatory strategy for the jurisdiction it covers. In such a context, rate setting could become an effective tool for coordinated policy implementation, particularly if such an agency also sought to forge links to PSROs for utilization and quality controls and to Health Systems Agencies for planning (Dowling and Teague, 1975).

Opportunities for synergism through the concentration of regulatory powers may be more apparent than real, however, since problems of noncommunication and bureaucratic rivalry can impede coordination among the separate offices within a single large agency almost as effectively as they do among the offices of separate agencies. For example, the 1975 Moreland Commission exposed an almost total lack of interchange between the nursing home inspection and the rate-setting divisions of the New York State Department of Health (New York State Moreland Act Commission, 1975).

Wherever the rate-setting function may be located within state government, certain endemic problems are likely to handicap its effective implementation. One is the familiar bricks-without-straw phenomenon, where state legislatures pass laws that require state agencies to perform new functions, but fail to pass the budgets that are needed for proper implementation. This was dramatically illustrated in New Jersey in 1971 where an unusually well-drafted law centralized a host of health regulatory functions, including hospital rate setting, in the State Department of Health—with no new funding (Somers, 1973). In consequence, for two years the department was able to assign only one full-time staff member to carry the rate-review responsibilities for New Jersey's 104 hospitals.

Currently, programs that promise to contain hospital costs have sufficiently high political visibility to make extreme underbudgeting of this kind unusual, but even now most state rate-setting executives feel severely handicapped by budget constraints. As noted in the paper by Cohen, the Maryland commission, after eighteen months of operation, has not yet been able to conduct rate reviews of all the Maryland hospitals. Looking ahead, with many state governments entering severe fiscal crises, one cannot be sanguine about funding continuity even at present levels.[3]

Another set of endemic problems arises from state civil service regulations governing job classifications, salary scales, recruitment, examinations, and promotions. In many instances these seem almost programmed to discourage the employment of rate-setting staff with capabilities to carry out the complex and important responsibilities with which they are charged. It is a tribute to the devotion and imagination of rate-setting program administrators that they manage as well as they do. However, most of the leaders in state rate-setting bodies today are unusual people, attracted by the challenge offered for developing programs in a new and important regulatory area. It is doubtful that many current incumbents will want to be at these same posts five years hence, and that replacements of the same caliber will be available. Again, looking to the future, one must speculate whether there is anything intrinsic to hospital rate regulation that is apt to make its long-run core staffing prospects much different from any other type of state regulatory body.

Even though state legislatures grant formal authority to rate-setting bodies, there are very real political constraints on the amount of power these bodies can actually exercise. If their actions prove to be sufficiently unpopular, laws can be changed, or already slim appropriations further cut. As the history of community battles over certificate of need has so well documented, constituents of legislators are markedly ambivalent about their community hospitals: they want costs to be controlled overall, but at the same time, they want their own hospital to be fully equipped and staffed to give them the care they need at the moment they need it. By the same token, they fight proposals for service closings.

---

[3]Rate-setting commissions can, if their enabling law permits, raise the revenue for their operations from special assessments on hospitals, which can then include them as costs allowable for reimbursement. This type of arrangement, endorsed by the AHA Guidelines, is criticized by some legislators because it removes the public accountability of the rate-setting body. One way out is to have assessments support the program but flow through a special state fund which can be used only with the approval of the legislature.

The problem appears to be common to other types of regulatory bodies as well. Noll, in a Brookings Institution report on regulation (1971), observes:

One measure of success of the [regulatory] agency is continued operation of the regulated sector. Widespread service failure is likely to be blamed on the agency, and is therefore to be avoided even if the cost exceeds the costs of the service failure.

Finally, there is the familiar problem of the capture of regulatory agencies by the industries they regulate. Noll offers the following explanations of this phenomenon:

There is little political gain in effective regulation. Once a regulatory agency has been established to deal with an issue of public concern, public attention is apt to shift to new issues. While the stake of the public may still be high, it is diffused.

[However] . . . most regulatory issues remain of continuing deep interest to the regulated industry. Its economic viability may rest on the agency decisions. The industry's motivation to fight unfavorable decisions is very high. . . .

[A] . . . measure of success is the failure of the courts or the legislature to override agency decisions on either procedural or substantive grounds. An agency that tries to minimize the chance of being overruled must, when the interests of the regulated firm and the public are at odds, be overly responsive to the interests of the regulated. It wants to be sure it cannot legitimately be accused of being unfair to the groups that are most likely to challenge its decisions.

According to this observer, whether the agency is independent or located in the executive branch of the government, or whether it is headed by a single administrator or is collegial, does not seriously affect its essentially pro-industry proclivities in the long run (Noll, 1971).

Hospital associations, however, sensitive to the political climate, usually recognize the importance of efficiency objectives to a greater extent than do their individual hospital members. Even if regulatory policy is dominated by the industry, Ginsburg observes (1975), this difference in perspective should result in a lower price than if there were no regulation.

Blue Cross Programs

Programs administered by Blue Cross have two large advantages over those administered by state government: they can usually command the budget, staff, and computer resources they feel to be necessary to implement their rate-review processes in an equitable manner, and they can be more flexible in the rate-setting processes they design. Program costs are paid for out of subscriber premiums. As long as the plan's board of trustees is satisfied that the program is cost effective, funding will continue. Furthermore, because Blue Cross programs are not subject to the job classification restraints of civil service, they can attract to their rate-review staffs people with intimate knowledge and understanding of hospital operations, such as ex-hospital controllers and accountants, who know what areas of inefficiency to look for and who can successfully defend their decisions during appeals. Finally, Blue Cross programs have much more flexibility than state programs. They are free to design rate-setting processes that incorporate various mixes of educational, negotiational, and formalistic approaches, and to modify these approaches over time in the light of subsequent evaluation.

On the other hand, the Blue Cross programs labor under their own special handicaps. In most states, participation is entirely voluntary; hospitals may decide not to participate at all. Or, once participating, if they feel the program is too strict, they may withdraw. (They have rarely done so, but this may only reflect their best guesses as to likely alternatives.) Second, lacking a legal mandate for their programs, Blue Cross plans may not be able to secure all the types of data they might wish from the hospitals on which to base their rate decisions. Finally, they are likely to receive scant recognition from their subscribers for their efforts. As with other types of cost-containment efforts by Blue Cross plans, the costs of running such programs inevitably appear in larger administrative budgets—making the plans open to charges of "inefficiency" by critics and competitors who assume no such responsibilities.

The Model of a Mixed Public-Private Structure

Since Blue Cross and state government rate-setting programs each have certain specific strengths and weaknesses, the possibility of their cooperation in carrying out rate-setting responsibilities offers an attractive alternative. In this model, the legal authority for hospital rate setting and for the securing of necessary data on which to base rate decisions comes from state laws, but the limited staff and budget usually available to state government agencies can be augmented by sharing implementation responsibilities with Blue Cross, which can bring a more appropriate level of resources to the task. This type of complementary activity is currently taking place in three of the nine states with rate-setting laws.

In Massachusetts, Blue Cross auditors are regularly detailed to work in the state rate-setting commission office to supplement the core staff; they review hospital costs reports and conduct a large proportion of the commission's hospital audits. In New York state, the Department of Health establishes the regulations that determine the rate-setting process for Blue Cross as well as for Medicaid, promulgates standard hospital reporting forms, and makes final decisions on all rates and rate appeals. But the department permits the eight Blue Cross plans to conduct their own analyses of member hospitals' costs and submit recommendations on future Blue Cross rates for member hospitals.

In Rhode Island, under state law the state director of the budget has final authority to approve hospital budgets, but Rhode Island Blue Cross staff conducts most of the analyses on which the budget negotiations are based. The Budget Office has access to all such analyses, as well as to the data on which they are based, and thus needs only a small staff with which to conduct monitoring activities and special studies. The budget director's staff representative participates in hospital budget negotiations side by side with Blue Cross officials.

These sorts of partnerships may serve to diffuse the heat of possible opposition to tough rate-setting decisions that might well weaken or destroy either of the partners were they to act singly. On the other hand, political risks always attend a state government agency's dependence on outside technical assistance.

Having noted these various types of structural constraints on currently operating rate-setting programs, let us examine their objectives and the mechanisms they employ to pursue them.

Rate-Setting Objectives and Processes

We saw earlier that third-party payers, legislators, and hospitals have looked to hospital rate setting as a means to accomplish different purposes. In the interest of space, we will not consider here the hospitals' goal of achieving fair share payments by third-party payers, but will confine our discussion to the goals of containing increases in hospital prices and of containing increases in overall expenditures for hospitalization without attendant sacrifice of access or quality.

The central issue is how to set rates in a manner that will neither underpay nor overpay, but will encourage each institution to increase the efficiency with which its services are provided. One overriding obstacle to accomplishing this is lack of any reliable way to define or measure the efficiency of most patient care services of hospitals. Another lies in the large number of hospitals to be regulated and their great diversity in patient mix; case severity mix; medical staff training levels; scope and quality of services; size, age, and characteristics of physical plant and equipment; financial reserves and endowments, and so on. So far, as we have already noted, many of these basic types of data are either not available or not used. Even when the required data become available, it will be some time before techniques to weigh and correlate the differences among hospitals are sufficiently refined to permit reliable judgments as to whether given levels of costs are justifiable or whether they reflect inefficiencies.

Thus, most rate-setting bodies must carry out their mandates to contain costs with few clearly defined notions of where specific spending excesses may lie. The tripartite mission of many hospitals—teaching and research as well as patient care—serves further to complicate their task. Finally, rates must be set in the realistic context of whether hospitals can, in fact, control many types of costs that rate setters may identify as unjustifiable. They soon come to recognize, for example, the very limited power of hospital administrators and trustees to change the cost-inducing behavior of their physicians.

These general problems underlie the rate setters' choice both of operational objectives and of the rate-review processes they employ.

Specific Cost Containment Objectives

The objectives to be pursued by rate-setting programs are usually set forth in state enabling laws and as part of preambles to Blue Cross contracts or contract amendments. Characteristically they state that:

- rates (or budgets, or charges) should be related to the efficient production of hospital services of good quality;
- excess hospital costs that may be associated with duplications of services and facilities should be discouraged.

Several also provide that:

- increases in hospital rates should be linked to increases in the prices of goods and services in the general economy.

Only in the 1975 Rhode Island experimental program under a Social Security Administration contract are rates set within the limits of some overall ceiling on an increase of total expenditures for hospital care in a geographic region. The rate-setting program and the hospital association arrive at the percentage figure for this statewide maxi-cap annually, through a strenuous process of negotiation some months before the hospitals submit their budgets for review. Subsequently, the reviewers negotiate each hospital's budget within the limit of the total increase—with the freedom to give higher increases to some and lower to others. Here, for the first time in the United States, rate-setting bodies are being forced to make choices in cost allocations among hospitals, rather than considering each case entirely on its own merits in an open-ended situation.

State rate-setting bodies usually have considerable latitude in translating the broadly stated objectives of enabling legislation into regulations and guidelines that either implicitly or explicitly specify particular targets for cost containment. Such regulations usually state certain intermediate rate-setting goals and set out mechanisms for achieving them that appear to be politically, administratively, and technically feasible in the context of their local environment. Blue Cross contract provisions, on the other hand, usually specify objectives explicitly and spell out the rate-setting process in full detail.

Almost all programs try to hold down capital costs through cooperation with certificate-of-need programs; their own major program efforts focus on the control of operating costs. Targets for cost containment usually include one or more of the following, in descending order of frequency:

- control of *increments to interest and depreciation* from unapproved facility construction or expansions;
- control of *increments to operating costs* from new medical programs, additions to personnel and supplies in existing programs and services, expanded fringe benefits, contracted services, and so on;
- encouragement of *improved management*, better internal budget and control systems;
- encouragement of the *phasing out of underutilized beds and services*;
- detection of *inefficiencies in base costs*, particularly in the hotel and support service departments;
- identification and *reduction of departmental cross-subsidies.*

Rate-setting programs may or may not explicitly spell out such target objectives. Often, their actual goals must be ascertained from interviews with program executives, from analysis of regulations or rate-review guidelines, and from observation of the rate-review process. Furthermore, there appear to be considerable differences in the intensity with which these various goals are actually pursued.

The types of containment *not* pursued through rate setting should also be noted. Only Rhode Island's program attempts to identify and reduce excessive lengths of patient stay. With this single exception, none of the programs uses its rate-setting power to reduce hospitalization costs that might be associated with inappropriate patient care management such as unnecessary surgery, unnecessary tests or drugs, or delays in treatment scheduling. Nor do the programs adjust rates to reward quality controls that minimize the extra hospital costs associated with complications resulting from hospital infections, from drug synergisms, or from other iatrogenic conditions. Again, although most program executives privately deplore the often six-digit remuneration of hospital-based physicians such as radiologists and pathologists, in this area too, controls are rarely attempted.

In short, as noted at the outset, rate setting rarely attempts to influence the huge segment of hospital costs generated by physician actions.

Scant effort is made through rate structure to promote hospital-based alternatives to inpatient care—such as day surgery units, home care programs, or preadmission testing. Widespread introduction of such services, designed to reduce overall expenditures for hospitalization and overall medical costs would, of course, force up the per diem or other unit costs for the more complex cases still more for the seriously ill patients requiring acute care inpatient services. If the rate-setting body is evaluated according to its success in moderating increases in unit prices, over the course of time such action would be counterproductive in terms of its own institutional viability.

Methods of Determining Rates

There is no established wisdom to guide hospital rate setting. Most programs are still struggling to develop a satisfactory process; they make changes in their methods almost yearly. Basically, however, in every program next year's hospital rates will in one way or another be based on this year's rates; modifications of natural trends will be relatively modest. No program starts the rate-setting process with the concept of zero budgeting.

Rate setters reach their decisions in one of a number of ways:

- special reviews of the costs, budgets, and volume of each individual hospital in the light of its own characteristics;

- interinstitutional comparisons;
- rate increases tied to movement of economic indicators;
- recommendations of planning agencies;
- some combination of these methods.

In all but a few programs rates are set annually, for all hospitals, either as of a given calendar date or at the beginning of the hospital's fiscal year.

Cost-Budget Reviews   The Blue Cross and hospital association programs tend to establish rates on the basis of cost and budget reviews that focus primarily on cost trends within the individual hospital. Reviews usually include line-item scrutiny of all budgeted additions to facilities, services, and personnel, and close analyses of cost trends in each hospital department. This rate-setting method reflects in part the preferences of hospitals, in part the belief that a strenuous but equitable review process itself serves to make hospital officials more cost conscious, to force the setting of internal priorities for expansion requests, and to motivate hospital managers to improve their own budgeting and to exercise better internal controls. Once the reviews have been conducted and budgets or rates approved, the hospital is usually free to make budget transfers within the bottom line amount. Most programs try to avoid infringing on management prerogatives.

Interhospital Comparisons   State programs tend to rely heavily on interinstitutional comparisons. Adopting one or another method of classifying hospitals into comparison groups, they perform analyses by service, department, and/or cost center. Employing screening methods, these analyses identify statistical outliers of preestablished parameters around the mean or median of each hospital group. Most programs then individually review the more costly outlier hospitals or hospital departments, giving opportunity for justification before establishing the final rates. Others, notably the New York state programs, automatically adjust the rates of outlier hospitals downward to the preestablished ceiling[4] (Bauer and Clark, 1974d).

---

[4] New York does not ask for budget projections from the hospitals. It calculates future rates solely on the basis of cost trends from the prior to the current year, and pro-

The same types of information are used for individual reviews and interinstitutional comparisons, although each program has designed its own report requirements to suit its own objectives and methods. Hospitals submit annually some type of uniform cost and budget report to the reviewing agency. At a minimum, this includes general statistical and financial descriptors of the hospital and counts and projections of its activity measures (patient days, clinic visits, and so on). At a maximum, the report may include detailed descriptors of medical staff, teaching programs, scope of services, contracts and leases, long-term capital budgets. The report packages run from twelve to forty-eight pages of schedules. As of December 1975, only one program (again, Rhode Island) sought any patient-related information on case mix or the age or sex of the patients for whom the hospital was caring. This program obtains standard reports derived from abstracts of the records of all patients discharged from Rhode Island hospitals each year, using the Professional Activities Study report system.

Limiting Rate Increases to the Rate of Inflation The New York, Massachusetts, and Western Pennsylvania programs explicitly tie hospital rate increases in allowable costs to corresponding wage and price trends in the general economies of their regions. Elaborate indices have been designed for use in making projections. Automatic adjustments are usually made at quarterly or six-month intervals during the rate year, to adjust the rates to the actual movement of the designated economic indicators. During the early years of the two New York programs affecting New York City hospitals, adjustments for underprojections were not routinely made. This was one of the several contributing causes of their widespread fiscal distress, documented by Rossman (Hospital Association of New York State, 1975).

Most of the other programs, while not employing formal economic projection indices, informally adopt some rule-of-thumb percentage increase in rate that they will consider to be reasonable in their budget reviews for the coming year, a target that serves the

jected inflation rates. Massachusetts employs this type of formula to set its Medicaid rates, but employs different methods to control charges for self-pay patients.

same purpose but that is more flexible. Hospitals that are dissatisfied may request special cost and budget reviews based on interinstitutional comparisons.

Increments to Operating Costs Budget increments for operating costs due to changes in facilities or services during the prospective rate year can be easily identified through the use of appropriately designed reporting forms. The problem lies in determining, on a line-item basis, whether or not the proposed new expenditures are necessary. Programs that conduct individual hospital reviews reach these decisions before setting the hospital's rates; in a formula system, they are reached after the rates have been set, through individual hospital appeals. In either case, decisions must ultimately be reached on the basis of subjective judgment of the reviewers. The process is almost always time-consuming and fraught with emotion, and is the source of the greatest tension between the parties at interest.

Decisions on adding to the rate the cost of interest and depreciation for new facilities are usually left to planning agencies; if a certificate of need or formal approval is forthcoming, the rate-setting agency usually agrees to make the necessary rate adjustment. Since in many areas the effectiveness of planning agency reviews is questionable, such controls are often more apparent than real. Some rate-setting programs, however, notably those of Washington, New York, and Rhode Island, work in close collaboration with planning agencies in mutually reinforcing arrangements (Bauer and Altman, 1975).

A few programs, such as Maryland's, reserve the right to make independent determinations on capital expansions, arguing that even though a community need for an additional hospital facility or service may have been found to exist, the capability to pay for it through the reimbursement rate may not. In such cases, the community and the hospital must raise the operating funds for the added service in addition to the necessary capital.

The New York state program is particularly stringent in regard to new services and facilities. In general, its formula for rate projection adjusts *only* for wage and price increases, except when new costs are authorized after a process of formal appeals. This assumes that the identical hospital product is to be produced in 1977 as was produced in 1970, when the cost control program began.[5] Even when appeals for changes in facilities or services are granted, since rate projections in New York are based solely on historical costs rather than budgets, support for a new program will not be fully included in the rate until several years have elapsed. In Massachusetts no new operating costs are recognized for one full year. Such refusals to subsidize start-up costs also discourage expansions.

Identifying Out-of-Line Costs in the Base Year Most rate-setting programs are fully aware that simply projecting a hospital's base costs forward to construct future rates provides license for the indefinite perpetuation of existing inefficiencies. A weakness of rate-setting methods that rely on statistical screens to identify hospitals for special review is that they have no means to detect inefficiencies in the hospitals that fall within their allowed cost parameters: that is, they assume that low costs are equated with efficiency rather than other factors such as case mix, quality differences, or exogenous factors. Individual budget reviews offer more possibilities, but most reviewers admit that with the kinds and quality of data and analytic tools presently available to them, their power to detect all but grossly out-of-line situations is severely limited. Only the university sponsored program in South Carolina employs industrial engineering consultants to work with hospitals to identify and correct specific areas of low productivity. (In both rate-setting and nonrate-setting states, however, individual hospitals are, on their own, increasingly using management science consultants to improve internal operating efficiency.)

Phase-Outs of Underutilized Beds and Services A number of programs try to attack the problem of continued low occupancy. Some, like those in Massachusetts and New York, impose rate penalties when average occupancy rates fall below preestablished minimum levels, for example, 80 percent for medical-surgical, 70 percent for pediatrics, and 60 percent for obstetric services. By establishing rates that fail to subsidize excess costs from underutili-

[5]Blue Cross plans in upstate New York, however, include a factor to allow for changes associated with new technology.

zation, they hope to encourage appropriate bed reductions. Other programs try to achieve this purpose indirectly through their inter-hospital comparisons of unit costs, to identify services where utilization is low but staffing remains high. To detect these kinds of inefficiencies requires that the true unit costs of direct services be compared. As the Maryland experience illustrates, this means that for purposes of the analysis, at least, the traditional cross-subsidization of services within hospitals, whereby revenues from departments like the laboratory make up losses from departments like the emergency room, must be eliminated. Also, direct costs are isolated for comparisons before indirect cost allocations are made.

Some Obstacles to Achieving Cost Containment with Equity

As we have seen in the foregoing section, the several different types of processes used in rate setting employ different types of methodologies and demand different types of information.

To reach decisions on new facilities and new medical programs requires guidelines and supporting data for determining community need, and reliable methods for projecting the capital and future operating costs attendant on hospital expansions. These problems are dealt with elsewhere in this volume.

To tie future hospital rates directly to the movements of wages and prices in the general economy of an area requires the development of an economic index constructed of items selected and weighed to reflect the particular types and mix of labor and supply items hospitals use to produce their services, and reliable data reported at frequent intervals for small areas. Although technical difficulties surround each of these tasks, the early 1970s have witnessed considerable progress (Gort et al., 1975; Berger and Sullivan, 1975). A major block to further refinement is the lack of Bureau of Labor Statistics wage and salary data for small geographic areas, since important variations in these factors may exist even within the boundaries of counties and of metropolitan areas. Inequities in projections that are inevitable during periods of rapid inflation can be compensated for by quarterly or six-month adjustments in rates during the prospective year. Unexpected factors over which hospitals have no control, such as the recent rise in malpractice insurance premiums and in fuel prices, can also be handled by periodic across-the-board rate adjustments.

The major problem with tying rate increases to inflation increases is that the mechanism does nothing to improve hospital operating efficiency. On the contrary, unless linked to a hospital review process as in the Western Pennsylvania Blue Cross plan, it protects and perpetuates any existing inefficiencies by projecting their costs into the future. At the same time, such formula projections make no allowance for innovations that may contain or reduce long-term episodes of illness and thus case costs if such innovations demand short-term expenditures that drive up the unit costs of particular types of patient services. Again, however, a sensitive review and appeals process, though cumbersome, can mitigate this danger.

Occupancy minimums designed to encourage hospitals to phase out underutilized services or effect mergers with other hospital services are easy to promulgate. But any hospital service reduction generates strong resistance by physicians since their livelihood may depend on continued access to that hospital. Therefore, unless utilization minimums are accompanied by moves toward opening up staff privileges and by regular feedbacks from effective utilization reviews, physicians can respond by ordering unnecessary volumes of care in order to avoid ceiling penalties. Again, the program may be able to demonstrate success in moderating unit prices, but the defensive actions taken may serve to increase the community's total expenditures for hospital care.

Whether the kinds of *indirect penalties on underutilization*, such as Maryland's, will work better remains to be seen. Much still remains to be learned about the complex art of volume prediction and volume adjustment; it is an area where hospitals can play many types of defensive games. In general, hospitals whose unit costs rise because of uncontrollable shortfalls from the predicted volume eventually obtain rate adjustments; those whose unit costs decline because of volume increases up to the limits of allowable parameters (if any), benefit.

To assess hospital efficiency calls for enormous leaps forward from where we stand today in our methodological capabilities.

Individual budget reviews, while offering important possibilities for achieving desired kinds of change in hospitals, are usually criticized for lacking objectivity, since decisions are reached on an ad hoc "best judgment" basis. Hospitals that can muster the accountants and physicians to plan an effective case, it is argued, have unfair advantage. However, the same criticism holds for the special reviews given to outlier hospitals identified by statistical screens. It also applies to the large volume of hospital appeals under a formula rate projection such as New York's. This is because rate setters under any method of review lack reliable standard performance measures on which to base their decisions. In the end, the reviewers must reach their decisions according to the plausibility of each particular case on the basis of the best evidence they can muster.

The lack of performance standards by which to measure hospital efficiency is the most intractable problem in rate-setting methodology. Most programs during their first years hopefully set out to develop such standards to guide them in setting rates that are "reasonably related to the efficient provision of hospital services of good quality." However, if one accepts a definition of "efficiency" to mean using the most economical, timely, and efficacious mix of labor, materials, and skills to generate a particular product of a given quality, the inherent problems these rate setters face in trying to develop standards become clear.

First, in the patient care services of hospitals it is usually impossible to identify, much less quantify, the actual product that is being produced, that is, specific degrees of improvements in health status and/or alleviation of suffering of the patients who come to the hospital for care. Even were these products to be defined, it is far from clear in many instances just what types, mixes, and timing of labor, materials, and skill inputs are efficacious in producing them (Cochrane, 1972). Finally, as we noted earlier, whatever monitoring of quality does exist, such as through medical audits and PSRO studies, is not reported to rate-setting bodies. Thus rate setters find themselves reduced to using surrogate measures of product, of process, and of quality—such as "patient days," "number of tests," and "accreditation"—measures whose inadequacies have long since been demonstrated (Berki, 1972; Haggerty, 1974; Rutstein, 1974). The pervasive temptation for rate setters simply to equate low cost per unit of service with "efficient production of hospital services of good quality" is only too understandable.

Lacking the ability to develop performance standards for patient care services, and reluctant to impinge on physician prerogatives, rate setters often content themselves with trying to control the more peripheral types of costs that are incurred in the hotel and maintenance departments of the hospital. Even here, however, few reliable performance standards exist. Again, the output measures are widely agreed to be unsatisfactory (Bauer, 1975). For example, when reviewers detect twofold differences between two hospitals' housekeeping costs per square foot, they may have spotted genuinely inefficient deployment of resources in the high-cost institution—but on the other hand, closer examination may reveal that the spread in costs reflects only differences in architectural layout, in building construction, and in traffic volumes. Management studies in individual hospital departments can indeed spot areas of inefficiency and develop standards that may point the way to savings (Hardwick and Wolfe, 1972). On the other hand, substantial cost containment from rates adjusted according to preestablished regionwide performance measures has yet to be demonstrated (Wolf, 1973; Elnicki, 1975).

Attempts to identify hospital inefficiencies by using interhospital comparisons have been fraught with several other types of difficulties. First, because of the wide diversity of hospitals, it is difficult to identify the key variables and to account properly for them in making comparisons. Second, both the scope and quality of the information reported from hospitals leave much to be desired.

For rate-setting programs that rely on comparative analysis to screen for inefficiency, *equitable selection of the comparison hospitals is essential.* There are various classification schemes by which to group hospitals (Bauer, 1974b). Most use only very crude variables such as size, urban versus nonurban location, and teaching status. This leads to considerable debate and special pleading during individual hospital reviews, as each institution brings forth data to show the many important respects in which it differs from its comparison group hospitals. In formula-type processes it leads to large volumes of appeals and lawsuits. Considerable refinement of grouping systems has been made in recent years, however. Some systems classify hospitals on the basis of detailed data on a few key variables, such as complexity of hospital services (Berry, 1973) or service complexity plus numbers and types of teaching programs (Shuman et al., 1972). The Shuman and Wolfe system has been successfully employed by the Blue Cross of Western Pennsylvania for several years.

Another approach, developed by J. Phillips at the American Hospital Association, captures and weighs a large number of both exogenous and endogenous variables through cluster analysis. A version of this more sophisticated grouping method is currently being used to group the 119 hospitals in the Washington State Hospital Cost Commission's program (Baker, 1975).

No rate-setting program yet classifies hospitals directly according to the complexity of the medical problems with which they deal.

Lack of patient-related data is the most serious single deficiency in the information available to rate setters. Without access to diagnostic case mix and operative procedure profiles, they risk the continual danger of setting rates too high for hospitals whose work demands low levels of input and of setting rates too low for tertiary care institutions. With the advent of patient discharge abstract data that must be generated for use by PSROs, this lack may soon be at least partially remediable. The New Jersey and the Maryland rate-setting programs plan to use such data to factor case mix into their rate decisions as soon as possible (Thompson et al., 1975).

Taking the methodology of case-mix analysis from the stage of research to application in rate setting will be difficult, however (Rafferty, 1971; Lave and Lave, 1971; Feldstein and Schuttinga, 1975). Diagnosis per se does not adequately reflect work-load demands in hospitals—the real problem lies in finding measures of case complexity. Few classification schemes to measure differences in patients' requirements for care that can be related to costs have yet been developed, although work is in progress (Diggs and Easter, 1974; Thompson et al., 1975; Cooney, 1974). In the absence of better measures, most programs take the teaching status of hospitals as a gross surrogate for both case mix and case complexity. Some, as already noted, also use complexity of services and composition of medical staff.[6]

Finally, *the quality of the cost and activities data* that rate-setting bodies receive in reports from hospitals is notoriously weak. Although the rate-setting bodies design standard schedules on which the data is to be reported, lack of uniform accounting and reporting practices in the hospitals usually make the resultant figures useless for comparative analysis. This problem, discussed in William Cleverley's paper, not only results in honest confusion, but offers able hospital controllers wide scope to exercise skills in "reimbursement accounting."

In a noteworthy exception to this general rule, the California Health Facilities Commission has over a considerable number of years developed first a detailed uniform accounting system, then a uniform reporting system, and finally a uniform budgeting system, each with very detailed accompanying manuals. Hospitals began to use the system for the first time in 1975. The states of Washington and Arizona have adopted the same system with slight modifications. While it is too soon to know what effects these systems will have on the quality of the data reported by the hospitals, it illustrates that progress is being made in a difficult and important area. Finally, under Section 1533(d) of P.L. 93-641 (the National Health Planning and Resources Development Act), the Department of Health, Education, and Welfare is charged with developing uniform accounting and reporting systems for the nation's hospitals. Criteria to guide such development have been formulated (Bauer, 1975), and work is under way.

In summary, the techniques for setting rates that will serve to contain hospital costs yet be equitable to both the public and the provider are still quite primitive. However, serious developmental efforts are being made to improve them.

---

[6]Lave and Lave (1971) found that institutional characteristics of size, teaching status, and a number of advanced services explained only about 25 percent to 45 percent of the variation in their case-mix measures and thus concluded that these could not be considered good surrogates.

Risks and Incentives

The degree of risk inherent in any program depends largely on the equity of its rate-setting process, the tightness of its rates, and the hospital's ability to secure additional revenue—whether from payers whose rates or charges are uncontrolled, from increased volume, or from favorable adjustments and appeals. As we have noted, all these factors vary considerably from one program to the next— depending on particular laws, regulations, or contract provisions.

A closer examination allows us to distinguish two quite separate types of risks: those to which the hospitals are deliberately exposed by the program to encourage them to contain costs, and those to which both hospitals and rate setters are unintentionally exposed from malfunctioning of the rate-setting process itself.

Deliberate Risks

The overall rationale for rate setting, as we have seen, is to put the hospital at risk for living within a rate calculated at a point that will discourage inefficient operation but that will meet the hospital's financial requirements for continuing to produce services at previous levels of quality and access.

If a given rate-setting methodology is sufficiently sophisticated to permit reviewers to identify the extent of excess costs stemming from inefficiencies in hospital operation, such as failure to adjust staffing to swings in occupancy, the presence of expensive "sweetheart" contracts with relatives of investor-owned hospital proprietors (or nonprofit hospital trustees), or failure to phase out underutilized services, rate adjustments can impose financial hardships on that hospital if it fails to mend its ways. Unless it can make up the rate difference from other revenue sources, the hospital will have to cut out its inefficiencies; the cost-containment objectives of the program will be achieved.

In real life, however, sources of inefficiency are rarely so clear cut, and, as we have seen, the reviewers have only limited means to detect them. In particular, with the present state of the rate-setting art, reviewers will discover many "out-of-line" situations, but hospitals will be able to explain most of them away. They will usually be able to show that their outlying costs have resulted from incomplete or unreliable data used in the rate reviewers' comparative analyses, or be able to point to real differences in patient mix, resource complexity, service quality, or one of many more legitimate explanatory variables. In consequence, most rate-review bodies after a few years of bloodletting experience devote most of their attention to limiting increments to hospital costs rather than to the much more difficult task of detecting on-going inefficiencies in the base of these costs.

Risks from an Inadequate Rate-Setting Process

The limitations of rate-setting methodology put both hospitals and rate setters at risk. First, and most obvious, the rate may underpay some hospitals, failing to meet their financial requirements for rendering services without detriment to the quality of or the access to proper patient care. This danger may be more apparent than real, however, since safeguards are usually available. A program's adjustment and appeals process is, of course, the principal means of mitigating the effects of inequitable rates. Some third-party payers such as Connecticut Blue Cross offer risk-sharing arrangements. They agree to make up some fixed percentage of a hospital's loss if its actual costs turn out to exceed its revenues from the prospectively established rates; in turn, the hospital agrees to share any savings that it might accrue under the rate. Other programs, such as those of Maryland and Indiana, allow hospitals to request rate increases at any time, rather than, as in most programs, confining reopenings to fiscal year endings. Finally, rate setters often informally sweeten the rate for a hospital's next rate year to make up for any justifiable losses in the prior year. In short, most programs employ a variety of means to relieve the plight of the hospital that can demonstrate that it is genuinely underpaid because of some weakness in the rate-setting process.

The risk of *overpaying* hospitals is equally real, but seldom discussed. Setting rates that are too high in relation to the type, quality, and appropriateness of services rendered brings cost consequences to the rate-setting program and the public that are especially serious because they are likely to remain undetected.

While the underpaid hospital can be counted on to make its case heard, offering a chance for rectification, the hospital that is overpaid through the processes of an inequitable system can be guaranteed to be silent. Common examples of overpayment are found in:

- hospitals with a less complex case mix than that of comparison group hospitals;
- hospitals whose case mix becomes progressively less complex over time;
- hospitals that were inefficiently operated when the rate-setting program began and thus started with an excessively high rate base;
- hospitals where the quality of care deteriorates;
- hospitals that deliberately inflate volumes of admissions, tests, procedures, patient days beyond what patients need in order to achieve low unit costs and thus avoid being caught as outliers in interhospital cost comparisons.

One can only speculate as to whether the cost savings effected from rate reductions for assumed or detected inefficiencies in some hospitals outweigh the overpayments to others.

A poor rate-setting process and methodology also expose a rate-setting body to political risks. First, its credibility is damaged since any adjustments it gives to unjustly underpaid hospitals tend to make its prospective reimbursement system look more and more like retrospective cost-based reimbursement. Thus, while in any given year the rate setters may be able proudly to show the public that they are keeping hospital cost increases down to a commendable X percentage increase, over a longer period of time subsequent rate adjustments will result in a quite different and less impressive overall record. In its own defense, any rate-setting body will want to keep its rates tight and its adjustments minimal, even at the expense of equity.

This in turn, however, exposes it to other kinds of risks—retaliations by hospitals, for whom revenues are lifeblood. Hospital retaliation can and does take the form of defensive accounting practices, lawsuits, cancellation or nonrenewal of Blue Cross contracts, and/or political action to change the enabling laws under which state rate-setting bodies function.

Incentives for and against Cost Containment

In examining the kinds of incentives that are set in motion by rate setting it is necessary to recognize two quite different classes. Some types of incentives, whether rewards or penalties, are expressly designed into a program to encourage greater hospital efficiency. Others, often perverse, emerge unexpectedly as unintended consequences of the program's own structure, or from its failure to recognize or deal with the special nature and goals of hospitals as organizations. It is useful to distinguish between structural and behavioral types of incentives.

As we have seen, early advocates of rate setting believed that hospitals would be motivated to increase efficiency by the possibility of retaining any savings they could effect by keeping spending under the allowed rates. In fact, hospitals do not respond to the possibility of making such windfall profits. Their financial officers quickly learn that their institution's future rates are calculated primarily on the base of its historical and current year spending; to reduce this spending base would, therefore, run completely counter to its long-run interests (Messier, 1975). Thus, in most programs, the true operative incentives are for each hospital to spend exactly to the limit of each year's allowed rates or budget—and as much more as it can reasonably expect to justify through the program's adjustment and appeals process.[7] Where group comparisons are made, it behooves them to calculate spending toward the top of the allowable spending parameter for their group. Over time, of course, this escalates the group average year by year.

Where penalties for underutilized services are imposed through downward rate adjustments, the obvious incentives are, as we have seen, for physicians to alter their admissions and ordering practices to keep beds filled. However, in services such as obstetrics where demand cannot be artificially stimulated, such controls may work

---

[7] It is possible that such counterincentives to improve efficiency may be less strong in rate-setting programs that pursue the objective of meeting total hospital financial requirements in each year's rate, allowing a reasonable margin of working capital and a factor for growth. Examples are programs in the state of Washington, the Cincinnati region, and Indiana.

well. In New York state, 483 obstetric beds were phased out in one period from January 1973 to March 1974 (Meitch, 1974).

As Dowling has explicated (1974), what kinds of incentives will be set in motion also depend on the type of payment unit the rate-setting program employs—per diem, per service, per case, and so on. Many of these incentives, unfortunately, run counter to the objectives of containing overall hospital expenditures. For example, as we have already noted, a tight per diem rate designed to keep unit costs low encourages increased lengths of stay and volumes of procedures, whether or not these are medically justified. In New York state, for example, where the tightest limits on per diem increases have been imposed, the average length of stay exceeds that of any other state in the nation. Unfortunately, although the shortcomings of per diem and charge payments are by now well recognized, most of the feasible alternatives also offer their own potentialities for establishing perverse incentives.

Most observers believe that the mere existence of hospital rate setting, regardless of type, has a positive effect on administrators and trustees, stimulating them to pay closer attention to hospital costs and to upgrade the quality of financial management. On the other hand, the advent of a new program often signals hospitals to make a hefty increase in rates before the program comes into effect, in order to maximize the base from which their future rates will be projected.

One possible source of future difficulty, already experienced by rate-setting bodies in some Canadian provinces, is a changed framework of incentives within which hospital labor negotiations take place. To the extent that the managers of individual hospitals feel they have nothing but trouble to gain from hard bargaining, either the costs of higher wages and increased fringe benefits will be passed through the new rate as "uncontrollable" costs, or the rate-setting body will find itself in the position of bargainer, since it alone has the authority to decide what final terms it will allow (Messier, 1975).

In general, the overriding emphasis on high utilization of hospital inpatient services, and lack of support in the rates for start-up cost of alternative forms of care, such as hospital-based home health services, militate against efforts of progressive hospitals to experiment with or move toward a changing role in their community health system. Fortunately, however, a few programs, such as Rhode Island's, actively encourage such system-improvement innovations.

Besides these structural types of incentives, intentional or perverse, most budget review programs regard their rate-setting process itself as a positive instrument for effecting behavioral change. The program's requests for detailed cost and budget data, its individual review sessions, and its cost and volume monitoring reports during the rate year are usually designed in some fashion to strengthen internal management controls in hospitals and to promote cost consciousness.

Case studies in Indiana and Cincinnati and the New Jersey program prior to 1975 indicate that the new visibility of their operations and the scrutiny by knowledgeable external reviewers may well motivate better management (Bauer and Clark, 1974a, b; Arthur D. Little, 1974e). Operating on the assumption that most administrators have strong personal concerns with job security and opportunities for promotion, these programs (largely designed by hospital associations) structure their rate reviews so that hospital managers are questioned on their performance by informed fellow administrators and by trustees, and thereby demonstrate their degree of professional knowledge and competence. Most such reviews are confined to costs directly under administrator control, in particular those for the hotel services of hospitals.

Some state programs also view the rate-setting process as a vehicle for inspiring organizational change within the hospitals. For example, the Washington program requires each hospital and each department head to submit a narrative account of its cost-saving management objectives for the coming year, with quantitative progress toward these objectives to be reviewed when the next year's budget is submitted.

State disclosure laws that expose hospital costs to public scrutiny offer another type of positive incentive for cost containment. Success depends on whether the press and consumer groups know how to ask the right questions from the cost data, how to interpret the answers, and how long they maintain their interest.

We have already noted the unanimity with which both Blue

Cross and state agency rate setters choose almost completely to ignore the influence of the hospital medical staff on hospital costs. To the author's knowledge, no program has made any attempt to gear incentives to raise the cost consciousness of physicians, to work with utilization review committees on problems of unnecessary utilization, or to bring the sacrosanct question of open staff privileges into rate-review discussions. Some rate-setting organizations appear to operate on the fiction that administrators and trustees could, if they only wanted to, take any necessary action to influence physician cost-affecting behavior. Other programs, however, consciously use the processes of rate-setting reviews to encourage modification of the traditional balance of power within hospitals. Few administrators and trustees themselves want to add unnecessary, loss-producing services, but are often pressured to endorse the wish lists of all their service chiefs rather than risk offense to any one of them. The requirements of the external rate-review system can provide a foil to force their medical staffs to order their new spending priorities and to cost out the consequences (Bauer and Clark, 1974c; Bauer, 1974a). Rate setters become the necessary scapegoats.

Requirements for five-year capital budgets from each hospital also force the setting of internal hospital priorities, and give rate setters and planning agencies an opportunity both to anticipate and to evaluate expansion requests in terms of population needs and the services already being provided by potential referral hospitals. If sensitively and judiciously applied, rate setting combined with other forms of external regulation could increasingly provide conscientious hospital trustees and managers with the muscle they need to make unpopular cost-saving management decisions—a substitute for the lever that the profit factor provides to corporate managers.

Conclusions

State and regional experience during the 1970s indicates that in and of itself, hospital rate setting is by no means the way to salvation. Federal policy makers were wise not to have prematurely rushed into this plausible-sounding route to cost containment. Setting rates for thousands of hospitals of diverse character at the point that will induce greater "efficiency" and that will at the same time protect the legitimate concerns of third-party payers, providers, patients, and the bill-paying public is easier legislated than accomplished. The methodology for implementing a task of this delicacy is still at a primitive stage. Worse, well-intentioned mistakes in designing either the structure or the processes of rate setting may be counterproductive; quite possibly they may actually stimulate increases in overall hospital care expenditures. This should not be surprising; it is the perennial risk associated with any new type of intervention in complex social systems.

At the same time, most rate-setting programs appear to be learning from their initial experiences. They are continually improving their methodologies and enlarging and improving the information base on which they are reaching rate decisions. Nevertheless, in the absence of a broader policy of health regulation, expectations of cost containment through most of the types of rate-setting programs currently in operation should be kept modest, commensurate with the modesty of the programs' own operational objectives, namely, to thwart the spiral of hospital inflation by discouraging duplicative expansions and overbedding, and to encourage types of potential cost savings in areas of hospital functioning not affected by physician decisions.

Rate-setting programs are not charged with responsibility either to identify or to control the vast bulk of excess hospital costs that spring from basic discontinuities in the system through which patients now obtain their health services. Nor can they be responsible for excess costs stemming from the ways in which society has chosen to organize and finance these services. In fact, rate setting per se is just a highly complicated tinkering operation, plugging up leaks in one small section of a rudderless ship that is cracking at the seams.

In the future, perhaps, it may play a far more powerful role. Continuing untrammeled health care costs may eventually force the nation to adopt some coherent overall health care policy to improve the processes of resource allocation in line with principles of cost effectiveness. Implementing such a policy will require new coordinated approaches and cooperative activities between and among organizations now providing care and those influencing its provision via planning, utilization review, quality monitoring, and payment. In preparing for such a role hospitals and rate setters have joint interests in developing far more refined methods of defining and measuring what hospitals do for the money they spend, and far more refined methods of accounting for that money.

The working links that have been forged between planners and rate setters vary in strength from one program to the next. The Rhode Island experience demonstrates that such a partnership can be used to promote system-wide objectives. Within the overall limit of hospital spending increases imposed by the annual maxi-cap, the rate-setting body approves spending for new programs in hospitals in strict conformance with written listings of priorities of statewide community need established by the planning agency.

As yet there are no similar links between rate-setting programs and utilization review and quality monitoring organizations such as PSROs. A national health policy designed to improve the cost effectiveness of hospital care would seem to call for their development. This would raise the sights of rate setters from narrow considerations of the unit costs of producing given types of hospital services to decision making enriched by information on the appropriateness, quality, and, one hopes, eventually the efficacy of those services.

Speculating on the possibilities of building these various types of cooperative relationships designed to improve the health status of the population while containing costs is a heady exercise. While acknowledging the possibility that in the real workaday world, the organizational and technical problems that inevitably accompany efforts to implement such new tasks may again turn to defeat the good intentions of those who pose the proposition, this approach still appears to be the best of any likely alternatives. Failure to move forward incrementally toward greater cost effectiveness of health care can only, by default, precipitate far cruder measures, such as across-the-board hospital rate freezes and cuts in health insurance benefits. Such solutions to the complicated problems of containing costs of the multibillion-dollar hospital industry would, of course, single out the ill and disabled citizens in our society to bear the consequences of reduced accessibility, comprehensiveness, and continuity of good quality medical care.

References

American Hospital Association
  1972   Guidelines for Review and Approval of Rates for Health Care Institutions and Services by a State Commission. Chicago.
Arthur D. Little
  1974a   The Prospective Reimbursement Program of Connecticut Blue Cross. Processed.°
  1974b   The Prospective Reimbursement Programs in the State of Colorado. Processed.°
  1974c   The Prospective Reimbursement Program of Blue Cross of Northeast Pennsylvania. Processed.°
  1974d   The Prospective Hospital Rate Review Program for Blue Cross of Wisconsin Payments to Hospitals. Processed.
  1974e   The Prospective Reimbursement Program of Blue Cross of Southwest Ohio. Processed.°
  1974f   The Prospective Reimbursement Program of Blue Cross of Northeast Ohio. Processed.°
Baker, F.
  1975   The Washington Hospital Commission's Method of Grouping Hospitals for Reimbursement. Washington State Hospital Commission, Olympia, Washington.
Bauer, K.G.
  1974a   The Combined Budget Review and Formula Approach to Prospective Reimbursement by the Blue Cross of Western Pennsylvania. Harvard Center for Community Health and Medical Care (April).°
  1974b   Classifying Hospitals for Purposes of Prospective Reimbursement. In fulfillment of contract SSA-PMS-74-336, United States Department of Health, Education, and Welfare, Social Security Administration (August).

°Copies may be secured at no charge from Office of Research and Statistics, Social Security Administration, Washington, D.C.

1975   Uniform Reporting for Hospital Rate Reviews: Criteria to Guide
          Development and Proceedings of a 1975 Conference. Pro-
          cessed.°

Bauer, K.G., and D. Altman
1975   Linking Planning and Rate Setting Controls to Contain Hospital
          Costs. Division of Resource Development of the Public Health
          Service, Department of Health, Education and Welfare, Region
          II, New York, New York (October).

Bauer, K.G., and A.R. Clark°°
1974a   The New Jersey Budget Review Program. Harvard Center for
          Community Health and Medical Care (March).°
1974b   The Indiana Controlled Charges System. Harvard Center for
          Community Health and Medical Care (March).°
1974c   Budget Review and Prospective Rate Setting for Rhode Island
          Hospitals. Harvard Center for Community Health and Medical
          Care (February).°
1974d   New York: The Formula Approach to Prospective Reimburse-
          ment. Harvard Center for Community Health and Medical Care
          (March).°

Berger, L.B., and P.R. Sullivan
1975   Measuring Hospital Inflation: A Composite Index for the Mea-
          surement and Determination of Hospitals in the Commonwealth
          of Massachusetts. Lexington, Mass.: Lexington Books, D.C.
          Heath & Co.

Berki, S.E.
1972   Hospital Economics. Lexington, Mass.: Lexington Books, D.C.
          Heath & Co. Pp. 31–77.

Berry, R.E., Jr.
1973   "On grouping hospitals for economic analysis." Inquiry 10
          (December): 5–12.

Cooney, J.
1974   Type of Medical Care Classification System. Chicago: Hospital
          Research and Educational Trust.

Cochrane, A.L.
1972   Effectiveness and Efficiency: Random Reflections on Health
          Services. London: The Nuffield Provincial Hospitals Trust.

°Copies may be secured at no charge from Office of Research and Statistics, Social
Security Administration, Washington, D.C.
°°Studies prepared for the Social Security Administration under grant No.
5–P16–HS00472 from the National Center for Health Services Research and Development.

Diggs, W.W., and J.A. Easter
1974   "Incremental hospital and nursing home pricing." Inquiry 11 (December): 300-303.
Dowling, W.L.
1974   "Prospective reimbursement of hospitals." Inquiry 11 (September): 163-180.
Dowling, W.L., and N. Teague
1975   Proposed Relationships among Regulatory Programs to Improve the Health Care System. School of Public Health, University of Washington.
Dunlop, J.
1975   New York Times (Sunday, November 9), p. 70.
Elnicki, R.A.
1975   "SSA—Connecticut hospital reimbursement experimental cost evaluation." Inquiry 12 (March): 47-58.
Evans, R.G., and H.D. Walker
1972   "Information theory and the analysis of hospital cost structure." Canadian Journal of Economics 5 (August): 405.
Feldstein, M.S., and J. Schuttinga
1975   Hospital Costs in Massachusetts: A Methodological Study. Discussion Paper No. 449, Harvard Institute of Economic Research, Cambridge, Mass.
Feldstein, P.
1968   "An analysis of reimbursement plans." In Department of Health, Education, and Welfare, Reimbursement Incentives for Hospital and Medical Care: Objectives and Alternatives. Washington, D.C.: Government Printing Office.
Ginsburg, P.B.
1975   Regulating the Non-Profit Firm: Hospital Price and Reimbursement Controls. Mimeographed. Department of Economics, Michigan State University.
Gort, M., et al.
1975   Report on the Hospital Price Index for Greater New York, prepared for the Associated Hospital Service of New York.
Haggerty, R.J.
1974   Advancing the Quality of Health Care: Key Issues and Fundamental Principles. Policy statement, Institute of Medicine. Washington, D.C.: National Science Foundation.
Hardwick, C.P., and H. Wolfe
1972   "Evaluation of an incentive reimbursement experiment." Medical Care 10 (March-April).

Hospital Association of New York State
  1975   Fourth Annual Voluntary Hospital Fiscal Pressures Survey. 15
          Computer Drive West, Albany, New York: Hospital Association
          of New York State (October).
Kovner, A.R., and E.J. Lusk
  1975   "State regulation of health care costs." Medical Care 13 (August):
          619–629.
Lave, J.R., and L.B. Lave
  1971   "The extent of role differentiation among hospitals." Health
          Services Research 6 (Spring): 15–38.
Meitch, George
  1974   Communication with Katharine Bauer (March 7).
Messier, E.A.
  1975   "Prospective reimbursement is no panacea." Hospital Financial
          Management 5 (September): 24.
National Advisory Commission on Health Manpower
  1968   Report. Washington, D.C.: Government Printing Office.
New York State Moreland Act Commission on Nursing Homes and Resi-
dential Facilities
  1975   Regulating Nursing Home Care: The Paper Tigers. Report No.
          1. October.
Noll, R.G.
  1971   Reforming Regulation: Studies in the Regulation of Economic
          Activity. Washington, D.C.: The Brookings Institution, pp.
          20–21.
Rafferty, J.A.
  1971   "Patterns of hospital use: An analysis of short run variations."
          Journal of Political Economy 79 (January–February): 154–165.
Rutstein, D.D.
  1974   Blueprint for Medical Care. Cambridge, Mass.: M.I.T. Press.
Shuman, L., H. Wolfe, and C.P. Hardwick
  1972   "Predictive hospital reimbursement and evaluation model." In-
          quiry 9 (February): 17–33.
Sigmond, R.M.
  1968   "Capitation as a method of reimbursement." In Department of
          Health, Education, and Welfare, Reimbursement Incentives for
          Hospital and Medical Care: Objectives and Alternatives. Wash-
          ington, D.C.: Government Printing Office.
Somers, A.R.
  1973   State Regulation of Hospitals and Health Care: The New Jersey
          Story. Blue Cross Reports, Research Series 11: 9.

Thompson, J.D., C.D. Mross, and R.B. Fetter
1975   Case Mix and Resource Use. Center for the Study of Health Services, Yale University Institution for Social and Policy Studies.
U.S. Department of Health, Education, and Welfare
1975   An analysis of state and regional health regulations, Health Resources Studies HRA No. 75-611: 2–4. Washington, D.C.
Waldman, S.
1968   "Average increase in costs—An incentive reimbursement formula for hospitals." In Department of Health, Education, and Welfare, Reimbursement Incentives for Hospitals and Medical Care: Objectives and Alternatives. Washington, D.C.: Government Printing Office.
Wolf, G.
1973   A Behavioral Analysis of the Connecticut Incentive Reimbursement Experiment. Mimeographed. Yale University Administrative Sciences (January).

An Empirical Analysis of
Several Prospective
Reimbursement Systems

FRED J. HELLINGER

Prospective payment systems have recently been established by state governments and Blue Cross plans in numerous states in an effort to control the pace of hospital cost inflation. Prices for selected health care services are fixed for a time period in the future under a prospective payment system in contrast with a retrospective cost-based system which reimburses hospitals on the basis of incurred expenses. Many observers of our health care system believe that retrospective cost reimbursement has been a major cause of the large increase in hospital costs, and that prospective payment systems are better able to control hospital cost inflation.

House Resolution 1 of the Social Security Amendments of 1972 stated (U.S. DHEW, 1972:80–81):

> . . . payment determined on a prospective basis offers the promise of encouraging institutional policymakers and managers, as well as the risk of possible loss inherent in that method to plan, innovate, and generally to manage effectively in order to achieve greater financial reward for the provider as well as a lower total cost of the program.

The Social Security Amendments of 1972 (P.L. 92-603, U.S. Congress, 1972:62) instruct the secretary of Health, Education, and Welfare to ". . . develop and carry out experiments and demonstration projects designed to determine the relative advantages and disadvantages of various alternative methods of making payment on a prospective basis to hospitals." There were, however, many prospective reimbursement experiments already in existence that were being operated by various state governments and Blue Cross plans. In an effort to assess the effectiveness of prospective reimbursement systems in controlling hospital costs, the Office of Research and Statistics of the Social Security Administration has funded contracts to evaluate several existing prospective payment systems. This chapter examines the findings of these evaluations of prospective payment systems in Western Pennsylvania, Rhode Island, New Jersey, and New York. We will not provide a detailed description of the mechanics of the operation for the four prospective payment systems because in-depth delineations of these and other experiments are contained in reports prepared for the Social Security Administration by Katharine Bauer and Arva Clark (1974b, c, and d). Also, a concise analysis of the operation of many of the prospective reimbursement experiments is provided by William Dowling (1974).

The primary concern of the evaluations is to determine the impact of the prospective payment system on the cost and quality of hospital care. In order to determine the effectiveness of a prospective payment system, we must know what would have been the behavior of hospitals in the absence of a prospective rate system. This, obviously, cannot be determined directly through an analysis of hospital cost data. But, to estimate the impact of prospective reimbursement, we may examine the rates of increase of hospital costs before and after the prospective rate experiment or we may compare the rate of increase of hospital costs in the state with the prospective rate system with the rate of increase of hospital costs in a neighboring state. Both of these approaches have major drawbacks. The before-and-after approach does not consider the effects of factors other than the prospective payment system which may have changed during the period. If the prospective payment system were implemented during the Economic Stabilization Program, it would be difficult to isolate and estimate the impact of the new reimbursement system. Comparisons among hospitals in different states implicitly assume that the different states possess comparable environments. Therefore, it is important to select control hospitals in a state which has similar market characteristics and similar standards for medical practice in order to isolate the effect of the prospective payment system. All of the evaluators analyzed the effectiveness of prospective reimbursement by comparing the behavior of hospitals which were operating within the prospective rate system with that of hospitals not in the system.

Evaluation Results

Western Pennsylvania

The Blue Cross of Western Pennsylvania (BCWP) has initiated and participated in numerous innovative experiments in the field of incentive reimbursement during the past twenty-five years. Beginning in 1950, the BCWP categorized hospitals in order to set maximum limits for per diem reimbursements (see Lave and Lave, 1970; Lave, Lave, and Silverman, 1973; and Hellinger, 1974, for an analysis of this BCWP incentive reimbursement experiment). The involvement with and commitment of the BCWP to new payment mechanisms are exemplified by the implementation in July 1971 of a prospective payment experiment. Five hospitals from rural Western Pennsylvania, one of which is a rehabilitation center, volunteered for the experiment. In July 1974, the system was included as an option for all Western Pennsylvania hospitals, and eleven hospitals entered the experiment.

The prospective rate is set by the BCWP for the hospitals according to a series of complex formulas. Essentially, the system is a budget review system but there are numerous controls on the approved per diem. The base year figures serve as the basis for the formula restrictions while the formulas determine the maximum allowable increase between the base and the current year. The maximum allowable rate of change is the average of the hospitals' and the groups' percentage increase over the previous three years. Hospitals are assigned to a group according to their location, teaching status, and bed size. The maximum allowable increase between the current and prospective year for each expense category is determined by applying various price indices. The final approved per diem rate may not be 12 percent above the groups' average per diem rate. The per diem rate for hospitals not included in the experiment is subject to a limit of 10 percent above the group mean.

Applied Management Sciences, Inc. (1975) has conducted the evaluation of the prospective reimbursement experiment in Western Pennsylvania for the Division of Health Insurance Studies, Office of Research and Statistics of the Social Security Administration. The appropriate selection of a control group was critical in order for the evaluators to be able to correctly identify the impact of the prospective payment system. Ten control hospitals were selected from the 120 hospitals in Western Pennsylvania. The percent of the population in a county living in a rural area, complexity of services, bed size, percent occupancy, ownership, and the existence of teaching programs were the factors considered in the selection of the control group.

The results of the cost study appear in Table 1 and in Figs. 1 and 2 (Applied Management Sciences, Inc., 1975:11-13). From this evidence, the evaluators concluded that the rate of increase in hospital costs is less under the prospective payment system than under the conventional incurred cost-based system of payment. Table 1 and Fig. 1 contain the total cost figures and the percent change in total cost figures for both prospectively reimbursed and control hospitals. Figure 1 indicates that the difference in the percentage change in total costs between prospectively reimbursed and control hospitals increased as the experiment progressed and the impact of the Economic Stabilization Program decreased. The experimental hospitals experienced a lower rate of increase in total costs for general service and routine patient care (that is, inpatient care) than did the control group. (See Fig. 2 and note that general service costs increased 75 percent for the control hospitals and 52 percent for the prospectively reimbursed hospitals.) The evaluators attributed this occurrence to efforts by the hospital administrators in the experimental hospitals not to curtail services which are important in keeping and attracting physicians (for example, ancillary

TABLE 1　Total Cost

Hospital Group	FY 1970	FY 1971	FY 1972	FY 1973	FY 1974	Pre P.R. (FY 70–71)	Intra P.R. (FY 72–74)
P.R. Hospitals							
Value	1,801,220	2,026,435	2,187,410	2,408,381	2,735,833	1,913,827	2,443,875
% change		12.5	7.9	10.1	13.6	12.5	10.5
Control Hospitals							
Value	2,010,481	2,282,837	2,492,154	2,772,114	3,277,316	2,146,659	2,547,194
% change		13.5	9.2	11.2	16.2	13.5	12.9
Other Western Pa. Hospitals							
Value	4,952,279	5,890,674	6,536,351	7,062,261	7,617,928	5,321,476	7,139,080
% change		14.9	14.9	8.1	10.7	14.9	11.2

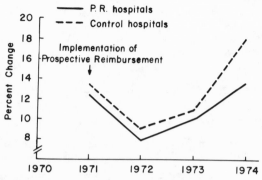

Fig. 1   Annual Percent Change in Total Cost

services). Their cost control efforts were directed to departments over which the administrators had control and which were not critical in attracting more physicians (for example, general services). In rural areas, each hospital has very few admitting physicians and there is considerable competition for their services.

The rate of increase in the inpatient cost per day was lower for the experimental than for the control hospitals. The number of patient days decreased during the first year of the experiment for both the experimental and control hospitals but increased for both groups during the last two years. Thus, the rate of increase for inpatient cost per day was inversely related to the volume trend. From this evidence the evaluators deduced that the cost per unit of output will increase at a slower rate under prospective reimbursement than under a retrospective cost-based system.

The consultation rate, net autopsy rate (deaths after forty-eight hours of admission), net mortality rate (deaths after forty-eight hours of admission), and postsurgical mortality rate were the indices used by the evaluators to detect quality changes during the experiment.

The consultation rates increased slightly for both the prospectively reimbursed and control group hospitals during the experiment (Applied Management Sciences, Inc., 1975:7.56-7.60). However, the increase for the prospectively reimbursed hospitals (2.6 percent) was greater than for the control group hospitals (2.1 percent). The

P.R. HOSPITALS

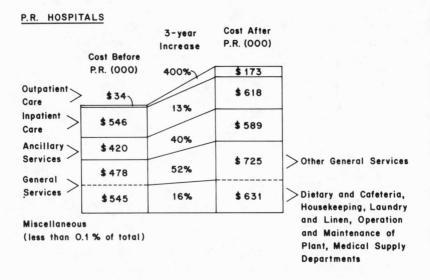

CONTROL HOSPITALS

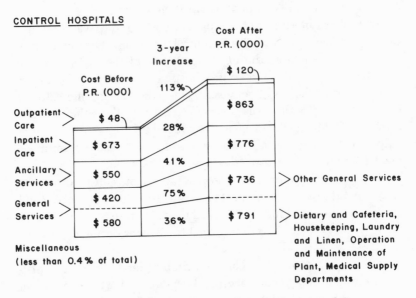

Fig. 2   Change in Direct Cost by Major Functional Category—
           Fiscal Years 1971-1974

net autopsy rate decreased 8.9 percent for the experimental hospitals and decreased 6.7 percent for the control hospitals between 1971 and 1973, a decrease indicating a general trend toward the omission of this procedure. There was a negligible decrease in the gross and net death rates for both the prospectively reimbursed and control group hospitals during the experimental period while the surgical mortality rate also exhibited an inconsequential decrease for both groups of hospitals. In conclusion, the evaluators inferred from this examination that the prospective reimbursement experiment in Western Pennsylvania did not have a deleterious influence on the quality of care.

Rhode Island

The Rhode Island prospective reimbursement experiment, like most others, was implemented in an attempt to find some way of containing the rapid increase in hospital costs and Blue Cross premium rates. Rhode Island Blue Cross in 1969 requested approval for a 24.5 percent increase in premium rates from the director of business regulation. The director, after lengthy discussions with state officials, directed Blue Cross and the hospitals to (Thornberry and Zimmerman, 1975):

1. Engage in a cooperative project with the Department of Health to examine the cost of operating hospitals in the hope that ways to contain costs could be found;

2. Engage experts to assist in the investigation of costs and to share costs among the participating groups;

3. *Reexamine, if not completely discard, the present reimbursement formula, and give serious consideration to a formula similar to the state of New York;*

4. Increase the use of joint purchasing and shared or consolidated services.

The hospitals feared the creation of a state rate commission and espoused a hospital-by-hospital budget review and negotiation with Blue Cross.

During the first few months of 1970, Lawrence Hill, the vice president for operations for Rhode Island Hospital, suggested to

**TABLE 2   Total Hospital Expenditures and
Percentage Increase, Rhode Island and United States,
1969–1972**

	Rhode Island Total Expenditure	R.I. Annual Percentage Increase	U.S. Annual Percentage Increase
1969	$ 86,863,187	16.4	16.7
1970	99,848,386	14.9	16.7
1971	114,603,013	14.8	15.4
1972	127,350,622	11.1	12.2

Blue Cross that a pilot project be implemented to test the feasibility of a prospective rate system based on budget review. Rhode Island Hospital, the largest hospital in the state, took the initiative in the summer of 1970 and entered into a prospective payment agreement with Blue Cross for fiscal year 1971. The remaining twelve voluntary hospitals in Rhode Island entered into a prospective reimbursement agreement with Blue Cross for fiscal year 1972. However, the remaining hospitals did agree to guarantee rates for fiscal year 1971 to cover expenses as they projected them. The guaranteed rates averaged to an increase of 15.8 percent over the rates for fiscal year 1970, which was about 3 percent above the 12.9 percent increase negotiated by Rhode Island Hospital.

Rhode Island Health Services Research was selected by the Office of Research and Statistics to conduct an evaluation of the prospective payment system in Rhode Island. Twelve hospitals in Massachusetts which subscribe to the Professional Activities Studies (PAS) were selected as the control group (all thirteen hospitals in Rhode Island utilize PAS). Only hospitals which participated in the PAS program were considered because the quality indices employed by the evaluators are devised from PAS data; PAS hospital data also permit a measure of case mix to be included in the cost function analysis.

The rate of increase in total costs, average cost per patient day, and average cost per admission were slightly lower for Rhode Island during the 1970–1972 period than for New England or the United States. From Tables 2 and 3 (Thornberry and Zimmerman, 1975:120–121), we note that the average cost per patient day and the average cost per stay are significantly higher than the national average.

TABLE 3 Adjusted Average Costs per Patient and per Patient Day

Adjusted Average Cost per Patient

	1969	1970	1971	1972
U.S. nongovernment not for profit	537.02	614.51	693.20	762.40
New England nongovernment not for profit	698.41	769.22	870.18	949.92
Massachusetts control hospitals	671.40	754.87	861.87	926.06
Rhode Island hospitals	699.26	750.04	828.34	904.08

Adjusted Average Cost per Patient Day

	1969	1970	1971	1972
U.S. nongovernment not for profit	65.49	74.94	85.58	95.30
New England nongovernment not for profit	81.19	91.96	106.00	117.02
Massachusetts control hospitals	70.56	80.63	94.16	102.80
Rhode Island hospitals	74.56	81.58	93.43	100.20

Sources: U.S. nongovernment not for profit adjusted (for outpatient activity) average cost is taken from *Hospital Statistics, 1972,* American Hospital Association (Chicago, 1973). New England average cost is taken from the same source and adjusted for outpatient activity by deflating average cost by the average U.S. nongovernment not for profit percentage of cost due to outpatient services. Massachusetts cost data are from Massachusetts Cost Commission form HCF400. Rhode Island cost data are from Blue Cross of Rhode Island audited cost reports. Utilization statistics for Massachusetts and Rhode Island are from PAS data tape supplied by the Commission on Professional and Hospital Activities, Ann Arbor, Michigan.

In order to test the hypothesis that the prospective payment system in Rhode Island has lowered the rate of increase in hospital costs, the evaluators utilized a cost function. Among the independent variables in the cost function were a measure of case mix, teaching status, and bed size (refer to Tables 4, 5, and 6, Thornberry and Zimmerman, 1975:147–151).

A dummy variable was contained in each equation and was set equal to one for hospitals which participated in the prospective reimbursement system (that is, hospitals in Rhode Island during the 1970–1972 period). In all equations which included the Massachusetts control group hospitals the coefficient for the prospective reimbursement variable was negative and insignificant. However, when we estimated the joint impact of the prospective reimbursement program and the Economic Stabilization Program (ESP began in August 1971) in the Rhode Island (1969–1972) equations, the coefficient for prospective reimbursement (the PR variable was set equal to one for 1971 and 1972 observations) was negative and significant. Consequently, we may not conclude that the prospective

TABLE 4   Identification of Variables

	Symbol	
Variable	Patients	Patient Days
Proportion:		
Under 14 years	A14	PA14
65 or older	A65	PA65
Operated on	Surg	PSurg
Infective and parasitic diseases	D1	PD1
Neoplasms	D2	PD2
Endocrine, nutritional and metabolic	D3	PD3
Diseases of blood and blood-forming organs	D4	PD4
Mental disorder	D5	PD5
Diseases of nervous system and sense organs	D6	PD6
Diseases of circulatory system	D7	PD7
Diseases of respiratory system	D8	PD8
Diseases of digestive system	D9	PD9
Diseases of genitourinary system	D10	PD10
Delivery and complications of pregnancy	D11	PD11
Diseases of skin and subcutaneous tissues	D12	PD12
Diseases of musculoskeletal system	D13	PD13
Congenital anomalies	D14	PD14
Certain diseases peculiar to newborns	D15	PD15
Symptoms and ill-defined conditions	D16	PD16
Injuries and adverse effects	D17	PD17
Teaching index	Teach	Teach
Bed complement	Beds	Beds
Occupancy rate	Occ	Occ
Mean length of stay	LOS	—
Prospective reimbursement dummy variable	PRD	PRD

reimbursement system in Rhode Island has lowered the rate of increase in hospital costs. Instead, our evidence supports only the position that the Economic Stabilization Program and the prospective reimbursement system have lessened the level of hospital cost inflation.

It should be noted that only two of the variables representing the proportion of cases in a given diagnostic category had significant coefficients in the average cost per day equations. In the average cost per stay equations, again only two of the seventeen variables representing the proportion of diseases in a given diagnostic cate-

TABLE 5 Hospital Inpatient Cost per Patient Day Regression Coefficients

	Linear Equations		Semilog Equations	
Variable	RI 69-72	RI-Mass. 71-72	RI 69-72	RI-Mass. 71-72
PA14	0.7819	-0.4022	0.008284	-0.005930
	(1.290)[a]	(0.522)	(0.913)	(0.567)
PA65	-0.0133	0.4677	0.000780	0.008273
	(0.047)	(1.104)	(0.185)	(1.438)
PSurg	0.0650	0.4938	0.001417	0.006414
	(0.367)	(2.775)	(0.534)	(2.656)
PD1	1.5149	-2.9613	0.020199	-0.040954
	(0.713)	(1.298)	(0.635)	(1.322)
PD2	-2.5221	-1.2854	-0.041687	-0.021111
	(2.375)	(1.465)	(2.623)	(1.772)
PD3	-0.6516	-0.1496	-0.010971	0.003261
	(0.496)	(0.091)	(0.558)	(0.145)
PD4	-4.2855	-3.6009	-0.062498	-0.050650
	(1.061)	(0.904)	(1.034)	(0.936)
PD5	-1.1599	-1.4454	-0.017526	-0.020241
	(1.062)	(1.606)	(1.073)	(1.657)
PD6	-0.1276	-0.2752	-0.003002	-0.006640
	(0.145)	(0.164)	(0.228)	(0.292)
PD7	-0.9338	-0.8789	-0.014953	-0.013144
	(1.337)	(1.185)	(1.431)	(1.306)
PD8	-1.2937	-1.3678	-0.018248	-0.018721
	(1.052)	(1.002)	(0.992)	(1.010)
PD9	-1.2055	-2.7696	-0.018048	-0.035944
	(1.013)	(2.014)	(1.013)	(1.927)
PD11	-1.6411	-0.7539	-0.022675	-0.008060
	(1.594)	(0.659)	(1.472)	(0.519)
PD12	1.9900	3.6080	0.028880	0.057172
	(1.134)	(1.651)	(1.099)	(1.927)
PD13	-0.7634	-1.3061	-0.011333	-0.012890
	(0.784)	(1.127)	(0.778)	(0.820)
PD14	6.4727	3.6626	0.094418	0.051574
	(2.165)	(1.046)	(2.110)	(1.086)
PD15	-18.2630	-3.9742	-0.335750	-0.066784
	(0.677)	(0.507)	(0.831)	(0.627)
PD16	0.4332	-0.2426	0.048449	-0.001247
	(0.402)	(0.203)	(0.300)	(0.077)
PD17	-1.1481	-0.5892	-0.016776	-0.007488
	(1.224)	(0.622)	(1.196)	(0.582)
Teach	2.0166	1.6273	0.032238	0.022849
	(2.843)	(3.165)	(3.037)	(3.274)
Beds	-0.0125	-0.0059	-0.000184	-0.000021
	(0.904)	(0.484)	(0.886)	(0.124)
Occ	-0.1711	0.0165	-0.002802	0.001035
	(1.185)	(0.065)	(1.297)	(0.302)
PRD	-1.6677	-2.5837	-0.031434	-0.037296
	(1.122)	(0.860)	(1.413)	(0.915)
Constant	162.7	121.6	5.665	4.782
	(2.160)	(1.486)	(5.026)	(4.303)
N	52	50	52	50
R^2	.907	.809	.896	.827
SEE	3.424	4.813	0.05123	0.06533

[a]Figures in parentheses are t-values.

TABLE 6   Hospital Inpatient Cost per Patient Stay
Regression Coefficients

Variable	Linear Equations RI 69-72	Semilog Equations RI 69-72	RI-Mass. 71-72
A14	-11.017	-0.020022	-0.006586
	(1.570)[a]	(2.053)	(0.695)
A65	-1.730	0.000775	0.001962
	(0.406)	(0.131)	(0.237)
Surg	4.411	0.006985	0.001634
	(2.138)	(2.436)	(0.630)
D1	11.154	0.018809	-0.026604
	(0.622)	(0.755)	(1.125)
D2	-8.248	-0.025702	0.009638
	(0.868)	(1.945)	(0.739)
D3	31.281	0.042327	-0.016195
	(2.313)	(2.253)	(0.546)
D4	-36.978	-0.038515	-0.205620
	(1.286)	(0.964)	(3.785)
D5	-2.636	-0.002999	-0.016427
	(0.245)	(0.201)	(1.176)
D6	5.518	-0.000924	0.007704
	(0.813)	(0.098)	(0.725)
D7	6.532	0.006767	-0.015230
	(0.785)	(0.585)	(1.336)
D8	7.186	0.013450	0.016422
	(0.672)	(0.905)	(1.183)
D9	-6.949	-0.008179	-0.007008
	(1.009)	(0.855)	(0.523)
D11	-0.547	-0.000289	0.009590
	(0.082)	(0.031)	(1.097)
D12	49.738	0.074868	0.071701
	(2.173)	(2.354)	(2.338)
D13	8.461	0.014172	0.008966
	(1.108)	(1.335)	(0.755)
D14	54.962	0.108600	0.067459
	(2.461)	(3.499)	(1.800)
D15	388.170	0.493150	-0.273590
	(1.526)	(1.395)	(1.338)
D16	-2.167	-0.008609	0.029860
	(0.270)	(0.771)	(2.354)
D17	16.101	0.023247	0.012881
	(1.682)	(1.748)	(1.337)
Teach	19.768	0.035652	0.025639
	(4.646)	(6.030)	(2.818)
Beds	0.032	-0.000018	0.000004
	(0.364)	(0.150)	(0.026)
Occ	-1.548	-0.002756	-0.005048
	(1.318)	(1.689)	(1.784)
LOS	41.847	0.080133	0.178620
	(2.872)	(3.958)	(6.446)
PRD	-37.865	-0.050832	-0.071272
	(2.687)	(2.595)	(1.620)
Constant	-193.50	5.098	4.919
	(0.328)	(6.225)	(7.548)
N	52	52	50
R²	.973	.979	.965
SEE	27.75	0.03856	0.04935

[a]Figures in parentheses are *t*-values.

gory were significant. The teaching variable was, however, significant and positive in every specification of both the average cost per day and average cost per stay equations. It is likely that the teaching variable reflects the more complex set of services provided by teaching hospitals as well as the greater expenditure of resources for a given case by teaching hospitals. Surprisingly, neither the bed nor occupancy variable have significant coefficients in any of the equations. Often, the bed variable will pick up the effect of a more complex set of services associated with large hospitals and enter into the cost equation with a positive coefficient. The bed variable may, however, be insignificant because of the strong correlation between bed size and teaching capacity.

In an effort to analyze the impact of prospective reimbursement on the quality of care the evaluators selected the following items from PAS data reports:

1. The percent of patients without minimum laboratory workup;
2. The percent of obstetrical patients without minimum laboratory workup;
3. The percent of obstetrical patients with hematologic examinations;
4. The percent of patients without admission white blood count;
5. The percent of operated patients over 4 without: electrocardiograms; chest x-rays, blood sugars; and blood nitrogen studies.

The researchers found that in almost all of the instances examined, the results in 1972 were more favorable than in 1970. It is not possible to determine what would have occurred if there had not been a prospective payment system instituted but it is unlikely that the results would have varied dramatically from those experienced under prospective reimbursement. The net autopsy rate dropped from 36.1 percent to 30.0 percent during the 1970–1972 period. However, we should note that the net autopsy rate also dropped for both the experimental and control hospitals in the Western Pennsylvania experiment. Thornberry and Zimmerman concluded (1975: 261), "If there is any empirical evidence of change from the data in the quality of patient care, it is in the direction of improved quality."

New Jersey

New Jersey was among the first states to limit reimbursement paid to hospitals. In 1958, through the authority granted in the 1938 Blue Cross enabling act, the commissioner of insurance imposed ceilings on Blue Cross rates of payment. These ceilings could be appealed to an advisory committee whose members were appointed by the commissioner. Each year the same large teaching hospitals filed appeals for adjustment of their rates that were generally successful. The advisory committee felt that rates would be better controlled if it reviewed each budget before it was put into operation. In the post-Medicare years in the late 1960s Blue Cross premium rates soared in response to the rapid pace of hospital cost increases, and legislation was approved which empowered the State Department of Health to review hospital per diem rates.

In 1971, the New Jersey legislature passed the Health Care Facilities Act, Chapter 136 of the New Jersey statutes, with the objective of establishing an administrative and regulatory structure to ensure the provision of high-quality care at reasonable costs. The advisory committee was given the responsibility of reviewing, before final approval from the commissioners of insurance and health, per diem rates for Blue Cross and state-supported patients. The gathering, preparation, and analysis of the hospital budgets was, however, performed by staff members of the Hospital Research and Educational Trust (HRET), which is a subsidiary corporation of the New Jersey Hospital Association. All the costs incurred by HRET in processing and preparing budget packages and deriving tentative per diem rates to be submitted to the advisory committee are borne by the hospitals. The advisory committee relies almost entirely on information provided by HRET staff members to evaluate the reasonableness of each budget. The commissioners of insurance and health, after hearing the opinion of the advisory committee, approve a per diem rate which is the maximum allowable per diem payment a hospital may receive from Blue Cross, Medicaid, and other state-supported programs.

If a hospital incurs costs less than its budgeted costs, the surplus must be rebated to the third-party payers. If, on the other hand, the hospital's actual costs exceed its budgeted costs, then the hospital

TABLE 7   Number of Certified
Cost Reviews Conducted

Year	Number of Reviews
1970	15
1971	25
1972	58
1973	53

Source: Bauer and Clark (1974c:57).

must absorb the loss or appeal. During the first four years of operation there have been over 150 appeals for cost reviews to the advisory committee (refer to Table 7).

Primarily because of the publication of *Bureaucratic Malpractice* (1974), a study produced by the Center for Analysis of Public Issues, which attacked the role of HRET in the budget review process, the budget preparations and workups for the advisory committee are presently conducted by state employees of the Department of Health. The new system has been in operation since the summer of 1974 and will not be analyzed in this section because of the absence of data from this period.

The analysis of the impact of prospective reimbursement on hospital costs in New Jersey that is presented in this section was produced by the author. The examination of the impact of prospective reimbursement on the quality of care in New Jersey was, however, developed solely by Geomet, Inc. (1974).

New Jersey hospitals volunteered for the prospective reimbursement experiment beginning in 1968, and all hospitals were included in the system by 1974. Many of the hospitals that first entered the program were high-cost hospitals which had filed appeals annually to the advisory committee. This type of self-selection bias imparts a positive bias to the coefficient of the prospective reimbursement variable because the prospective reimbursement variable is positively correlated with the error term. In this case, the prospective reimbursement variable will reflect the fact that hospitals with unusually high costs entered the experiment and will not be an accurate measure of the impact of the payment system. If we assume that the rate of increase in costs for high-cost hospitals is, ceteris paribus, equal to the rate of increase in costs of low-cost hospitals, then including the lagged value of average cost as an independent variable will allow us to obtain a better estimate of the impact of prospective reimbursement on hospital costs. There is evidence, however, that high-cost hospitals have a slower rate of increase in costs than low-cost hospitals (Lave, Lave, and Silverman, 1973). This suggests that our estimate of the coefficient of the prospective reimbursement variable will have a negative bias (that is, we will overestimate the cost-saving influence of prospective reimbursement).

We have estimated a cost function for all New Jersey hospitals with pooled data from 1969, 1970, 1971, 1972, and 1973 in the following form:

$$AC = \frac{TC}{PD} = f(\text{constant: Beds, Teaching Status, Scope}$$
$$\text{and} \qquad \text{of Services, Percent of Patients over 65,}$$
$$\frac{TC}{ADM} \qquad \text{Wage Rate, PR, Percent Surgical,}$$
$$\text{Time }_i, AC_{t-1})$$

where TC = total cost
           PD = patient days
           ADM = admissions
           AC_{t-1} = average cost in the previous period.

Teaching Status = 1, if hospital has an intern or residency
                     program
                  0, if not

PR = 1, if hospital participated in PR program
        during the year
     0, if not

Time$_i$ = 1, if the observation was from period i
          0, if not

Scope of Services = weighted sum of services (see Roemer, Moustafa, and Hopkins, 1968)
            Wage Rate = total labor costs/number of employees
We have also estimated the above function with a case-mix variable

TABLE 8   The Effect of Prospective Reimbursement on
Hospital Costs in New Jersey

Independent Variables	Average Cost Per Day	Average Cost Per Admission
Constant	17.616	456.745
Beds	.003	.008
	(.632)[a]	(2.147)
Occupancy	.080	-.704
	(.758)	(.385)
Teaching	4.051	88.516
	(2.021)	(1.270)
Time$_{70}$	.543	-48.355
	(.366)	(.824)
Time$_{71}$	1.506	-60.791
	(.868)	(.916)
Time$_{72}$	2.625	6.024
	(1.378)	(.084)
Time$_{73}$	1.887	89.849
	(.911)	(1.255)
Wage Rate	-.000	.001
	(.000)	(.554)
Percent Surgical	-.045	3.386
	(.898)	(1.685)
Over 65	-.134	-.267
	(2.001)	(.100)
Scope of Services	.022	1.595
	(.701)	(1.256)
AC_{t-1}	1.058	.753
	(33.288)	(9.857)
PR	-1.346	57.041
	(1.001)	(1.270)
R^2	.912	.404

[a]The numbers in the parentheses are t-scores.

which is composed of seventeen separate measures of the percentage of cases in each of seventeen diagnostic categories.

The empirical results appear in Table 8 and indicate that prospective reimbursement has a negative, yet insignificant impact on the average cost per patient day and a positive, insignificant effect upon the average cost per admission (we found essentially the same results when the case-mix vector was included). Under a prospective reimbursement system with a fixed reimbursement rate per day we expected the intensity of care to lessen and the length of care to increase. The evidence suggests that prospective reimbursement systems based on a per diem reimbursement rate should be careful not to allow increased lengths of stay to wipe out savings gained through decreases in the average cost per patient day.

The research design selected by Geomet utilized an analysis of three tracer conditions: pneumonia, tonsillitis and adenoiditis (T and A), and acute myocardial infarction. The protocols for each diagnosis were based on existing criteria developed by health care facilities, Experimental Medical Care Review Organizations (EMCROs), medical care foundations, medical specialty groups, and several research projects. Geomet staff members analyzed ninety patient records from each of fifty-six institutions (twenty-eight in the greater Philadelphia area and twenty-eight in New Jersey) and assigned a numerical score for the quality of care received by each patient. An examination of the numerical quality scores indicated that prospective reimbursement has not affected the quality of care in New Jersey.

New York State

The state of New York and the state's Blue Cross plans operate the only prospective reimbursement system in the nation that sets prospective rates solely on the basis of formulas and has no automatic retroactive adjustment. Because of the magnitude of the program and the unique nature of the experiment, there has been an active interest among health care researchers in the effect of the program on the cost of hospital care in the state. The New York prospective rate system does not include any review of hospital budgets or analysis of their internal operations, but does, however, permit a hospital to file an appeal for the adjustment of its prospective rate after the rate is set.

The state legislature in Albany reacted swiftly to rapid increases in state payments for Medicaid during the late 1960s and passed an amendment in 1969 to the state's Medicaid enabling act, freezing the rates of Medicaid payments for three years at their 1969 levels. After a hectic period of meetings and debates, a counterproposal, the Cost Control Law of 1969, was passed with the support of the state's two hospital associations. The new law, superseding the amendment that froze the Medicaid rates, outlined criteria for the state Department of Health to follow in reviewing and certifying hospital rates. Prospective reimbursement was not mandated in the Cost Control

Law of 1969 but was required by the superintendent of insurance, who with the aid of the state Department of Health regulates the seven upstate and one downstate Blue Cross plans. The law required that hospital rates be reasonably related to the cost of the "efficient" production of hospital care.

There are presently three different rate-setting programs in New York state, setting reimbursement levels for Blue Cross patients in upstate New York, for Blue Cross patients in downstate New York, and for state Medicaid patients. The state Department of Health operates the program for Medicaid recipients; the Associated Hospital Services (AHS), the downstate Blue Cross plan, sets rates for Blue Cross patients in the seventeen lower counties of New York state; and the seven upstate Blue Cross plans jointly operate the prospective rate system that handles Blue Cross patients in the upstate region.

The state Department of Health, the AHS, and the seven upstate Blue Cross plans have each developed formula-based prospective rate programs that are remarkably similar in content and process. Each system relies on base year (two years before the year for which the prospective rate applies) costs, which are subject to a ceiling derived from the per diem charges of a group of similar hospitals and a trend factor. (The trend factor is a three-year moving average of several price indices.) None of the three systems provides for an automatic, retroactive adjustment, but they all permit appeals and they vary considerably in their appeals procedures. Each of the seven upstate Blue Cross plans conducts an appeals process, all of which allow a hospital to appeal a certified rate on the basis of events beyond the hospital's control. The state Department of Health and the AHS do not provide for appeals on that basis, but instead require that "Any request for prospective modification of a certified rate shall be accompanied by financial, statistical and program evidence sufficient to demonstrate a substantial change in economic status and an expansion of services, a necessary improvement in the quality of care, anticipated improved efficiency, or projected long-term cost savings" (Part 86, State of New York, Department of Health, Administrative Rules and Regulations, Reporting and Rule Certification for Medical Facilities).

The Office of Research and Statistics of the Social Security Administration has awarded the University of Washington a contract to evaluate the impact of prospective reimbursement on the cost and quality of care provided by downstate New York hospitals. The project director for the contract is Professor William Dowling. The estimates of the cost functions in this section were performed by the University of Washington under the evaluation contract. At this time, there are no results available from the contractor in charge of the evaluation of the upstate prospective rate systems.

A cost function of the following form was estimated for the downstate and control-group hospitals:

$$AC = \frac{TC}{PD} = f \text{ (constant: Beds, Teaching Status, Scope of Services,}$$

Occupancy Rate, Time_i, Area Dummy, Prospective

and Reimbursement (PR))

$$\frac{TC}{ADM}$$

$$TC$$

where TC = total cost

PD = patient days

ADM = admissions

Teaching Status = 1, if a hospital is a member of the Council
      of Teaching Hospitals
      0, if not

Scope of Services = a count of the number of services as reported
      by the American Hospital Association in the
      Guide Issue

Time_i = 1, if the observation was from period i
      0, if not
PR = 1, if a hospital was involved in the prospective rate
      program during the year (i.e., all New York hospitals
      beginning in 1970)
      0, if not

Area Dummy = 1, for all downstate New York hospitals
0, all other hospitals (i.e., control-group hospitals)

The data were collected for all hospitals in downstate New York, Cleveland, Philadelphia, and Chicago for the years between 1968 and 1973. Data for the teaching status and scope of services variables were obtained for all hospitals from American Hospital Association data tapes. All other data for the downstate New York hospitals were acquired from uniform financial reports that all hospitals submit yearly to the state Department of Health. The control group includes all hospitals in Cleveland, Philadelphia, and Chicago; Medicare cost reports were used to gather their data.

A dummy variable, denoting a New York hospital, was included in each equation and set equal to 1 for all downstate New York hospitals, regardless of the year of the observation. The prospective reimbursement dummy variable (PR) was set equal to 1 for all observations from hospitals in downstate New York starting in 1970, and was set equal to 0 for all observations for downstate New York hospitals in 1965 and 1969 and for all control-group hospitals in every year. The area dummy variable was included to estimate and isolate the impact of the high cost level in the New York area on the cost level of hospitals in that area.

The results from estimated cost functions for the downstate New York and control-group hospitals appear in Table 9 and support the hypothesis that the prospective reimbursement program in downstate New York has lowered hospital costs per patient stay. From Table 9, equations (1) and (2), we find evidence which suggests that the prospective reimbursement program in downstate New York has lowered the average cost per patient day by 4.5 or 5 percent. In addition, results of equations (3) and (4) indicate that the average cost per hospital stay is about 8.5 percent lower because of the prospective reimbursement program. The coefficients of the teaching status, scope of services, and occupancy variables possess the expected sign and almost all variables are significant. The explanatory power of the equation (that is, R^2) is about .5, which is low compared to some average cost equations estimated in other studies, but relatively high for the average cost per stay equations. The

TABLE 9   The Effect of Prospective Reimbursement on Hospital Costs in Downstate New York

Independent Variables	Log (Average Cost Per Patient Day)		Log (Average Cost Per Patient Stay)	
	(1)	(2)	(3)	(4)
Constant	3.817	3.560	5.312	5.163
	(45.271)a	(54.297)	(42.716)	(62.126)
Log Beds	-.046	.121	.169	.183
	(3.116)	(11.790)	(7.575)	(12.630)
Teaching Status	.275	.279	.414	.414
	(15.093)	(15.050)	(15.070)	(15.083)
Log Occupancy	-.168	-.153b	.098	.006 b
	(3.480)	(2.375)	(1.880)	(1.784)
Time$_{70}$	-.048	-.043	.0980	9.843
Time$_{71}$	.123	.129	.172	.171
	(5.070)	(5.265)	(4.717)	(4.688)
Time$_{72}$	.220	.225	.233	.228
	(8.964)	(9.030)	(6.330)	(6.220)
Time$_{73}$	.212	.223	.214	.230
	(8.388)	(8.670)	(6.064)	(6.028)
Area Dummy	.201	.201	.277	.280
	(9.985)	(9.859)	(9.108)	(9.210)
Log Scope of Services	.148		.019	
	(6.747)		(.543)	
Prospective Reimbursement	-.045	-.051	-.086	-.084
	(1.838)	(2.057)	(2.312)	(2.238)
R^2	.512	.494	.473	.472

aThe numbers in the parentheses are t-scores.
bThe occupancy rate was used as the dependent variable in these equations, rather than the logarithm of the occupancy rate.

estimated cost function may possess some simultaneity bias because of the inclusion of independent variables that are influenced by hospital activity (beds, occupancy rate, teaching status). But attempts at developing a simultaneous equation model for a hospital have been unsuccessful because of the difficulties in precisely defining a model for hospital behavior.

In addition to the impact of prospective reimbursement determined through cost function analysis, the study of downstate New York hospitals examined the time trends of several cost measures. The impact of prospective reimbursement was determined by looking at the rate of increase in costs before and after prospective reimbursement in New York and by comparing this with the experience of the control group. The evaluators adjusted the cost figures for outpatient visits and the difference in input prices among regions and found a substantial downward impact on the average cost per patient day and a moderate downward impact on the average cost per case attributable to the prospective rate program in New York. After differences attributable to input price differences and the number of outpatient visits were factored out, the average cost per patient day rose 21 percent for downstate New York hospitals as compared with a rise of 39 percent for the control hospitals during the 1968–73 period. And during this period, the average cost per case in downstate New York increased 17 percent while the average cost per case in control hospitals rose 20 percent.

Summary

We have reviewed the findings of four evaluations of different prospective reimbursement systems—in Western Pennsylvania, Rhode Island, New Jersey, and New York—sponsored by the Office of Research and Statistics of the Social Security Administration and described the operation and background of each system.

In Rhode Island and New Jersey, participation in the prospective reimbursement system to determine Blue Cross, Medicaid, and state-supported rates was essentially mandatory. All Rhode Island and New Jersey hospitals participated in the experiments and both systems are budget review systems. In Rhode Island and New Jersey, as in all states, Blue Cross premiums soared in the late 1960s in response to enormous increases in the cost of hospital care. Hospitals in both states espoused a budget review system, not because of a firm conviction in the soundness of this process, but more because they felt that any system was preferable to a strict formula system.

Estimation of the impact of prospective reimbursement in Rhode Island and New Jersey was accomplished through the use of a cost function. A prospective reimbursement variable was included among the independent variables and was set equal to 1 for hospitals that participated in the experiment and 0 for those not in the prospective reimbursement system. In regression equations from both states explaining variations in the average cost per day and the average cost per admission, the coefficient of the prospective reimbursement was always found to be insignificant. Only when we estimated the joint impact of the prospective reimbursement program and the Economic Stabilization Program in Rhode Island did we find a significant negative coefficient. The results support the hypothesis that the prospective reimbursement systems in New Jersey and Rhode Island have not significantly lowered the cost or quality of hospital care.

In both the New Jersey and Rhode Island experiments the prospective rates were derived through budget review. Rhode Island hospitals negotiated with the state Blue Cross association in order to arrive at the prospective rate, while the advisory committee in New Jersey proposed rates which were sent to the commissioners of health and insurance for approval. The modest impact of these systems on hospital costs may reflect a basic deficiency in the system of hospital-by-hospital budget review. In face-to-face contact or in the appeals process hospital representatives are better prepared to defend price increases because of their intimate knowledge of the daily operations of the hospital. Review committees with dozens of hospital budgets to process may be reluctant to refuse a price increase for a hospital whose budget they have only quickly reviewed. A formula system that automatically sets the prospective rates obviates the need for a complete review of each hospital's budget and allows rate-setting authorities to concentrate on a few hospital budgets.

The Blue Cross of Western Pennsylvania's prospective reimbursement experiment included only five hospitals, one of which is a rehabilitation center. All five hospitals voluntarily entered the program and all were high-cost hospitals in their groups. (Hospitals are grouped by BCWP according to teaching status, bed size, and location.) Lave, Lave, and Silverman (1971) have found that high-cost hospitals in each BCWP group had lower rates of increase in costs than the lower cost hospitals in the same group. In evaluating the BCWP experiment Applied Management Sciences, Inc. (1975) found that the experimental hospitals experienced a slower rate of increase in their average cost per patient day and their average cost per admission than did the control group hospitals. The cost impact of prospective reimbursement seems to have been on services most directly under the influence of hospital administrators (dietary, nursing, maintenance, housekeeping) rather than on physician-controlled services (pathology, radiology, surgery). The evaluators rejected the hypothesis that prospective reimbursement has led to a deterioration in the quality of care, which is the same conclusion they arrived at for New Jersey and Rhode Island.

The prospective rates in Western Pennsylvania are determined by a combination budget review and formula system. The formula restrictions ensure that the approved budget for a hospital is not out of line with the approved budgets of similar hospitals. In addition, the formula restrictions ensure that the approved budgets as a sum do not represent an increase which varies significantly from the increase in certain price indices for the previous year. Primarily because of the small number of participating hospitals and the problem of self-selection bias, the results of this experiment must not be considered as the final word on the effectiveness of a combination budget review–formula method of prospective reimbursement. It is likely that the five hospitals which entered the experiment were among the hospitals which were best able to effectuate cost decrease. Under these circumstances, we would expect the cost increases for these hospitals to be less than for the control group of hospitals. In any case, further evaluations of this type of prospective rate review system should be conducted with a considerably greater number of participating hospitals.

The prospective rate program in New York state does not set rates through a hospital-by-hospital budget review process. In fact, there is no analysis or comparison of hospital budgets by the rate-setting authorities prior to the certification of the prospective rates. The system sets rates by a formula; a trend factor to account for increased prices in the prospective period is added to a hospital's per diem costs in the period two years prior to the prospective year. There are no automatic retroactive adjustments after the year but dissatisfied hospitals may appeal their rate.

Although, the New York system does not directly restrict hospital expenditures, it appears that controlling hospital revenues has brought about a decrease in costs. Critics of the program maintain that a program which controls only hospital revenues will produce not lower hospital costs, but merely insolvent hospitals. The critics are only partially correct. New York hospitals are becoming less solvent; however, it also appears that hospital costs have been increasing less rapidly because of the squeeze on hospital funds.

New Events

Since 1973, a number of new prospective payment systems have been started that have not yet been evaluated. As of August 1975, nine states had enacted state prospective payment and rate-review legislation. In three of these states (Washington, Connecticut, and Massachusetts) special commissions have been specifically organized to perform these functions. In the remaining six (New York, New Jersey, Arizona, Rhode Island, Maryland, and Colorado) this same power is vested in previously existing public agencies.

State rate-setting systems vary in their organizations, procedures, and control; yet every state rate-setting system has changed considerably the substance and form of its program after a few years of operation.

These kaleidoscopic systems adapt quickly to the changing requirements of their states' political, economic, and social environment and alternatively cajole, beseech, urge, and demand compliance with their wishes without causing major upheavals or dislocations. Most state rate-setting programs conduct a hospital-by-hospital budget review in order to set rates. This permits each hospital to present its case to the rate-setting body and thus increases the equity of the regulatory process.

A Request for Proposal (RFP) was issued on September 30, 1975, by the Office of Research and Statistics, SSA, which solicited responses from state agencies that encouraged the respondents to develop either a formula-based or budget-review-by-exception approach. Several contracts have recently been awarded to state rate-setting agencies, and presently the Office of Research and Statistics is funding rate-setting efforts in Maryland, New Jersey, Massachusetts, Connecticut, Western Pennsylvania, and Rhode Island. Although an evaluation of these experiments and other ongoing state programs is not available, there is some preliminary evidence that suggests that recent state efforts to lessen the pace of hospital cost inflation have been effective.

The most significant feature of the Rhode Island rate-setting program is the statewide maxi-cap. The maxi-cap is an outside guarantee on the aggregate gross operating expenses of the voluntary hospitals in Rhode Island. The maxi-cap for the past two fiscal years (13.85 percent for 1975 and 11.5 percent for 1976) has been significantly lower than the rates of increase in total hospital expenditures for the nation (17.6 percent in 1975 and 14.8 percent in 1976).

Arizona operates a rate-review program that mandates a review of hospital budgets by the Department of Health Services, but relies on voluntary compliance. Recent evidence shows (Arizona Health, 1977:4):

> that since the beginning of the state's rate review program in 1972, hospital charges in Arizona have increased at a lesser rate than the national average. For example, a recent study of the impact of hospital rate regulation showed that during the period 1972–1975, the annual percent change in hospital expenditures per capita in Arizona was 11.4 percent. The comparable percent change in seven sample states without a rate review program was 14.4 percent.

The Maryland Health Services Cost Review Commission is comprised of seven members and is an independent commission within the Department of Health and Mental Hygiene. The commission was established in 1973 to review and certify rates established by health care institutions. Data from the Bureau of Labor Statistics indicate that hospital charges in Maryland have increased 14.8 percent during the period 1974–1976, which is about half the rate of increase for the nation. In addition, the commission has recently evinced evidence that demonstrates that the average cost per patient day during 1976 rose 11.78 percent for Maryland as compared to 14.87 percent for the nation.

In the summer of 1977, a contract was awarded to evaluate the effectiveness of various state rate-setting commissions. From this evaluation we should learn more about the impact of the new state rate-setting commissions on the cost and quality of health care.

Overall, however, firm conclusions concerning the dampening effect of prospective reimbursement on hospital inflation in the four experiments reviewed are not easily drawn. Lack of statistical significance in some cases, and possible specification biases in the cost functions employed, cloud any definitive interpretation of the potential and magnitude of cost savings.

Some lessons of experience that highlight those factors critical to an effective system are, nevertheless, noteworthy:

1. The ability of a rate-setting authority to function is conditioned by numerous political, legal, and economic influences;
2. Uniform hospital accounting and budget information are essential for prospective rate setting;
3. There is a need to coordinate health planning and rate-setting functions;
4. System focus should be on total hospital expenditures and cost per case rather than restricted to a per diem cost basis (that is, allow for the impact of changes in utilization);
5. Prospective reimbursement systems should involve the active participation of all third-party payers, including commercial insurers;
6. Less costly and more flexible statistical measures (for example, conceptually appropriate formulas) as well as reasonable exception processes must evolve.

Finally, there are many other existing approaches to prospective reimbursement in the United States that require evaluation. Such evaluation may generate somewhat harder data on the potential for prospective reimbursement to lessen the pace of cost inflation. It will certainly be an important component of the continuing effort to make our health system more cost-conscious in the future.

References

Applied Management Sciences, Inc.
    1975   Analysis of Prospective Reimbursement Systems: Western Pennsylvania. Prepared for the Office of Research and Statistics,

Social Security Administration, U.S. DHEW, under Contract No. HEW-OS-74-226.

Arizona Health
1977   Volume II, No. 9, January.

Bauer, K.G.
1974   The Combined Budget Review and Formula Approach to Prospective Reimbursement by the Blue Cross of Western Pennsylvania. Harvard Center for Community Health and Medical Care.

Bauer, K.G., and A.R. Clark°
1974a   New York: The Formula Approach to Prospective Reimbursement. Harvard Center for Community Health and Medical Care.
1974b   The Indiana Controlled Charges System. Harvard Center for Community Health and Medical Care.
1974c   The New Jersey Budget Review Program. Harvard Center for Community Health and Medical Care.
1974d   Budget Review and Prospective Rate Setting for Rhode Island Hospitals. Harvard Center for Community Health and Medical Care.

Center for Analysis of Public Issues
1974   Bureaucratic Malpractice. Princeton, N.J.

Dowling, W.
1974   "Prospective reimbursement of hospitals." Inquiry 11 (September): 163–180.

Geomet, Inc.
1974   The New Jersey Hospital Prospective Reimbursement Study. Gaithersburg, Md.

Hellinger, F.J.
1974   "A comment on a proposal for incentive reimbursement for hospitals." Medical Care 12 (February): 186.

Lave, J., and L. Lave
1970   "Hospital cost functions." American Economic Review 60 (June): 379–395.

°Studies prepared for the Social Security Administration under grant No. 5-P16-HS00472 from the National Center for Health Services Research and Development. Copies may be secured at no charge from Office of Research and Statistics, Social Security Administration, Washington, D.C.

Lave, J., L. Lave, and L.P. Silverman
1973   "A proposal for incentive reimbursement for hospitals." Medical Care 11 (March–April): 79–90.
Roemer, M., A.T. Moustafa, and C.E. Hopkins
1968   "A proposed hospital quality index: Hospital death rate adjusted for case severity." Health Services Research (Summer): 96–118.
Thornberry, H., and H. Zimmerman
1975   Hospital Cost Control: An Assessment of the Rhode Island Experience with Prospective Reimbursement, 1971 and 1972. Rhode Island Health Services Research. Prepared for the Social Security Administration, U.S. DHEW, under Contract No. HEW-OS-74-197.
U.S. Congress
1972   U.S. Senate Committee on Finance. Public Law 92-603, 92d Congress, House Resolution 1, Section 222 (October): 62.
U.S. Department of Health, Education, and Welfare
1972   Medicare Report Number 92-23. In House Resolution 1, Social Security Amendments of 1972.

Experiences of a State Cost Control Commission

HAROLD A. COHEN

There has been much discussion in recent years concerning the application of prospective rate setting to the hospital industry, especially through a public utility-type pricing model (Sattler, 1975; Hanft and Rettig, 1975).

Let us briefly describe the public utility model and make some institutional observations that relate the economic rationale behind the model to the hospital industry. Observed divergencies will, in turn, lead us to observe differences in the expected institutional conduct and performance as individual hospitals react to regulations (Scherer, 1970).

We shall then discuss the formation of Maryland's Health Services Cost Review Commission (HSCRC) and outline its duties and responsibilities. The Maryland commission was the first to attempt public utility-type regulation of hospitals; similar commissions have been established in Connecticut and Washington (Lewin and Associates, Inc., 1975).

The major part of this study relates problems and experiences regarding the HSCRC's attempt to meet its responsibilities. Many, if not all, of these experiences could have been predicted after reading Stigler (1971) and Pauly and Redisch (1973).

The Public Utility Model

The economic rationale for the development of regulated monopoly generally includes at least the following points (from Kahn, 1970):

1. That the service provided is important. This importance is associated both with a sizable share of GNP and with inelasticity of demand;

2. That there is a prevalence of "natural monopoly" such that costs are lower if there is a single supplier;

3. That for some reason or other, competition does not work well.

There is considerable current concern because of the high and growing share of health care in GNP. Hospital care is the most costly part of health care. Much evidence also points to a low price elasticity of demand for hospital care. While hospital care may not be as "important" in an input-output model as most conventional public utilities are, its importance to the public is clear.

A large body of literature suggests that hospitals are not natural monopolies in large markets, but rather that all significant economies of scale have probably been realized by 200 beds and that the optimal scale is probably no larger than 400 beds.

There are various reasons why competition does not appear to work well. These include consumer ignorance, the not-for-profit nature of the industry, the prevalence of insurance, the major cost-based reimbursers, and so on. (Cohen, 1968).

Since market price has not acted as an efficient allocator of resources into and within the hospital sector, establishment of prices by governmental units, using the public utility model as a rate-setting device, might be a significant improvement. Yet given the existence of price inelasticity of demand, especially for heavily insured individuals, the major behavioral reactions to altering the way rates are set are expected to come from the industry.

The public utility pricing model is often a matter of applying a formula concerning fair value, fair return, expenses, and the rate level:

$$\text{Rate of return} = \frac{\text{revenues} - \text{expenses}}{\text{fair value}} .$$

The model reflects average cost pricing in that marginal cost pricing leads to losses for natural monopolies. In hospitals of most sizes in Maryland (the average size is 250 beds—the majority are between

200 and 600), long-run marginal cost is probably very close to average cost. Once the rate of return, the rate base, and prospective expenses are determined, the above formula is solved to yield the required revenues, or the rate level.

The remaining question is how to generate the required revenue. This is a matter of the rate structure and includes such questions as whether prices should be higher during peak use, whether bulk buyers should receive discounts, whether sidelines should be priced according to full costs or differential costs, what are sidelines, and so on.

This is, of course, a very cursory discussion of the utility model. The reader is referred to Kahn (1970, 1971) for a more complete exposition.

The absence of a profit motive and equity capital in almost all Maryland hospitals has effectively reduced the utility pricing model to:

$$\text{revenues} = \text{cost.}$$

Many of the experiences that follow refer to attempts to define costs as well as attempts to reach an equitable rate structure. Furthermore, the absence of natural monopoly and of the profit motive makes the control of capacity especially difficult.

Several writers have suggested that hospitals attempt to maximize output subject to a budget constraint. Moreover, the nature of hospital reimbursement, particularly the inclusion of depreciation as a cost for Medicare, Medicaid, and Blue Cross, has guaranteed that any profits or donations spent on capital expansion will be largely recovered through payments for hospital services.

Since hospital buildings are very expensive (in part because of prevalent reimbursement methods) and have few alternative uses, there is good reason to be wary of entry that diverts business from an old but still useful facility. On the other hand, since there are no significant economies of scale, regulators should be sure not to favor existing firms when it comes to either serving expanded needs or replacing outmoded facilities where the capacity is needed.

In sum, then, the economic rationale for at least attempting

public utility-type regulation exists. The absence of natural monopoly requires special consideration. Many states have attempted to
regulate capital expenditure under certificate-of-need laws. The
consensus seems to be that such control has not worked well
(Havighurst, 1973).

Unlike the model visualized in the National Health Planning and
Resources Development Act (P.L. 93-641), Maryland has established
one agency, the HSCRC, to review rates and another, Comprehensive Health Planning (CHP), to review capital projects.

It might be pointed out at this time that the hospital industry
differs markedly from power companies, though less so from water
and transportation companies, in the existence of a quality difference, the difficulty of quality measurement, and the threat of quality
deterioration. Much of the responsibility for guarding against quality deterioration as a reaction to rate control is in the hands of
Maryland's various PSROs. Thus, hospital rates, capital expenditure,
and quality are all reviewed by different agencies. This paper
concentrates on experiences of the rate-review agency, with some
discussion of its relations to CHP.

Background

Attempts to create a commission began in 1967 when Representative Rosalie Abrams, a former nurse, introduced a three-part
legislative package. The parts concerning Comprehensive Health
Planning and facility licensure were enacted, but the part concerning rate control was not. A rate-control bill was introduced every
year, but it was not until 1971, when the Maryland Hospital Association decided to support the idea, that Abrams (now senator) was
able to amass enough support, including strong backing from the
governor, to have such a bill enacted into law.[1]

Maryland's hospitals had two main reasons for supporting state
rate regulation. First, they feared rate regulation by the federal
government, especially if that regulation was bureaucratically re-

[1] The bill was cosponsored by Senator Abrams, a trustee of Sinai Hospital, and
Senator McGuirk, a trustee of South Baltimore General Hospital.

lated to one of the government payment programs. Second, and more important, they hoped to get Maryland Blue Cross to pay a share of charity and bad debts.

Maryland Blue Cross reimbursed hospitals on the basis of cost elements that were almost identical to Medicare's and Medicaid's. Blue Cross pays somewhat more than Medicare or Medicaid because it pays charges rather than costs for covered outpatient services (mostly accident-related emergencies and some diagnostic services) and because it pays the average per diem plus 10 percent for private room days. These divergences are designed, if inadvertently, to help the rich suburban hospitals while squeezing the older inner city hospitals, which have fewer private rooms and more bad debts.

Blue Cross tried to block the creation of the commission, but while it was unable to do so, it was able to get modifications in the law which, it thought, would protect it. We will see to what extent the hospitals and Blue Cross have been successful.

Blue Cross's main concern has been with the differential afforded it relative to charges made to patients covered by its competitors— the commercial insurance companies. Any spreading of bad debts lessens the differential and makes it easier for the commercials to compete on a price basis. In Maryland, Blue Cross has been paying an average of 86 to 90 percent of charges statewide. The importance of this discount cannot be overemphasized. In large part, it is the reason the commission was created and has Hospital Association support. The discount's size contrasts with the other states that have all-inclusive rate control, Connecticut and Washington, where Blue Cross paid approximately 98 percent of charges before regulation. Group Hospitalization, Inc. (GHI), the Blue Cross plan in Washington, D.C., which covers the Maryland suburbs of the District, reputedly pays more lucratively.

Maryland's hospital industry perceived its bad debt problem and the public perceived problems associated with rising costs. The commission's enabling act gives it responsibility to eliminate all inequities, including those caused by the way the costs of uncompensated care are covered, and to eliminate unreasonable costs and rates (including those caused by previous payment mechanisms).

Powers and Duties

The commission has authority regarding certain health care institutions—hospitals and nursing homes.[2] Here we emphasize its authority regarding hospitals.

Public Disclosure

The commission is to cause the public disclosure of the financial condition of hospitals. Toward this end, it has developed a Uniform Accounting and Reporting System (ARS). Annual reports have been circulated detailing such data as operating and bottom line "profit," gross revenue, percentage occupancy, cost per equivalent inpatient days,[3] and so on. In addition, all files are open. The public, including the press, is encouraged to review the data bank and files.

The most significant aspect of the ARS is that functions are uniformly defined and statistics defined for reporting work load. Thus, the data bank includes arrays by hospital of each function. For example, the public can see what the direct costs are for different hospitals to perform diagnostic x-rays according to the American College of Radiology's Relative Value Units (including and excluding any money the hospital pays the radiologist).[4]

An example of a policy problem in relation to disclosure is one hospital that appeared to be in serious financial trouble and was attempting to arrange loans, delays in paying withholding taxes, and so on. Public disclosure of this condition might harm the hospital's ability to resolve it; that is, any public attempt by the commission to help with the problem might actually make it unresolvable. Creditors might descend en masse and demand payment or bankruptcy

[2] This originally included domiciliary homes that provide no real nursing care. Some homes for alcoholics were also covered, but no purely ambulatory centers. The commission sponsored legislation in 1977 that eliminated all institutions except hospitals and nursing homes from its jurisdiction.

[3] EIPDs are a weighted sum of inpatient and outpatient activity. The ratio of outpatient visits to inpatient admissions in Baltimore is among the highest in the country (see any AHA annual statistical report).

[4] The use of these arrays by the staff in cost review will be discussed below.

proceedings. Yet the commission, by law, must "keep itself informed as to whether the financial resources of each institution are sufficient to meet its financial requirements and to concern itself with solutions when resources are inadequate" (Annotated Code of Maryland, Article 13, §568H). To date, the commission is keeping itself informed and seeking solutions quietly.[5]

Rate Review

The commission is charged with assuring the public that (1) an institution's total costs are reasonably related to the total services offered; (2) an institution's aggregate rates are reasonably related to its aggregate costs; and (3) rates are set equitably among all purchasers or classes of purchasers without undue discrimination. Further, the commission must approve prospectively rates that permit an efficient and effective nonprofit institution to remain solvent and allow an efficient and effective proprietary institution to earn a fair return on fair value.

For their part, institutions cannot charge any rate other than that approved by the commission (Article 13, §568U). The commission-approved rate is both a maximum and a minimum. This latter aspect is not dictated by some economic theory. The hospital industry, in drafting the bill, included it so that, for example, Blue Cross could not bargain with individual hospitals for discounts, without having to convince the commission both that it was entitled to unique consideration of some type, and that the proposed discount was equitable for all classes of purchasers.

The problems associated with implementing this portion of the commission's responsibilities are discussed below.

Trustee Disclosure

Following a series of articles in the Washington *Post*, a section was added to the law requiring trustees of nonprofit hospitals and nursing homes to submit annual reports detailing all business trans-

---

[5] Seeking solutions does not necessarily mean maintaining the solvency of the institution, which was very inefficient.

actions conducted among themselves or between their firm and the institution.[6]

It is important to note that the law does not assume anything is wrong. Many times lending institutions require board membership as a prerequisite to granting a large loan. (Several oil companies do not have a friend at Chase Manhattan—they have a director.) Many lawyer-trustees donate free services to the institution.

Some of the most interesting problems involve physician-trustees. I received a call from a radiologist-trustee who had a contract with the hospital. Under that contract, he was paid one-third of departmental gross billings. The trustee asked if there was any potential conflict to report. (Both his contract and departmental billings were subject to board approval.) The commission recently held a public hearing concerning a pathologist-trustee whose contract called for 20 percent of the gross or 50 percent of the net billings for both pathology and radioisotopy. His income under the contract as the hospital's sole pathologist was budgeted at $433,000 for fiscal year 1976 (In re Union Hospital of Cecil County). During the hearing, commission Vice-Chairman Mancur Olson, an economist at the University of Maryland, questioned the two hospital board members who testified as to whether their decision and discussions were influenced by the physician's being on the board. One board member testified that the physician had telephoned other board members in support of his contract.

The commission, then, has three broad areas of responsibility: public disclosure of financial conditions, rate review, and trustee disclosure. While the disclosure aspects have generated some interest, most has been concentrated on rate review.

Experiences and Problems in Areas of Rate Review

The commission's rate-review proceedings can begin in two ways. Either a hospital applies for a change in its rates or the

---

[6] No report is required if the dealings are worth less than $15,000 or if the trustee-firm relationship is marginal. For example, a trustee would have to be beneficial owner of 3 percent of the stock in AT&T before having to be concerned with reporting the volume of business.

commission orders an investigation of the hospital's existing rates. The first and most difficult task for the commission is to determine reasonable costs for the services offered.

Service-Cost Relationship

After development of the Uniform Accounting and Reporting System the major concern was to develop the budget review system. The commission's staff reviews budgets on the basis of its guidelines and recommends dollars to be disapproved and/or issues for a public hearing. In performing its budget review by exception, the commission's staff uses two types of screens. Each hospital's direct costs for the various functions are compared with those of other hospitals and with the prior year's approved or actual cost for internal inflation. Costs are reviewed prior to any allocation.

The commission, with the aid of a federal contract, is moving toward absolute cost standards. Relative comparisons do not catch widespread inefficiencies.

The exceptions picked up by the external, interhospital comparative screens are hospital cost centers above the eightieth percentile in their group—urban, rural, or teaching. When an exception is noted, the staff asks for an explanation and recommends either approval, disapproval, or modification of the amount over the eightieth percentile. A hearing may well be called for on the issues so noted.

The eightieth percentile criterion is applied to direct costs in patient care areas other than physician costs,[7] which are reviewed separately. The costs of hospitals with large house staffs should not be compared with costs of those without unless house staff costs are isolated. Furthermore, hospitals that pay, for example, radiologists or pathologists on a percentage or salary basis cannot fairly have their total departmental costs compared with those in a hospital where the physician bills directly. The commission has isolated physician costs and reviews them individually. As was mentioned

[7] The commission has used restraint in challenging nursing costs because the current measure of output, the patient day, is so poor. Regulations were recently published requiring the submission of case-mix data so that the burden of illness brought to each daily patient care center can be more accurately measured.

above, the commission's authority extends only to the hospital's (or nursing home's) rates. Thus, physician charges are regulated only when the physician is on salary or when the physician gets a percentage of hospital billings.

Certain hospital-based physicians—most notably pathologists and radiologists—are granted an exclusive franchise or monopoly by the hospital. Once in a hospital (which itself is almost never chosen by the patient, but by the attending physician), the patient has no choice of radiologist or pathologist. The commission believes that the way in which this service is billed is a matter of form and that the substance of the arrangement is one of monopoly. The commission has introduced legislation to extend its authority to such services regardless of how the patient is billed, but those efforts have failed. Several hospitals have recently requested and received lower rates in radiology as their radiologists have shifted to direct billing— and thus avoided both the public disclosure and rate-review aspects of the commission's law.

The inflation screen is developed for each hospital by applying specific hospital-based weights to inflation factors calculated by the staff. Separate factors are maintained for labor (relevant CPI) and other supplies. Fuel and malpractice insurance increases have been treated as a pass-through. Hospitals must explain any increase in inflation which exceeds the screen developed for them.

The budget or rate-review system develops costs as defined and prescribed by the commission. Thus, the costs that are subject to the exception review process are developed somewhat differently than they are by Medicare and Medicaid.

Treatment of capital costs In developing the ARS, the commission determined to abandon traditional depreciation accounting. Depreciation may be fine for some purposes, but is not appropriate for rate making. What historical cost-based depreciation can lead to is exemplified by applying it to one of Baltimore's hospitals that was built, free of debt, with a gift of $17,000,000. Given a forty-year life, depreciation would be $425,000 per year. If the money was invested, at, say, 8 percent, then at the end of forty years, the hospital, as a tax-exempt institution, would have assets of $110,100,000 in its building fund (whether the hospital was needed or not and whether $17,000,000 was excessive or not). This potential accumulation of capital appears unreasonable.

The commission has substituted a new system of determining reasonable capital costs for purposes of rate approval. First, replacement cost depreciation is used for equipment in the capital-intensive areas. Hospitals are not driven to the capital or lease markets for equipment. Second, an allowance per bed is approved for general equipment. This amount was based on auditing a sample of hospitals. The allowance is inflated to represent replacement cost. This aspect of the system has come under heavy criticism from hospitals even though the formula allowance is high—on average much more than the Medicare payment.

The main argument and the legal challenge have involved the building portion of the Capital Facilities Allowance (CFA). Hospitals are expected to enter the capital market for major replacements.

Capital costs are calculated as being the greater of two options. The first is cash needs to pay existing mortgages; the second is an amount of money sufficient to provide a down payment (currently 20 percent) on the current replacement value of the target beds calculated for the hospital.

The first computation is clear. The second requires elaboration. Current replacement value is developed by financial consultants to the commission. The figure (currently around $50,000 per bed) has been under heavy criticism from the industry—especially since many hospitals were built at much higher cost.[8]

Target beds are also calculated by the commission. Target beds represent average occupancy plus reasonable standby capacity. The target is developed separately for each patient care area in the hospital. For purposes of developing reasonable standby capacity (or the reasonable number of average empty beds), patient care areas are grouped with all others within fifteen minutes' accessibility, a Poisson distribution is assumed (which overstates the variability in areas with elective admissions), and reasonable extra beds in

---

[8] It is the nature of depreciation, of course, to put more money into richer communities that provide themselves with more costly hospitals—whether reasonably or not.

the area are determined as equal to three standard deviations. These extra beds are then allocated back to the hospital under review, based on its share of the area market.[9]

This situation clearly puts the commission somewhat in the planning business and it also raises issues concerning closed physician's privileges.

When a hospital is paid according to the down-payment option, the dollars must be funded in the accounting sense, that is, the institution must account for them; it need not store them. The funding target is offset by the currently available building fund.

It is important also to note that when a hospital budgets at occupancy below the minimum target level, the commission may well approve rates at what costs would be at the minimum occupancy level. In the Union Memorial case (1974), the sum of $198,900 was disapproved on the basis that the projected pediatric utilization was too low and the resultant budgeted cost of $191 per day was much too high.

The hospitals have challenged the CFA. A group of twenty-five hospitals took us to court, and Judge Proctor, in his opinion, stated that the CFA was unlawful (Franklin Square et al., 1975a).[10] The order states that hospitals could choose between depreciation and the CFA (Franklin Square et al., 1975b). Even though Judge Proctor believed the CFA to be unlawful, he felt hospitals could choose it when they wanted. The 1975 Maryland legislature, at the request of

---

[9]Assume hospital X is within fifteen minutes of hospitals A, B, C, and D and has an average pediatric census of 15, hospital A, 25, hospital B, 20, hospital C, 21, while hospital D has no pediatric service. Then the guidelines for the target pediatric beds in the region defined by hospital X is 108. (15 + 25 + 20 + 21 = 81; square root = 9; 81 + 3(9) = 108.) The recommended pediatric portion of the CFA for hospital X would be based on twenty beds. This derives from the following:

$$\frac{\text{average census of Hospital X}}{\text{average census in region}} \times \text{target beds}; \ 15/81 \times 108 = 20.$$

(HSCRC, 1975.)

[10]It might be noted that Judge Proctor thought the CFA was based only on replacement of average occupied beds, but the commission thought effective utilization meant 100 percent occupancy. He labeled, among other things, the description of using the Poisson distribution to calculate reasonable standby capacity as "gobbledygook" (Franklin Square et al., 1975a). The lower court decision has recently been reversed.

the commission, revised the law so that the CFA is not unlawful and can probably be applied when the commission deems it to be the reasonable basis for rate approval. This law is yet to be tested.

One question raised by the hospitals is "What about money for expansion and for new devices?" First, patients should not have to pay for services they are not receiving, and second, regulatory commissions should not assume that new markets or expanded needs should be met by existing firms rather than entrants. As discussed earlier, the hospital business is not a natural monopoly and start-up costs can be capitalized. There is more on this subject below.

Treatment of contracts and labor settlements The commission holds that the existence of a contract does not prove reasonableness or efficiency. For example, in a case in Cumberland, Maryland, the staff challenged the pathologist's income (In re Sacred Heart). Two pathologists and a lab technician were under contract to receive $300,000. The evidence indicated that the technician was receiving about $15,000. The commission approved a total of $180,000. The hospital has appealed in part on the basis of the existence of a valid contract. One of the commission's arguments is that the contract has not been abridged. The hospital can still pay the $300,000, but it cannot charge *patients* any more than $180,000, that is, the part found to be reasonable by the commission.

In the Union Hospital of Cecil County case, previously discussed, the commission challenged a physician's contract that was renegotiated downward prior to the hearing. The pathologist was to earn $433,000 but the renegotiated contract called for $293,000, of which $25,000 was for equipment and an unspecified amount was for hiring another pathologist. The commission, after a hearing, allowed $185,000. The hospital did not appeal. It is important to note that Blue Cross, Medicaid, and Medicare paid all these amounts without question.

There is little unionization in Maryland hospitals. Only eight have unions, all in the greater Baltimore area and mostly in the inner city. The bargaining unit does not extend up to practical nurses except in the case of one hospital.

A few unionized hospitals in Baltimore did have a short strike before a wage agreement was signed. Other hospitals gave wage increases to meet (or beat) the union. After the strike, the union employees won an increase of approximately 12 percent. In the one hospital where LPNs were covered, the percentage increase was less because the agreement was for an across-the-board cents-per-hour increase.

Baltimore County General, a suburban Baltimore hospital, gave its employees a 12 percent across-the-board increase—administrators, RNs, LPNs, and so on. The commission found $90,000 of the increase to be unreasonable. The hospital appealed. The court remanded the case on procedural grounds but the judge indicated that based on the current record, he would reverse (Baltimore County General, 1975). He argued that the hospital had a right to give across-the-board increases. The commission, while questioning the wisdom of the increases, does not deny the hospital's right to grant them; it questioned the size of the increase. If the case is reopened for public hearing, much testimony will be put in the record to show that hospital employees are no longer underpaid relative to other industries. The existence of a contract does not make reasonable all payments it requires.

The commission reviewed wage increases given employees in Bon Secours Hospital (1975). The hospital had hired a consultant who provided data on relative salaries and listed two possible wage policies. The less costly would have the hospital meet the wage rates in the community; the higher one would allow it to meet the wage rates in other hospitals. The hospital chose the second. The commission order allows Bon Secours to meet its current costs, but did not give it any money for wage increases to meet future inflation.

House staff costs It is clearly incorrect to compare per diem costs of a hospital with a house staff with those of one without. The commission appointed two committees (made up mostly of physicians)—one for teaching hospitals and one for nonteaching hospitals—to review physician coverage cost and make recommendations. The commission received much useful data but no guidelines for review.

At the same time, the Board of Medical Examiners, a group of physicians appointed by the medical society, determined that preceptorships would be terminated. At the national level, a determination was made, again by physicians, that many residencies and internships in nonteaching hospitals would be terminated.

With this background in mind, the commission began the review of Baltimore County General Hospital, a 188-bed hospital. The hospital had budgeted an increase from $340,000 to $860,000 for providing nonemergency room coverage. It had signed contracts for physician coverage, including substantial pay for on-call time, and so forth. In testimony two chiefs of services, both of whom admitted fee-for-service patients to the hospital, testified that the coverage was needed. In cross-examination, it was apparent that neither the physicians nor the hospital's administration knew how much work was being done for the dollars.

The commission found $470,000 of the $860,000 to be unreasonable. In his obiter dicta, however, the judge indicated that on the basis of the evidence he would reverse. The commission, he said, must put on a positive case, not just show that the hospital could not prove reasonableness. Furthermore, he indicated that it would take the preponderance of the evidence to dispute a professional's testimony. The commission had not put explicitly into the record the degree of self-interest on the part of the hospital's witnesses. Building a record appears to require all-out adversary-type hostility or else the hospitals will win their appeals. The commission's staff had anticipated this need and had lined up three witnesses, a physician, a nurse, and a health planner specializing in manpower needs. All three were advised not to testify by their employers just prior to the staff's taking of depositions.

An interesting sidelight to the Baltimore County General case is that the attending medical staff has threatened not to bring any patients to the hospital unless they have full coverage. The doctors apparently have other places to bring their patients. Yet the hospital has recent CHP approval to build an entirely new facility totaling 242 beds. It is not clear at this writing whether there will be further hearings in this case.

The treatment of working capital The commission treats the reasonable cost of financing accounts receivable as a legitimate cost element. In order to distribute those costs equitably, the commission adds 2 percent to all hospital bills to represent the cost of working capital. Hospitals must give a 2 percent discount to any purchaser who either pays upon discharge or provides an advance equal to the payer's average outstanding balance. A 1 percent discount is provided for payment within thirty days. The commission has ordered some hospitals to charge interest of 1 percent per month on late accounts. Several hospitals have requested that this be made optional and the commission has approved the request.

It should be noted that public utilities are expected to invest working capital and are allowed a return on that investment. Similarly, the commission allows in rates enough money to maintain an adequate working capital position. This allowance differs from that provided by Medicaid only to the extent that hospitals' working capital advance is other than their average outstanding balance. It differs from Medicare's PIP program in that PIP expects hospitals to finance three weeks of receivables.

The services hospitals provide are costly. As discussed above, the commission reviews the reasonableness of budgeted cost in its relationship to budgeted service volumes. The costs are developed in a uniform manner and include important departures from Medicare and Medicaid. The most significant differences are the treatment of capital costs and the treatment of working capital. Having determined reasonable costs, the commission must approve aggregate rates that are reasonably related to those costs.

Cost-Revenue Relationship: The Rate Level

The commission's rate-review system recognizes "other financial considerations." These are adjustments to costs that are taken into account in determining reasonable rates. The major adjustments relate to nonpatient care revenues, especially endowment income, charity and bad debts, and losses from nonpatient care activities.

The commission has indicated that it is not exercising any authority over rates for nonpatient care activities. Hospitals can alter nursing school tuitions, cafeteria rates, or rental rates on physicians' offices without prior approval. The prime concern is that patients are not asked to subsidize those activities unduly.

As to endowment income, the commission holds that it cannot be allowed to subsidize inefficiency and ineffectiveness. The hospital must indicate how it intends to use its indowment income, and the commission reviews the plan for reasonableness. Endowment income has been used as an offset to rates unless CHP has given permission to build. Then endowment income can be accumulated to offset approved construction costs.

The commission has not applied endowment corpus unless it was volunteered by the hospital. In the case of Children's Hospital (with an annual budget of approximately \$4.7 million and endowment funds of approximately \$7.1 million), the hospital applied for a 61 percent rate increase on grounds that its costs were above its charges (1974). Maryland Blue Cross does not allow carry-over of such "losses" so the hospital wanted to charge rates high enough in the latter part of the fiscal year to avoid having charges below cost for the fiscal year settlement. During the course of the proceeding, the hospital volunteered to offset rates not only by the income from its endowment fund, but by \$250,000 of the corpus. The commission approved a rate increase slightly above the level of cost, about a 25 percent increase.

In the Sinai case, the hospital willingly pledged over \$1,000,000 in endowment fund income to offset costs of charity care, education, and research (1975). A witness for Sinai argued that unless capital donations were matched by depreciation, the future of such donations was in jeopardy. That witness indicated that in his collection efforts for universities, he never had problems because tuition did not cover depreciation.[11]

Two other cases, Suburban Hospital (1975) and Church Hospital (1975), indicate the importance some hospitals place on this issue.

Suburban Hospital (annual budget \$16.1 million, total endowments \$13.7 million) has, for the past several years, been the most profitable hospital in the state. Its endowment funds are apparently almost entirely made up of previous patient revenues. In June 1974, just before the commission began to regulate but after the guidelines

[11] I do not look upon the prospect of lessening donations for hospital capital projects as a terrible thing.

were distributed, the hospital spun off a foundation under the IRS code. The foundation was given $5.9 million. The hospital claimed it had no control over the dollars and challenged the commission's right even to get information about the fund. The information was subpoenaed and the hospital provided the needed information while still claiming that none of the income could be used to offset rates. Since the hospital has permission from CHP for a $15 million expansion and indicated the money would be used for construction, no offset was made other than for the small amount of charity the hospital had budgeted.

Church Hospital took other legal steps. Before rate review Church Home and Hospital of the City of Baltimore Corporation ran a hospital and a nursing home, and had endowments (very little, if any, from patient profits). Then the corporation spun off the hospital and the nursing home but kept the money. In its testimony, relative to a review designed to approve rates beginning December 1, 1975, the hospital stated that it had not received any money from Church Home and Hospital during the past fiscal year and did not expect to receive any during the next fiscal year. The commission used the entire $180,000 income as a rate offset.

The other major question in this area regards "profits" or money for "growth." Overall, the commission believes that a reasonable relationship between costs and revenues is for a prospective break-even budget. In determining that position, accounting-type profit and loss statements are irrelevant. Rather, reasonable expected uses of funds should balance with expected sources of funds to maintain the solvency of an efficient and effective hospital.

A hospital's reasonable expected uses of funds must, of course, reflect reasonable reactions to inflation. The commission's staff believes the treatment of inflation is one of the most important aspects of the review system. It introduces incentives by way of lengthening regulatory lag and provides general guidelines for hospital cost behavior. It minimizes the commission's involvement in management decision review. The system basically works as follows.

The rate-review system develops cost for projected volumes at factor prices that prevailed at the close of the fiscal year. Indices are maintained for labor (based on CPI), food (based on CPI and WPI series), and other supplies (WPI adjusted). Fuel and malpractice insurance have been treated as a pass-through. Replacement cost is monitored for equipment. The above factors are applied to fiscal year-end costs to project cost as of when rates are approved.

The rates approved are prospective. This normally requires a projection of inflation but that is avoided by the commission's system. Rather, the costs at factor prices as of approval are increased by 3 percent. Inflation is then monitored. Whenever inflation reaches 6 percent, the hospital has broken even and receives a 6 percent increase to again put it 3 percent ahead of current factor costs. Through this method, any hospital that can live within the inflating adjustment can avoid a review. If hospital costs had not been increasing so much faster than the CPI, no commissions would have been formed.

The commission's enabling act requires it to review each hospital individually. Furthermore, Blue Cross should be given an opportunity for objection before being asked to pay a larger share of any hospital's approved costs. The commission as of June 1977 had reviewed and approved rates for all general hospitals in Maryland. Medicare and Medicaid began paying on the basis of those rates on July 1, 1977.

Undue Discrimination, or the Rate Structure

The commission approves rates that are binding upon individual purchasers. While all-inclusive rates are sufficient for determining Blue Cross, Medicare, or Medicaid reimbursement, they may not be for individual patients.

One of the trickiest jobs for a commission like the HSCRC is to walk the line between protecting the public and allowing management discretion. We have determined that the appropriate level of involvement in rate approval is the average charge per some statistic in the revenue centers. Unless sound reasons are presented, each patient care area is expected to be self-supporting, that is, patients pay the costs of their own treatment. We have allowed cross-subsidization primarily of clinics and emergency rooms. In the short run, subsidization of obstetrical and related services has been allowed (though not to its previous extent).

Clinic subsidies are permitted for several reasons. Charging rates equal to costs would increase charges but not increase net revenue. Many clinic users are receiving worse care than that generally given in physicians' offices. Burdening those patients, almost all of whom are quite poor, with full allocated costs seems unfair. Further, there is considerable question as to whether any faith should be put into the allocation of joint costs, especially to sidelines such as clinic care. The commission has not allowed clinic rates to go below average direct cost (Faulhaber, 1975).

The primary reason for allowing subsidization for obstetrical and related services is the existence of poor insurance coverage. The commission will shortly begin approving rates that reflect the cost of those services. Hospitals have kept the public from knowing the true cost of the excessive duplication in these services; for instance, many hospitals offer services yet average less than three births a day.

Further, the losses in labor and delivery rooms have typically been made up in radiology and pathology—those monopolized areas where some physician is often getting a percentage of gross billings. Many hospitals have raised radiology rates $3 to get $2 to cover obstetrical losses. The third dollar went to the physician. The commission allocates any· approved subsidization throughout the hospital but often does not allocate any to a center in which there is a percentage contract without an operative limit.

One of the most interesting experiences regarding cross-subsidization arose in the Children's Hospital case. The hospital requested that its clinic charge of $3.40 be increased to $34. The commission approved an increase up to costs ($17) and announced a hearing as to whether rates should be approved above costs to make up for earlier losses. At the hearing, the hospital next requested that its clinic charge be $5 with the losses to be made up in medical-surgical. It developed that certain attending physicians at the hospital were using the clinic in lieu of a private office. Their patients were happy with the $3.40 charge but not with $17. The physicians had the hospital request the reduction and reallocation. The commission eventually approved rates slightly above direct cost, or about $10 per visit.

Several hospitals have attempted to apply a version of the theory of option demand. They argue that any rate structure makes sense because all services offer standby value so all patients could legitimately be charged for any portion of the hospital's reasonable cost.[12] The commission has not accepted that interpretation of option demand.

Baltimore County argued that all patients benefited from blood banking and wanted a low rate for transfusions. Losses were to be subsidized elsewhere. The hospital argued that it would rather receive blood than money and the lower subsidized rate would encourage more people to give blood. The commission, in its opinion, pointed out the hospital's error.

The commission has determined, through regression analysis and expert testimony, that the costs of certain functions are better explained by the number of admissions than by the number of patient days. The commission has assigned much of those costs to an admissions cost center and has approved an admissions charge for Maryland's hospitals.

Several insurance companies have refused to pay the admissions charge, though they would clearly pay the approved costs if they were in the room rate. The commission also wanted all central supplies below $50 to be included in the room rate along with the overhead for central supplies. Only high-cost supplies would be itemized and then only at invoice cost. Unfortunately, one Medicare intermediary in the state would not allow Medicare to pay for supplies without specific supply charges. It is clear that putting more rationality into the rate structure is not without major problems.

A final question, and one that has taken an inordinate amount of commission and staff time, is whether certain third-party payers are entitled to a differential. The Court of Appeals of Maryland is currently deciding whether Blue Cross is a class of purchaser (Blue Cross of Maryland, 1975). The commission is attempting to pool funds from Blue Cross and the Health Insurance Association of America to finance a study that will help determine an appropriate differential, if one is legal. Currently a tentative 4 percent differen-

---

[12] See the testimony in Suburban Hospital for a discussion of Weisbrod (1964) and others.

tial is available for any insurer offering a particular package of services. Many commercial carriers meet all the requirements except open enrollment. They have indicated that open enrollment costs more than 4 percent. (Blue Cross receives 4 percent from the commission and an additional 2 percent through its exception from the premium tax.)

Blue Cross argued that it should not pay for any nonsubscriber's bad debts. The commission's staff has argued that, with regard to bad debts, there are two relevant classes of patients—those who pay and those who do not. Clearly equity requires charging bad debts to the second class. Unfortunately, this does not generate the needed revenue. The commission, in attempting to get governmental support of these costs, has had little success. Meanwhile, hospitals under commission orders are charging all paying patients, including Blue Cross patients, for a percentage of bad debts. The percentage included an allocation of what Medicaid and Medicare did not pay. Effective July 1, 1977, when Medicare and Medicaid began paying 96 percent of commission-approved charges, rate orders were sent out reducing rates on average by about 2 percent.

The commission's rate structure includes, then, some cross-subsidization among services and some price differentials among classes of payers. Blue Cross argues that the rates it pays under commission orders represent discrimination against it relative to all other payers. Other insurance carriers and the hospital association argue that Blue Cross may be discriminated against relative to Medicare and Medicaid, but is favored relative to commercial carriers. The commission hopes to develop the data to determine which party is correct.

Relations with the Comprehensive Health Planning Agency and the Maryland Health and Higher Educational Bonding Authority

The HSCRC does not have authority regarding certificate-of-need or prior approval for capital expenditures. Those responsibilities have been given to the Maryland Comprehensive Health

Planning Agency, which has jurisdiction over all institutions subject to the HSCRC (plus others). Since, in the long run, a major key to reducing costs in hospitals is eliminating underutilized nursing stations, curtailing excess capacity, and promoting efficiently designed structures, the decisions of CHP are of paramount importance.

Maryland CHP has been in existence since 1968. After a few years, CHP came under heavy criticism because it had not developed a plan, nor has it yet. Meanwhile, new federal legislation (P.L. 93-641) gives much responsibility for plan development to the Health Systems Agencies.

Still, primary decisions regarding capital expenditures rest with the state's planning agency. The commission has urged CHP to develop a plan so that rate review can be used to shape the industry accordingly. The commission's staff has also made estimates of the extent of excess beds in Maryland and has urged CHP to adopt a moratorium on new beds, at least until a plan is developed.

The commission also has had the opportunity for input into certificate-of-need decisions, yet there is little evidence that any decisions have been significantly influenced by that input.[13] The following examples indicate differences in philosophy in some cases. They indicate the importance of coordinating data submissions in other cases.

In 1971, three organizations applied for permission to build a 200-bed hospital in Howard County. Two were existing Baltimore hospitals, Bon Secours and Lutheran, and one was the Hospital Corporation of America (HCA). After reviewing the financial data, the commission reported a clear preference for HCA, with Bon Secours second and Lutheran third. Since there was no plan, each hospital made its own estimate of the amount of demand. CHP did not indicate which estimate was correct. The estimated number of births, for example, varied widely. The regional agency eliminated HCA largely because it would not allow local citizens control over their investment. It is unreasonable to expect proprietary institutions

---

[13] CHP has called on some hospital applicants to reduce their cost estimates on the basis of commission comments. Selected regional units, or "b" agencies, have based decisions in greater part on financial impact data.

to allow consumers great influence in internal decision making—certainly not veto power over decisions of the investors. Bon Secours was chosen, but with the condition that the (Catholic) hospital assure that abortion services were available, although it did not have to perform them. When the hospital refused, Lutheran was awarded the certificate.

In 1974, the prior existing hospital in Howard County applied for expansion, and that request was granted. Lutheran's project, though approved in 1972, is currently in jeopardy because of zoning problems.

In September 1974, the commission publicly questioned the cost of two approved expansion plans. This led to considerable consternation in the industry. One hospital, Franklin Square (1974), argued that over half of its project cost was for outpatient facilities and the commission should not have complained about its inpatient costs. The facts turned out in the hospital's favor. The hospital had so significantly underbuilt in the beginning that after expansion the hospital would have 850 square feet per bed and would have been constructed within the commission's guidelines of approximately $50,000 per bed. The key finding here is that hospital clinics are truly expensive and are not marginal capital outlays (Franklin Square CHP application, 1974).

The second hospital decided the commission was correct and revised its architectural plans. They resubmitted to CHP an estimated cost considerably below that which had previously been approved (Baltimore County CHP application, 1974).

A final example involved Saint Agnes Hospital (1974, 1975), which applied for permission to offer a Home Health Care Service. It projected approximately 2,500 visits the first year at a cost of about $25 per visit. CHP approved the application. The hospital then applied for rates, projecting 1,000 visits and a cost of about $80 per visit. The hospital requested a rate of $28, with the remaining cost subsidized through the medical-surgical rate.

After notifying CHP and examining the hospital, the commission approved the requested home care rate but refused to raise any other rate for subsidization. Rather, the hospital was told that the opening losses would be capitalized and included in rates during the following four years if volume achieved that projected in the CHP application.

A final point regarding entry regulation involves competition from new industries. That regulatory agencies tend to extend their jurisdiction to new forms of competition threatening "their industry" is a well-known phenomenon. Pressure to do so usually arises from the industry.

Maryland's hospital industry followed this pattern in requesting that the commission regulate Health Maintenance Organizations (HMOs). The commission stated its support for HMO development and a policy of "hands off." The argument in support of HMOs is that they have the proper internal incentives to be efficient. Any test of that hypothesis would be destroyed if they were made subject to detailed external cost and rate control.

Pressure to extend regulation also came from Maryland's CHP agency. In 1974 and 1975 CHP attempted to add to the definition of regulated health care providers ambulatory care centers, HMOs, surgicenters, and home health agencies. The commission argued that these institutions should be excluded from rate review.[14]

Through its reglationship with the Maryland Health and Higher Educational Loan Authority, the commission has become more involved in capital expansion decisions. That agency was created to float tax-exempt revenue bonds for nonprofit hospitals and colleges. The authority has indicated that it will not attempt to market revenue bonds without prior indication from the commission that the amortization costs will be approved as reasonable rate elements. The commission is still groping for an appropriate response. Its members are, naturally, concerned with issuing orders that might appear to be binding on future commission members (member terms are four years—most of the bonds have thirty-year terms).

---

[14]Several commissioners, as well as myself, question whether nursing homes should be subject to our jurisdiction. Since over 70 percent of nursing home business in Maryland is paid for by Medicaid and competition exists for self-responsible payers, such regulation appears undesirable. If Medicaid, which must pay nursing homes on the basis of reasonable costs beginning July 1, 1976, accepts our rates, then such regulation might become desirable. The commission is currently being sued to begin regulation of nursing homes.

The authority has devised its instruments in light of commission preferences and has, in my opinion, given the commission an important and appropriate entry into the capital market.

Conclusion

It is much too early to say whether public utility-type regulation of hospitals can work. Since the commission began reviewing hospital rates, Maryland's have increased at an annual rate slightly above 7 percent. During the same period, costs per equivalent inpatient day have risen at a rate slightly above 10 percent per annum.

It is clear that many problems have surfaced; that many parties are not anxious for a shift in power. It is also clear that any group interested in trying to regulate the hospital industry, with its entrenched favored parties, must anticipate legal battles. Yet the current system cannot be "fine tuned." It must be completely overhauled if costs are to be contained. The utility model remains an overhauling worth trying.

References

Cohen, H.A.
   1968   The Rationing Ability of Price in the Market for Hospital Services. Federal Programs for the Development of Human Resources, Washington, D.C.: U.S. Government Printing Office.
Faulhaber, G.R.
   1975   "Cross subsidization: Pricing in public enterprises." American Economic Review (December).
Hanft, R.S., and P.C. Rettig, eds.
   1975   Controls on Health Care. Washington, D.C.: National Academy of Sciences.
Havighurst, C.C.
   1973   "Regulation of health facilities and services by 'certificate of need.'" Virginia Law Review 59 (October): 1143–1232.

Health Services Cost Review Commission
1975   Guidelines for Commission Staff Rate Review, unpublished.
Kahn, A.E.
1970   The Economics of Regulation: Principles and Institutions, vol. 1,
        Economic Principles. New York: John Wiley & Sons, Inc.
1971   The Economics of Regulation: Principles and Institutions, vol. 2,
        Institutional Issues. New York: John Wiley & Sons, Inc.
Lewin, L., and Associates, Inc.
1974   Nationwide Survey of State Health Regulations. Washington,
        D.C., Social Security Administration.
Pauly, M., and M. Redisch
1973   "The non-for-profit hospital as a physician's cooperative." Amer-
        ican Economic Review 63 (March): 87–99.
Sattler, F.L.
1975   "Hospital prospective rate setting, issues and opinions." Wash-
        ington, D.C.: Social Security Administration.
Scherer, F.M.
1970   Industrial Market Structure and Economic Performance. Chi-
        cago: Rand McNally & Company.
Stigler, G.J.
1971   "The theory of economic regulation." The Bell Journal of
        Economics and Management Science 2 (Spring): 3–21.
Weisbrod, B.A.
1964   "Collective consumption services of individual consumption
        goods." Quarterly Journal of Economics (August).

Court Cases

Baltimore County General Hospital v. Health Services Cost Review Com-
    mission, in the Circuit Court for Baltimore County at Law, Misc.
    Docket 10, Folio 79, File 5655, 1975.
Blue Cross of Maryland, Inc., et al. v. Franklin Square Hospital, et al., in the
    Court of Appeals of Maryland, September Term, 1975, Case No. 53.
Franklin Square Hospital, et al., v. Health Services Cost Review Commis-
    sion, in the Circuit Court for Baltimore County, Docket 104, Folio 293,
    File 82047, 1975a Order, 1975b Opinion.

Administrative Cases

Before the Health Services Cost Review Commission:
    Baltimore County General Hospital, Docket 1975, Folio 5, Proceeding
    29RC.

Bon Secours Hospital, Docket 1975, Folio 20, Proceeding 44R.

Children's Hospital, Docket 1975, Folio 7, Proceeding 31T.

Church Hospital of the City of Baltimore, Docket 1974, Folio 10, Proceeding 10C.

Mercy Hospital, Docket 1975, Folio 8, Proceeding 32C.

Sacred Heart Hospital, Docket 1975, Folio 2, Proceeding 26R.

Saint Agnes General Hospital, Docket 1975, Folio 13, Proceeding 37R.

Sinai Hospital, Docket 1974, Folio 8, Proceeding 8RC.

Suburban Hospital, Docket 1974, Folio 3, Proceeding 3C.

Union Hospital of Cecil County, Docket 1975, Folio 40, Proceeding 64R.

Union Memorial Hospital, Docket 1974, Folio 4, Proceeding 4C.

Before the Maryland Comprehensive Health Planning Agency:

Baltimore County General Hospital, Registration No. 70-03-0014.

Franklin Square Hospital, Registration No. 74-03-0225.

Saint Agnes Hospital, Registration No. 74-24-0282.

Certificate-of-Need Legislation and Hospital Costs

DAVID S. SALKEVER
AND THOMAS W. BICE

Introduction

Controls on capital investment and services are presently the cornerstone of state and federal policies for containing costs of health care. The principal rationale for these controls is that the availability of facilities and services affects utilization and costs of health care. Accordingly, limiting the availability of inpatient beds and specialized equipment and services is expected to constrain the volume of inpatient admissions and days and the use of specialized diagnostic procedures, resulting in savings in both capital and operating costs.[1] Also, it is frequently argued that uncontrolled capital and service expansion leads to duplication of facilities and services and to underutilization of capacity, which, in turn, result in higher unit costs and low quality of care. Controls on investment and services that prevent duplication are therefore deemed desirable whether or not they reduce the overall volume of services used.

Beginning in the mid-1960s, states and the federal government have adopted various forms of investment and services regulation.

[1] Note that this conclusion is tenable even if one rejects "Roemer's Law" and accepts the argument that additional beds and equipment do not directly stimulate additional demand (Newhouse, 1974:n. 2). Although controls may not reduce demand growth, they may necessitate rationing as demand expands while capacity is limited and thereby may reduce the total volume and costs of services.

The general approach taken is modeled after restrictions imposed on regulated public utilities and common carriers that require firms to secure certificates of convenience and public necessity before altering their service capacities. In the health sector two main types of control are exercised—direct and indirect—each of which requires health care institutions to obtain prior approval from designated agencies of their plans for capital expenditures and/or changes in service capacities. The approaches differ primarily with respect to the types of sanctions incurred by institutions that implement unapproved or disapproved capital expenditure projects. Direct controls through state certificate-of-need (CON) laws usually specify legal means to prohibit institutions from carrying out disapproved projects (for example, denial or suspension of operating licenses). Indirect controls levy only economic sanctions whereby third-party payers may refuse to reimburse institutions for costs associated with investment projects and/or service changes that fail to receive prior approval from designated agencies (Lewin and Associates, Inc., 1974).

At present, both forms of control are widespread in the United States. As of 1974, either or both direct and indirect controls were in effect in all states except Texas, Vermont, and West Virginia.[2] The first CON law was adopted in 1964 by the state of New York; by 1974, some version of CON was in force in twenty-four states, and proposals were under legislative consideration in seven others. Indirect controls are applied in thirty-seven states that participate with DHEW in so-called Section 1122 review programs. Under Section 1122 of the 1972 Amendments to the Social Security Act, reimbursements authorized by Titles V, XVIII, and XIX for depreciation, interest, and other costs associated with investments of at least $100,000 may be withheld if approval is not obtained. Similar provisions known as "conformance clauses" link Blue Cross reimbursements for capital costs to project review and approval by designated agencies in areas within nineteen states.[3]

[2] Data in this section are from a study by Lewin and Associates, Inc. (1974), which is current as of April 1974.

[3] It should also be noted that investment subsidy programs frequently require project review and approval, although sanctions are not levied on unapproved projects. All

Although direct and indirect controls are directed to the same ends and pose similar theoretical and policy issues, the present study focuses primarily on CON. Two considerations warrant this emphasis. First, it is likely that CON controls will supplant other types of investment and services regulation as the National Health Planning and Resources Development Act of 1974 (P.L. 93-641) is implemented. Section 1523 of this law requires states to enact CON statutes to be eligible for federal subsidies to support statewide and regional health planning. With this strong incentive for universal adoption of CON, it is reasonable to expect that indirect control programs will become redundant and either fall into desuetude or be merged with CON programs. Second, since CON has been in effect in sixteen states since at least 1971, we have more experience with CON than with the various forms of indirect controls. Although there is a paucity of evidence as to the functioning and efficacy of any form of investment and services regulation, the shortage is most severe with respect to the more recently appearing indirect controls.

Content of Certificate-of-Need Controls

Although CON laws are generally similar in intent, their content varies widely among states. Variations are found in (1) types of facilities covered, (2) types of changes requiring certification, (3) thresholds for review, (4) standards for review, (5) sanctions, and (6) the nature of the review process.[4]

Facilities Covered

Most CON laws cover hospitals, nursing homes, and other facilities such as outpatient clinics and laboratories. Over time, amendments to CON statutes and more recently enacted laws favor

states tie eligibility for capital investment subsidies from the Hill-Burton program to prior approval from designated agencies, and forty-two states require such endorsements for assistance from their construction finance programs.

[4]Information in this section is from Lewin and Associates, Inc. (1974). Other summaries are in Curran (1974) and Havighurst (1973).

broader coverage. Only one state (Michigan) regulates only hospitals, and only one (Oklahoma) confines CON to nursing homes. In addition to Michigan and Oklahoma, two states (Colorado and Washington) and the District of Columbia exempt other facilities; according to the review by Lewin and Associates, Inc. (1974), of CON laws, Georgia's and Wisconsin's statutes are "unclear" regarding coverage of other facilities.

Changes Requiring Certification

Three broad types of changes are subject to review: changes in physical plant (facilities), equipment, or services. As with the types of facilities covered, the trend in CON statutes has been toward broader inclusion of types of changes requiring certification. Among the twenty-three states with CON in 1974 that covered hospitals (that is, excluding Oklahoma), fifteen imposed review on facilities, equipment, and services; six others attended to facilities and services. Six of the states considering CON laws in 1974 proposed to review all three types of changes, and the other intended to cover facilities and services.

All states require certification for new construction in covered facilities, although many exempt projects below a specified minimum. The clear intent of CON is thus to prevent overinvestment in new facilities, equipment, and services. However, three CON programs currently in force and five of the seven proposed bills also mandate that proposed discontinuances of services be reviewed.

Thresholds

CON laws differ significantly with respect to magnitudes of changes requiring certification. For hospital facilities and equipment changes, these so-called thresholds are typically expressed in dollar amounts or as percentages of operating costs or assets. Dollar thresholds for changes in facilities range from $15,000 in Arizona to $350,000 in Kansas; thresholds for equipment changes range from $10,000 in Colorado to $100,000 in seven states. The modal threshold for facilities and equipment changes is $100,000.

Thresholds for review of bed capacity are typically more

restrictive than for other types of changes. Twelve states presently require and three more propose certification for either any increase in or change of bed stock, and five others specify maximum changes allowable without certification. Changes and expansions of scope of services requiring certification are specified, albeit often vaguely, in ten CON laws.

Standards of Review

The language of CON laws as to standards is highly varied. Several statutes are silent on this point, but most mention that decisions must be derived in some manner from state or areawide health plans. As Curran (1974) notes, however, few laws are specific as to what a plan should include. Oregon's statute is uniquely detailed in this regard, listing various types of evidence that must be considered in CON reviews.

Sanctions

In all but two states, agencies' refusal to award certificates results in states' denying applicant institutions licenses to operate the proposed facilities. California prohibits implementation of the plan for one year; thereafter, institutions that implement disapproved projects are ineligible for reimbursement for associated capital costs under MediCal. Florida's law specifies no sanctions. However, as its CON provisions are virtually identical to those employed in Section 1122 review (in which Florida participates), denial of a certificate of need results in levying Section 1122 sanctions (the withholding of capital costs for Medicare, Medicaid, and Maternal and Child Health services).

Nature of the Review Process

CON involves various types of agencies in the review process. In most states, it includes the agencies that ultimately grant certificates. States differ, however, in the number of formal review steps that precede a final decision. Most employ either a two- or three-step process, beginning with an initial review by areawide Comprehensive Health Program (CHP[b]) agencies leading to final reviews and decisions by state departments of health or human services, state health commissions, or statewide CHP(a) agencies. Among the twenty-one CON states with CHP(b) agencies, seventeen vested in them responsibilities for initial reviews of applications. Four states employ no local agencies in the review, while two others allow local agencies to make final decisions.

The Political Economy of CON Regulation

As with other forms of economic regulation, the rationale for CON controls rests on assumptions about behaviors of regulatory agencies and of regulated firms. What Noll (1975) terms the "public interest theory of regulation" holds that agencies charged with administering controls are both able and willing to identify outcomes that serve the public interest and to take decisions in accordance with them. Furthermore, imposition of controls is assumed not to evoke among regulated suppliers responses that would militate against the desirable effects of regulation or, worse, exacerbate the problems it is intended to ameliorate. Were these assumptions even approximately realized in practice, one would expect CON programs successfully to contain health cost increases, to improve utilization of current service capacity, and to prevent duplication and underutilization of specialized services and facilities.

Doubting the validity of assumptions underlying the public interest theory, several critics of economic regulation in general and of CON programs in particular have recently offered alternative perspectives to explain behaviors of regulatory bodies and regulated firms. They observe that the political economy of the regulatory process creates political pressures, incentives, and constraints which cause regulatory agencies to deviate substantially from practices postulated by the public interest theory and to evoke perverse responses from providers.

Without necessarily endorsing the largely negative conclusions of critics of CON programs, we believe they offer several insights into the behavior of regulators and health providers and interactions among them that are useful when interpreting empirical data. Therefore, before presenting research findings, let us consider several of the major arguments.

The Capture Theory

The most extreme counterargument to the public interest theory of regulatory behavior is the capture theory. It asserts that regulatory bodies will generally be concerned primarily with the welfare of the regulated industry rather than with the public interest; in short, it holds that regulators are "captured" by producers. Such capture might result from overt political pressures by producers or from attempts to "buy off" regulators. As Havighurst (1973) observes, however, capture may also occur as a consequence of more subtle and pervasive forces. He suggests (p. 1119) that

> . . . even if the balance of power in an agency belongs to reasonable men, it is natural for them to develop a belief in the services rendered by the industry and sympathy for its problems, which will usually appear as obstacles to the continued improvement and wider availability of those services. In those circumstances, the compromises reached within a multimember agency will usually be in keeping with industry interests.

That regulated producers have often strongly supported and vigorously lobbied for the legislation under which they are regulated lends credence to the capture theory (Stigler, 1971). Producers' demand for regulation presumably reflects the confident expectation that their interests will be advanced by the regulatory agency. In this regard, it is noteworthy that several state hospital associations actively supported adoption of CON programs as cost control mechanisms, particularly when laws assigned major roles in the regulatory process to voluntary planning (CHP) agencies (Macro Systems, 1974:vol. 2).

Some observers note that voluntary planning agencies that implement CON programs are particularly vulnerable to provider capture. In most states CON reviews are conducted by agencies that include among their members representatives of hospitals who have access to agency personnel and influence over agency policy (Lave and Lave, 1974:168). Furthermore, hospitals often are an important source of financial contributions required for agency survival and growth, and agency staff and consumer members must rely in the review process upon providers for information and expertise (Havighurst, 1973:1183–1184).

The major implication of provider capture of the CON process is that regulatory agencies will disapprove applications for new facilities, thereby protecting existing providers from the competition of new entrants into the market. Similarly, if agencies identify with the interests of particular groups of providers (for example, nonprofit hospitals), they will discriminate against proposals from other providers (for example, proprietary hospitals or HMOs). A recent study of CON and Section 1122 controls by Lewin and Associates, Inc. (1975) lends support to these expectations. Specifically, they report that regulatory agency personnel frequently express biases against for-profit providers and are especially opposed to "outsiders" entering local health care markets. These biases are reflected in higher disapproval rates for proprietary facilities. Agency bias against HMOs, surgicenters, and other alternatives to inpatient care is less common.[5]

Although provider capture may result in discrimination against potential entrants into health care markets, it does not follow that capture precludes effective control of investments proposed by *existing* providers. Controls such as CON may actually be welcomed if they limit competition among existing providers (Posner, 1974) and enhance hospital administrators' bargaining positions vis-à-vis their medical staffs.[6] By holding that they are powerless to prevent CON agency disapproval of investment plans to which they attach low priorities, administrators gain the power necessary to forestall such plans (Schelling, 1963).

---

[5]Of course, the ability of CON agencies to act in accordance with these biases and blatantly to discriminate against new or other disfavored providers can be limited by procedural requirements. Well-defined standards and public disclosure of reasoning behind each decision presumably constrain agency discretion. Such procedural constraints appear to be minimal at present (Lewin and Associates, Inc., 1975).

[6]Curran's (1974) observation that medical societies, unlike hospital associations, have not been strong advocates of CON controls is of interest in this context.

The Political-Economic Theory

Dwelling exclusively on pressures and tendencies that lead regulators to serve the interests of regulated firms, the capture theory presents a rather narrow refutation of the public interest theory. An alternative perspective on regulatory behavior, which Noll (1975) terms the "political-economic theory," holds that regulation may fail to serve the public interest even if regulatory agencies are not tools of the industries they regulate. This perspective assumes

> . . . that regulators try to serve some concept of the general public interest, rather than act as conduits for the interests of regulated firms. The problem regulators face is to identify this general public interest in a milieu in which information is uncertain, expensive, and biased, and in a society which contains numerous groups whose interests are conflicting rather than harmonious [Noll, 1975:29].[7]

Being unable clearly to identify the public interest and to defend their actions by reference to precisely articulated standards, agencies respond to political reward structures. Specifically, they seek to avoid costly conflicts[8] and highly visible failures while striving to produce clearly visible successes.

In the case of CON regulation, such behavior has important implications for the manner in which controls are applied. Without question, CON agencies typically lack well-formulated standards upon which to base decisions, a deficiency that stems from the inadequacy of routine data-reporting systems, the primitive state of the art of health planning, and a scarcity of resources for acquiring information. Although most CON laws identify state or local plans as the desired sources of standards for CON review, the reality is that few planning agencies have produced long-range, comprehen-

---

[7] The possibility that agencies may attempt to serve *both* the interests of regulated firms and the public interest should also be considered. This notion is consistent with Posner's (1971) thesis that agencies induce regulated providers to engage in unprofitable "public interest" activities by protecting them from competitive pressures.

[8] Hilton (1972) refers to this as the "minimal squawk" principle.

sive plans in sufficient detail to serve as criteria for the conceivable variety of proposals that could emerge (Cohen, 1973). For instance, a review of planning agencies by the U.S. General Accounting Office found:

> Less than half of the 163 health planning agencies . . . indicated knowledge of 1972 needs for types of inpatient and extended and ambulatory care facilities and beds. . . . The number knowing 1975 beds was even lower. . . . Most knew the number of existing health facilities [Comptroller General of the United States, 1974:18].

A more recent study of investment controls in twenty states found agencies relying extensively on Hill-Burton plans for bed-need standards, "which are viewed as inadequate and based on obsolete data." Standards for reviewing special services, equipment, outpatient services were generally nonexistent (Lewin and Associates, Inc., 1975:ch. 3).

Lacking comprehensive plans and systematic information about needs for and use of services and having limited personnel and funds, CON agencies are unable to base each review decision on equally thorough analysis. Because agencies desire to avoid costly conflicts and to maintain credibility and legitimacy among their sponsors and constituents, political and economic considerations are brought into their decision-making processes. Large, politically powerful institutions willing to devote considerable resources to defending their proposals through appeals, legal action, or legislative attempts to override agency decisions threaten to deplete agency resources and, if successful, tarnish the agency's public image of an effective and fair regulatory body.[9] This would suggest that CON controls will be applied selectively, with the likelihood of disapproval being inversely related to the economic and political

---

[9] The experience of the Massachusetts CON program demonstrates that the dangers of agency denials triggering judicial and political conflict are real. Most striking is the fact that within the four-year history of the program two agency decisions were reversed by special legislation. These are described by Reider, Mason, and Glantz (1975). Another instance of political conflict surrounding a CON decision in Maryland is detailed by West (1975).

power of the applicant institution.[10] Similar reasoning leads to the expectation of higher disapproval rates for projects that pose competitive threats to established providers, such as plans to build new hospitals or to provide lower cost alternatives to hospital care (for example, surgicenters). On this point the capture and political-economic theories agree.

Another type of selectivity deriving from the political-economic theory is the likelihood of more stringent control over the expansion of bed supplies than over new services and equipment. To some extent, this is implied by the bias against entry of new providers. However, the most compelling arguments for this hypothesis stem from the lack of review standards and information about use of and needs for services, which is especially severe with respect to new services and equipment. Although data on the supply and use of beds and estimates of bed needs are often unreliable and out of date, they are at least widely available. By contrast, information about the supply, use, and costs of special equipment and services is generally sketchy, and consistent review standards are virtually nonexistent (Lewin and Associates, Inc., 1975:ch. 3).

This informational asymmetry implies a corresponding asymmetry in the reward structures confronting CON agencies. External evaluators and legislative oversight committees concerned about the costs of acquiring information needed for developing standards and for conducting reviews tend to confine their assessment of agency effectiveness to the ability to limit growth of bed supplies.[11] In consequence, agencies are rewarded more for controlling beds than for stemming the proliferation of special services and equipment. The consequences of erroneous approvals of additional beds—

[10] The Massachusetts experience (Reider, Mason, and Glantz, 1975) demonstrates that large institutions do not have a monopoly on political power. Community hospitals that serve well-defined population groups may effectively mobilize popular support for expansion plans (partly because these population groups bear only a fraction of the costs of expansion under existing third-party payment schemes) and translate this support into direct pressures on the CON agency or intervention by elected officials.
[11] An example is the recent evaluation of Florida's CON program by the state legislature. The sole criterion upon which the evaluation is based is the extent to which the program limited bed growth to the Hill-Burton agency's need estimates (State of Florida, n.d.).

empty beds and low occupancy rates—are clearly visible indicators of agency failure; consequences of erroneous disapprovals (for example, longer waits for elective admissions) are less so (Pauly, 1974:158–159).

These considerations suggest that CON agencies will be predisposed to disapprove proposals for new beds and to invest considerable time and resources in reviewing them. By contrast, we expect a more lenient attitude toward proposals for new services and equipment. Moreover, since costs of acquiring information about new services or equipment proposals are high while the political rewards for building convincing cases against them are low, CON agencies have little incentive to subject such plans to careful review.

This expectation of leniency toward new services and equipment proposals is reinforced by several political and legal considerations. First, while the costs of thorough review and analysis may be prohibitive, the practice of denying such proposals after only cursory review opens the CON agency to charges of capriciously denying citizens the fruits of medical progress. Second, disapprovals may arouse hostility toward CON agencies among groups of physicians who find their hospitals unable to offer new diagnostic or treatment technologies while colleagues with admitting privileges at other hospitals have access to them. Finally, there are significant limitations in the coverage of new services and equipment under CON laws. As we have noted, although most CON statutes require certification for new construction and for significant increases in bed capacity, other potentially important types of investment are not controlled. Several states exempt all projects below a minimum capital expenditure, and in several states expenditures for equipment or expansion of existing services or renovations that do not involve increases in beds are excluded from review.

The expectation that CON agencies will exercise strict control over bed growth while generally approving proposals for new services and equipment without detailed review is supported by several descriptive studies. Data reported by Reider and his associates (1975) and by Bicknell and Walsh (1975) show that in Massachusetts proposals for facility improvements not involving new beds were approved more often than were proposals to expand bed capacity. Furthermore, Bicknell and Walsh (1975) observed that proposals not involving new beds usually did not "attract the closer, technically more sophisticated scrutiny . . . normally reserved for bed-related applications" (p. 1057). Similar differences in approval rates under CON and Section 1122 review programs in seventeen states were found by Lewin and Associates, Inc. (1975:ch. 4). It should be noted, however, that approval rates are an imperfect index of the stringency of controls, for agencies often employ informal means to screen out projects that are likely to be disapproved prior to their formal submission. Nevertheless, these findings provide at least qualified support for our hypothesis.

Perverse Provider Responses

Several authors have noted that establishment of a CON program causes providers to alter investment plans. It is not clear, however, whether providers' responses would create more or less rapid capital expansion. Bicknell and Walsh (1975) hold that adoption of CON would reduce planned expansion, arguing (p. 1079) that

. . . a certificate-of-need program, merely by its existence, may discourage construction and capital expenditures by causing an anticipatory reaction on the part of providers.

Others note that CON controls are similar to franchising and posit the opposite effect. According to Havighurst (1973:1171, n. 104), for instance,

[t]here would seem to be a danger that the certificate-of-need process may actually stimulate hospital construction by causing applicants to accelerate their plans in order to pre-empt others.

This reasoning is also applied to decisions about costly innovations in services and facilities (Roth, 1974). Being the first hospital in an area to install a $400,000 brain scanner becomes especially important if the chances of approval of second and third requests are nil.

To the extent that the pre-emptive response outweighs the discouragement effect, provider responses will be perverse; that is, they will tend to increase health care costs. The possibility of a substantial perverse response appears especially probable if, as the preceding discussion of regulatory behavior implies, CON controls are applied in a selective fashion. For example, both the capture theory and the political-economic theory suggest that certain providers and groups of providers are likely to receive especially favorable treatment from CON agencies, specifically, less stringent controls over their own investments and protection from competition for patients or for donor capital. It seems reasonable to conclude that these favored providers will react by increasing their capital expenditure plans.

The expectation that investments in new equipment and services will be less stringently controlled than expansions of bed supplies also points to perverse provider responses. If the preferences of hospital trustees, administrators, and medical staff for the growth of their institution cannot be satisfied by the addition of new beds, alternative expressions of their preferences will be found among the less regulated investment options (that is, new equipment and services). An especially pessimistic view of this possibility has been expressed by Noll (1975:44):

> Controlling the number of beds will simply turn the attention of hospital administrators to other, perhaps even less desirable expenditures. Thus is the regulatory tar-baby conceived. Regulators will find their attempts to force efficiency upon a recalcitrant industry as leading only to even more detailed and expensive regulation, prohibiting a lengthening string of unnecessary expenditures, but with no apparent long-run success in dealing with the general problem of rising costs.

Implications for the Effectiveness of CON Controls

At the outset of this section we noted that the rationale for CON controls as an effective anti-inflationary device is based on the assumptions (1) that the public interest theory accurately describes behaviors of the regulatory agencies that administer CON regulations and (2) that the imposition of these controls does not evoke a substantial perverse response by providers. From our review of the capture and political-economic theories and the limited evidence pertaining to them, we believe there are reasons to doubt these assumptions. Without prejudging ultimate effects on costs of health care, experience recorded to date lends credence to the major conclusion of the capture and political-economic theories, namely, that CON controls will be applied selectively. Investment by existing providers will be less tightly controlled than will be entry of new providers. Further, we would expect more stringent controls on additional beds than on investment in services and equipment. Finally, this pattern of selective controls seems likely to stimulate perverse provider responses manifested in increased investment planning for services and equipment projects.

Whether these patterns of investment effect changes in average per diem hospital costs and total hospital expenditures depends, of course, on their cumulative effects on operating and capital costs and utilization patterns. Trade-offs between bed expansion and investment in services and equipment could increase average per diem costs as a result of higher intensity or wider scope of services while lowering the volume of inpatient days. These two factors exert opposing influences on total costs. In consequence, without detailed examination of the quantitative effects of CON on costs and use, it is impossible to predict whether CON will attain the ultimate end of controlling hospital costs.

Effects of Certificate-of-Need Controls on Hospital Investment, Costs, and Use and on Health Care Costs

Although control of health care costs is not the sole purpose of CON regulation (Reider, Mason, and Glantz, 1975), the language of most CON laws clearly indicates that it is a major objective.[12] Therefore, analysis of CON programs' impacts on hospital and

[12] However, Lewin and Associates, Inc. (1975), report that relatively few staff members of agencies administering CON regulation consider cost control the most important objective of these controls.

other health care costs is a relevant means of assessing their effectiveness. Two strategies have been employed by researchers to study this question: a descriptive approach and an analytic approach.

The descriptive approach, illustrated by the work of Bicknell and Walsh (1975) and Lewin and Associates, Inc. (1975), focuses on the regulatory process, describing the types and numbers of applications submitted to CON agencies and the decisions taken by agencies. Although such studies provide valuable insights into health care institutions' investment priorities and CON agency behavior, they cannot directly assess CON controls' effects on investment patterns and costs. Estimates of savings based on the total costs of projects disapproved by CON agencies fail to account for projects that might have been undertaken in the absence of a CON program but for which applications were not filed because a rejection was anticipated.[13] Failure to record such projects leads to underestimates of savings effected by CON programs. Another deficiency of the descriptive approach is that it ignores program effects on types of investments that do not require agency approval. Of course, the most serious limitation of this approach is that it inevitably leads to the conclusion that CON controls reduce investment. No account is taken of the possibility of perverse provider responses.

The analytic approach estimates impacts of CON regulation by examining its effects on investment patterns and costs while statistically controlling effects of other factors that influence investment. To date, only one extensive study employing this approach has been concluded.[14] In this section we summarize its methods and findings and interpret these in light of the competing theories of CON regulation and findings from other studies of CON processes and impacts.

[13] Lewin and Associates, Inc. (1975), attribute the high rates of agency approval of applications partially to agencies' screening-out proposals that are highly likely to be disapproved before they reach the formal review process and to negotiations between agency staff and applicant institutions in the formulation of proposals.

[14] As of this writing, only the analysis of investment patterns is in published form (Salkever and Bice, 1976a). The results of the overall study are in Salkever and Bice (1976b).

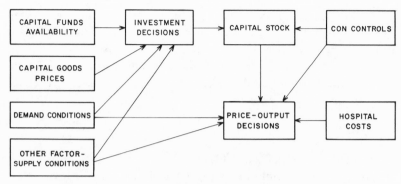

Fig. 1   *Conceptual Framework for Hospital
Cost Determination*

Evidence from our study shows that CON controls have no appreciable impact on total investment by hospitals but encourage a redirection of investment from bed expansion to growth of new services and facilities. This, in turn, leads to lower rates of utilization and somewhat higher hospital and total health care costs. In sum, CON controls do not bring about lower costs but may actually exacerbate health care cost inflation.

These conclusions derive from analyses of CON programs' effects on variables depicted in Fig. 1. We reasoned that hospital costs are affected by hospitals' capital stock and price-output decisions, both of which may be influenced by CON regulation. The former, which specify the size of a hospital's bed complement as well as the types and numbers of equipment and other capital facilities, are determined (in an environment without regulatory controls) by the availability of capital funds, prices of capital goods, demand conditions, and other factor-supply conditions (Ginsburg, 1970; Muller, Worthington, and Allen, 1975; Pauly, 1974). Price-output decisions, which determine the prices and volumes of services rendered during a specified period, are affected by demand and factor-supply conditions and the capital stock in place during the period in question (Davis, 1973; 1974). Finally, given the nonprofit nature of the hospital industry, the aggregate price-times-volume figures will closely approximate the costs of rendering hospital services.

Following the order implied by the conceptual framework, we first examined the impact of CON controls on capital stock; next we estimated the direct effects of capital stock and CON controls on costs. By combining the results from both stages in the analysis we then computed the total (direct and indirect) effects of CON controls on costs.

Methods

Estimates of impacts of CON controls were derived from cross-section and pooled multiple regression analyses of investment, costs, and utilization of nonfederal, short-term general and other special hospitals. The data pertain to the forty-eight contiguous states and the District of Columbia and cover the period from 1968 to 1972, a period chosen because it included some exposure to CON controls in several states and was relatively free of confounding effects of Section 1122, federal price controls, and Blue Cross conformance clauses adopted subsequently.

Estimates of CON controls' impacts were obtained by two procedures. First, we specified models in which changes in dependent variables were regressed on sets of predictors specified by the conceptual framework, including a variable measuring exposure to CON controls.[15] The regression coefficient associated with the CON variable was interpreted as CON programs' direct effect on the dependent variable under investigation. A second approach estimated effects of predictors other than the CON variable, using data from non-CON states only; these estimates were then applied to data from CON states to obtain predicted values for the dependent variable. Differences between observed and predicted values were interpreted as estimates of CON programs effects. Finally, results from the regression analyses were translated into estimates of the

---

[15] For analyses of investment patterns, which examined a single cross-section of state data on changes in capital stock from 1968 to 1972, the CON variable was operationally defined as the fraction of that four-year period during which CON regulation was in effect. For analyses of costs and utilization, which employed pooled cross-sections of annual state data for the years 1968–1972 (or 1967–1972 in some cases), the CON variable was set equal to one if a state had a CON program in effect for two or more quarters during the year, and was zero otherwise.

magnitudes of changes in dependent variables attributable to CON controls.

Findings

Hospital Investment Hospital investment was measured by three variables: changes in total plant assets, in total beds, and in plant assets per bed from 1968 to 1972. Changes in total plant assets represents the total dollar value of investment; changes in plant assets per bed may be viewed as an indicator of increases in the sophistication or capital-intensiveness of facilities.

In addition to the CON variable, predictors included measures of changes in demand variables (population size, income, insurance), capital funds availability factors (net revenues, Hill-Burton allocations), and factors influencing capital goods costs (construction wages). Most predictors were measured as changes for the lagged period from 1964 to 1968 as well as for the 1968–1972 period.

Results of analyses based on several specifications of the regression model showed a consistent pattern. CON coefficients for changes in total plant assets were positively signed but were generally not statistically significant, indicating that CON controls did not reduce total investment. Analyses of changes in beds and plant assets per bed revealed, however, that CON programs had a significant impact on the composition of investment. Specifically, they clearly restricted investment in new beds while encouraging investment in other services and facilities that resulted in increases in plant assets per bed. Magnitudes of these effects were relatively large. The estimated effects for the CON controls in force for the entire 1968–1972 period were a reduced growth in beds by 5.4 to 9.0 percent and a rise in the increase of plant assets per bed by 15.2 to 19.7 percent.

Findings from the second analytic approach confirmed these patterns. Eliminating the five states where CON regulation had been in effect throughout 1971 and 1972 (California, Connecticut, Maryland, New York, and Rhode Island) and deleting the CON variable, we reestimated the investment equations and used the resulting coefficients to predict changes in the dependent variables for the excluded states. Results from several specifications of the regression model showed that in almost all cases actual increases in beds in the five CON states were less than predicted increases, and actual increases in total plant assets and plant assets per bed exceeded predicted changes.

These patterns strongly suggest that investment in new equipment and facilities is substituted for expansion of bed supplies when the latter is controlled by CON regulation. The observed limitation of bed expansion is consistent with critical analyses of CON programs that point to provider domination, limitations in the coverage of CON laws, and the likely response of CON agencies to the scarcity of resources and to the asymmetry of rewards they face. Less obvious, however, is the cause of the relatively higher rate of growth in plant assets per bed in CON states. This may be due to the franchising aspect of CON controls that encourages pre-emptive investment or to the added protection from competition that regulation affords existing providers. Given the strong pressures operating within hospitals to expand services and facilities and to upgrade their quality, control of one type of investment rechannels expansionist preferences into areas not subject to stringent control.

Hospital Costs and Utilization   Having found that CON regulation affects investment patterns (and thereby capital stock), we examined the second type of effect specified by the conceptual framework, namely, the direct influence of CON regulation and capital stock on price-output decisions. Estimates of these effects were combined with those measuring CON programs' impacts on capital stock to obtain measures of the total (direct and indirect) effects of CON regulation on hospital costs.

Although CON regulation may conceivably directly influence hospitals' price-output decisions, it is not clear what specific responses will occur. Hospitals might tend to set prices lower and run higher occupancy rates in order to be in a better position to justify proposals for expansion. Alternatively, they might set prices higher and provide a lower volume but a higher quality of services because they are protected from the competition of potential new entrants. Indeed, lower occupancy rates may facilitate blocking of entry since CON agencies will be more reluctant to permit any increases in bed supply in the market area.

To assess outcomes of CON programs' impacts on price-output decisions, several analyses were carried out in which hospital costs per capita were regressed on determinants of demand for services and factor prices, as well as on descriptors of existing capital stock (beds and assets per bed). Parallel analyses of other indicators of costs (inpatient costs per inpatient day, outpatient costs per capita) and utilization (inpatient days per capita, inpatient admissions per capita) were carried out to give a more complete picture of CON programs' impacts and to provide a check on the reasonableness of the estimates.

As in the investment analyses, estimates of CON programs' effects were derived from two different methods. First, coefficients for the CON variable and for capital stock variables were estimated for all states, and these were combined with estimates of CON programs' impacts on capital stock to calculate the average overall impact of CON regulation on the dependent variables. Second, regression equations based on data from non-CON states were combined with predictions of the 1972 levels of capital stock variables in the absence of CON in four CON states (New York, Connecticut, California, and Rhode Island) in order to obtain predicted 1972 values of the dependent variables in these states. As before, these values were compared with observed values to determine whether actual cost levels in these three CON states are different from predicted levels. If CON regulation were an effective cost control mechanism, actual costs would be less than predicted levels.

The hospital costs per capita regressions showed that increases in capital stock—beds and plant assets per bed—led to higher costs and that CON regulation also had a positive but less significant direct effect. Since increases in both capital stock variables were associated with increasing costs and CON controls affect them differently, the net indirect effect of CON regulation reflects the balancing of competing tendencies. CON controls indirectly lead to lower costs via their reducing bed expansion while contributing to cost increases by stimulating other types of investment. Adding various estimates of these indirect effects to the estimate of CON programs' direct effects resulted in a range of estimates of overall impacts on per capita costs. Using the smallest estimates of CON programs' effects on capital stock, the estimated overall influence of a CON program over the 1968–1972 period was to raise a typical state's per capita costs in 1972 by 1.54 to 2.44 percent; corresponding estimates based on the largest capital stock impacts showed reductions of per capita costs by 1.09 to 1.85 percent. Clearly, CON regulation did not substantially lower per capita costs and may have increased them slightly.

The overall effect of CON regulation on the volume of inpatient services was to reduce utilization. The direct impact of CON controls was found to be consistently negative (but not always statistically significant) for both indicators of utilization—inpatient days per capita and admissions per capita. Through its restrictions of bed expansion CON regulation led to lower utilization of inpatient services, though to a lesser extent its stimulation of other types of investment had the opposite effect. The estimated net result of these influences in combination was to lower inpatient days in a typical state having CON regulation (from 1969 to 1972) by 2.15 to 8.30 percent and to lower admissions per capita by 4.92 to 8.30 percent.[16]

To supplement analyses of CON controls' effects on hospital costs per capita, their impacts on costs of services covered by Medicare were examined. For this purpose, we employed dependent variables measuring reimbursements for inpatient services under Part A as well as total Medicare reimbursement under both Parts A and B. Results of these analyses were similar to those found before. CON controls' direct effect was slightly positive (but not statistically significant), and influences of capital stock changes were positive but slightly smaller than those estimated for per capita

[16] Inspection of deviations of predicted costs per capita based on effects of capital stock and other predictors derived from analyses of non-CON states with capital stock variables set equal to their predicted values for CON states confirmed these results. Overall, 1972 costs in the four CON states were consistently higher than predicted values. To allow for the possibility that these deviations may have reflected stable characteristics rather than CON effects, we also examined residuals for the pre-CON years from three states (Connecticut, California, and Rhode Island). The fact that these residuals were always either negative or positive but smaller than the 1972 deviations confirmed our conclusion of a positive CON effect on costs.

hospital costs. Adding the indirect and direct effects of CON regulation results in the prediction that CON controls over the 1968–1972 period would have increased total Medicare reimbursements by 1.44 to 4.01 percent in the typical state. Because of imprecisions in the methods employed in generating these estimates, they should not be taken as conclusive proof than CON controls raise costs. However, the pattern observed across several indicators of costs clearly provides no support for the widely held presumption that these controls have reduced costs.

Results from Other Studies

Although we are not aware of other econometric studies of CON impacts on costs to which our own results could be compared, there have been several recent analyses of CON impacts on investment which should be mentioned.

Hellinger (1976) used cross-sectional state data for 1973 to estimate the impact of CON controls on total plant assets in short-term hospitals. His finding that CON did not have a significant effect is similar to our own result for total investment. In similar analyses with 1971 and 1972 data, he found that investment increased in the year in which a CON law was passed and interpreted this as the result of hospitals' efforts to undertake additional investment before the implementation date of controls. However, the results of this study must be viewed with some skepticism because of several problems with the econometric methods employed. For instance, Hellinger's regression equations incorporate the doubtful assumption that the magnitude of the CON impact is the same in all states regardless of size. It would seem more reasonable to assume that this impact varies positively with the size of the hospital industry in the state.[17] Hellinger's use of the ordinary least squares estimation technique is also problematic, since his regressions are based on a proportional adjustment model and therefore include the dependent variable lagged one year as a predictor. It is well known that ordinary least squares will yield biased coefficient estimates when a

---

[17] In our own total investment equations, the impact of CON on plant assets in 1972 is specified as proportional to the magnitude of plant assets in 1968.

lagged dependent variable is used if (as is likely) autocorrelation is present.[18] Because of these and other problems in Hellinger's analysis, his findings do not provide strong corroboration of our results.

Abt Associates, Inc. (1975), used cross-sectional regression analyses of 1973 state data to estimate the impact of CON on investment in ten specialized services. Results indicated that in three cases (x-ray therapy, cobalt therapy, and radium therapy), the percentage of hospitals within a state offering a particular service was significantly reduced by CON. Although this finding seems to contradict our own evidence regarding changes in assets per bed, it may be questioned on the ground that most hospitals offering these services did so even before CON laws were in effect in their states. In other words, CON may merely be serving as a proxy for other preexisting factors omitted from the analysis. It would be interesting to test for this possibility by replicating the analysis with current data on the CON dummy variable and data for other variables from an earlier year (in the late 1960s, for example) when CON laws were nonexistent (except in New York). If this replication also revealed a significantly negative CON coefficient, its role as a proxy for preexisting factors would be confirmed.[19]

Conclusions, Limitations, and Suggestions for Further Research

Our analyses of impacts of CON regulation yield a pattern of findings that support critical arguments about the possible deleterious consequences of imposition of such controls. Contrary to expectations of the public interest theory, our findings suggest that CON controls contributed to cost increases during the 1968–1972 period. CON regulation did not deter total investment in the

[18]The high probability of bias due to positive autocorrelation in Hellinger's results is revealed by the extremely low estimates for his speed-of-adjustment parameter. Most of his estimates range between .068 and .022, implying an average lag time for investment in excess of ten years.

[19]For an example of this replication procedure in a related context, see May (1974).

hospital sector; instead, it altered its composition by discouraging expansion of beds and thereby encouraging (or at least facilitating) expansionist urges of hospitals to find expression in investment in new equipment and facilities. Such findings are consistent with observations from descriptive studies of the CON process (Bicknell and Walsh, 1975; Lewin and Associates, Inc., 1975), which reveal that CON agencies lack information and standards to guide decisions about needs for new equipment and facilities and often—because of limitations of coverage of CON controls—lack authority to review them. Under such circumstances, it is likely that equipment and facilities will diffuse among hospitals until providers themselves determine that there is no longer need for additional expansion.

Although findings from our study conform to a set of plausible predictions and are consistent with observations from other studies, several limitations of our analyses must be mentioned. First, they pertain almost exclusively to hospital services. Additional studies of other types of services such as long-term and ambulatory care and further exploration of comprehensive cost measures are required to obtain firm conclusions about CON controls' influences on health care costs. Second, our findings pertain to changes in investment and costs measured at the state level. Since CON regulation is directed initially at planning regions within states, studies of state-level impacts should be replicated for smaller geographical units to determine their possible sensitivity to the level of aggregation employed.

Furthermore, we should stress that our results pertain to a period when other approaches to cost control were not widespread. Our largely pessimistic conclusions about CON regulation may therefore apply only to situations in which CON controls were the sole or principal regulatory constraint on costs; their relevance for cases where CON regulation acts in combination with other now widely applied controls (such as PSROs and state rate-setting programs) is unknown. We would strongly suggest, however, that faith in the ameliorative possibilities of a multifaceted attack on the cost inflation problem which incorporates investment controls should not obscure the fact that this form of regulation is potentially exacerbating. Further research on the critical question of how CON regulation interacts with other controls is needed.

The reader should also note that the usefulness of our findings for predictive purposes may be further limited by selection biases resulting from systematic differences between states which adopted CON laws and those which did not. We cannot be assured that impacts of CON controls on hospital investment, costs, and use revealed in our analysis will be repeated in states that adopt CON controls in order to participate in the planning program mandated by P.L. 93-641.

Of course, there are other research questions concerning the effects of CON controls which deserve investigation. For instance, research is needed to determine whether CON programs affect the structure of the health sector by blocking entry of new competitors, retarding the growth of HMOs, and discouraging investment in less costly alternatives to hospital care. Finally, there is a need for more descriptive studies of the review process, such as those carried out by Bicknell and Walsh (1975) and Lewin and Associates, Inc. (1975), to aid in the interpretation of econometric results and to generate new hypotheses about agency behavior.

Policy Implications

In view of our finding that the failure of CON agencies to curtail hospital cost inflation is largely attributable to their inability to control investment in new equipment and facilities, one might be tempted to conclude that CON programs can be made more effective by tightening existing controls and extending them to cover most (if not all) investment projects (Abt Associates, Inc., 1975:125). The wisdom and feasibility of this approach, however, are by no means self-evident. Careful review of all certification requests, including the additional ones generated by extending the scope of CON regulation, would require large additions to agency resources. Conceivably, resources required for review might exceed costs of investment projects being reviewed. Without additional resources, simply extending the coverage of CON laws over additions to equipment and facilities makes it less likely that agencies will be able consistently to render decisions in the public interest. As we have already noted, CON agencies lack adequate information and standards for review of these additions. Burdening agencies with the responsibility of developing standards for a larger universe of conceivable projects would only exacerbate this problem.

Other seemingly straightforward options for restraining investment in new equipment and facilities may be undesirable because they are either politically infeasible or at variance with CON controls' putative objective of deterring *unnecessary* investment. For instance, CON agencies could adopt the general policy of denying certification for equipment and facilities except in cases where extreme and urgent need is demonstrable. Alternatively, substantial submission fees or even taxes on investment could be employed to discourage hospitals and other institutions from seeking certification. Although such measures have the superficial appeals of simplicity and economy, they are not particularly discriminating between needed and unneeded investments. Furthermore, they would most likely favor the large, wealthy institutions' interests even more than does the process currently in use.

Several alternative possibilities for increasing the effectiveness of CON controls are suggested by our previous discussion of the political economy of regulation. Increases in CON agencies' resources, for example, may permit more detailed reviews of proposals for new equipment or facilities and the generation of additional data relevant to these reviews. With a more substantial factual basis, agencies' decisions should be more difficult to contest and their willingness to risk conflict with providers by denying certification should therefore increase. Furthermore, the generation and promulgation of better data on the supply, costs, and use of various specialized facilities and equipment items may diminish the tendency of external evaluators to focus strictly on control of bed supplies and thereby enhance the CON agencies' incentives to control equipment and facilities investments.

Another policy option involves altering administrative procedures used in reviewing investment proposals. Presently, CON agencies render decisions in an open-ended context where, except for competing applications for the same equipment and facilities, reviews of investment plans of different institutions are treated as independent events. Placing a ceiling on allowable investment expenditures within regions and requiring agencies to select from among applications submitted during specific periods might dramatically alter the politics of the review process. Different providers, each seeking a share of the limited supply of funds, could be inclined to view others' proposals critically and to expend some effort in documenting these criticisms. In this event, agencies would have at their disposal a more complete and balanced information base for each proposed project than is typically the case at present. The use of an investment ceiling could alter the role of nonproviders as well. Decisions on the level of the ceiling, which could be made by the CON agency or another governmental body (for example, the legislature), would probably attract the participation of broad-based citizens' groups, elected officials serving large constituencies, or public agencies whose programs might be affected (for instance, Medicaid agencies). In contrast, under the current piecemeal approach, nonprovider participation frequently takes the form of one or two neighborhood or community groups lobbying for new services in their locality. Moreover, consideration of slates of competing proposals might also stimulate greater public participation in the planning process, since attention would be focused not merely on reviewing a trail of seemingly unrelated projects, each addressed to particular segments of a population, but rather on deciding which alternative means of achieving community priorities will be adopted.

While we have thus far discussed various strategies for increasing the effectiveness of CON controls, it must be acknowledged that a very different sort of policy response is also consistent with our empirical findings. Presuming that the evidence of CON's ineffectiveness reported here reflects the inevitable result of this type of regulation, one might argue for more limitations on its scope and use if only to reduce its undesirable side effects. In this spirit, Frech (1975) and Havighurst (1973) suggest exempting HMOs and other nonhospital facilities from coverage under CON laws to forestall the possibility that hospital-dominated agencies will block entry of facilities providing lower cost alternative sources of care.[20] For the same reason, critics of CON have suggested that the risk of provider capture may be reduced by alterations in the arrangements for program administration (such as placing the CON program in the control of a state agency which also has responsibility for rate regulation or for purchasing medical care under public insurance programs). Of course, the most preferred policy option for these critics is the abolition of all CON controls, although this is recognized as highly unlikely and in fact contrary to recent trends in national health policy.

Finally, we suggest that the desirability of extending CON controls should be considered within the total context of health sector regulation. Investment controls have been supplemented nationally by utilization review programs under PSROs and in several states by rate-review programs. By controlling the volume and unit costs of services (and thus total costs), these additional programs in combination may obviate the need for expanded investment controls and even make desirable their diminution or elimination.

In sum, available evidence as to the effectiveness of CON programs suggests that this form of control is not likely to bring about lower rates of cost inflation. However, research conducted to date has barely touched the range of policy questions and options advanced by proponents and critics of CON controls. Much of the reasoning employed by proponents and critics alike stems from thus far unsupported assumptions about responses of regulatory agencies and regulated firms to the political context that accompanies imposition of regulatory programs. Until the incentives created by regulatory devices such as CON programs are better understood, we will be in the position of legislating in the hope that the public interest is necessarily served by more regulation.

---

[20] Another effect of this exemption is to encourage movement of certain activities from hospitals to ambulatory facilities and thus beyond the reach of regulation. However, one suspects that this phenomenon may be limited by the fact that insurance coverage is still considerably more complete for inpatient services than for ambulatory services.

References

Abt Associates, Inc.
   1975   Incentives and Decisions Underlying Hospital Adoption and
            Utilization of Major Capital Equipment. Cambridge, Mass.: Abt
            Associates, Inc.

Bicknell, W.J., and D.C. Walsh
   1975   "Certification-of-need: The Massachusetts experience." New
            England Journal of Medicine 292 (May): 1054–1061.

Cohen, H.S.
   1973   "Regulating health care facilities: The certificate-of-need process
            re-examined." Inquiry 10 (September): 3–9.

Comptroller General of the United States
   1974   Comprehensive Health Planning as Carried Out by States and
            Areawide Agencies in Three States. Washington, D.C.: Govern-
            ment Printing Office.

Curran, W.J.
   1974   "A national survey and analysis of state certificate-of-need laws
            for health facilities." In C.C. Havighurst, ed., Regulating Health
            Facilities Construction. Washington, D.C.: American Enterprise
            Institute for Public Policy Research.

Davis, K.
   1969   "A Theory of Economic Behavior in Non-Profit, Private Hospi-
            tals." Ph.D. thesis, Rice University.
   1973   "Hospital costs and the Medicare Program." Social Security
            Bulletin 36 (August): 18–36.
   1974   "The role of technology, demand and labor markets in the
            determination of hospital cost." In Mark Perlman, ed., The
            Economics of Health and Medical Care. New York: John Wiley
            & Sons, Inc.

Feldstein, M.S.
   1971   "Hospital cost inflation: A study of nonprofit price dynamics."
            American Economic Review 61 (December): 941–973.

Frech, H.E.
   1975   "Regulatory reform: The case of the medical care industry."
            Paper presented at the Conference on Regulatory Reform,
            American Enterprise Institute, Washington, D.C., September
            10–11.

Ginsburg, P.B.
   1970   "Capital in non-profit hospitals." Ph.D. thesis, Harvard Univer-
            sity.

Havighurst, C.C.
   1973   "Regulation of health facilities and services by certificate-of-need." Virginia Law Review 59 (October): 1143-1232.
Hellinger, F.J.
   1976   "The effect of certificate-of-need legislation on hospital investment." Inquiry 13 (June): 187-193.
Hilton, G.
   1972   "The basic behavior of regulatory commissions." American Economic Review 62 (May): 47-54.
Lave, J.R., and L.B. Lave
   1974   "The supply and allocation of medical resources: Alternative control mechanisms." In C.C. Havighurst, ed., Regulating Health Facilities Construction.
Lewin, L., and Associates, Inc.
   1974   Nationwide Survey of State Health Regulations. Washington, D.C., Social Security Administration.
   1975   Evaluation of the Efficiency and Effectiveness of the Section 1122 Review Process. Washington, D.C.
Macro Systems, Inc.
   1974   The Certificate of Need Experience: An Early Assessment. Silver Springs, Md.
May, J.J.
   1974   "The impact of regulation on the hospital industry." Unpublished working paper, Center for Health Administration Studies, University of Chicago.
Muller, C., P. Worthington, and G. Allen
   1975   "Capital expenditures and the availability of funds." International Journal of Health Services 5 (Winter): 143-157.
Newhouse, J.P.
   1974   Forecasting Demand for Medical Care for the Purpose of Planning Health Services. Santa Monica, Cal.: The RAND Corporation, R-1635-OEO (December).
Noll, R.G.
   1975   "The consequences of public utility regulation of hospitals." In Controls on Health Care. Washington, D.C. National Academy of Sciences, Institute of Medicine.
O'Donoghue, P., and Policy Center, Inc.
   1974   Evidence About the Effects of Health Care Regulation. Denver: Spectrum Research, Inc.

Pauly, M.V.
1974   "The behavior of nonprofit hospital monopolies: Alternative
        models of the hospital." In C.C. Havighurst, ed., Regulating
        Health Facilities Construction.
Posner, R.A.
1971   "Taxation by representation." The Bell Journal of Economics
        and Management 2 Science (Spring): 22–50.
1974   "Certificates of need for health care facilities: A dissenting
        view." In C.C. Havighurst, ed., Regulating Health Facilities
        Construction.
Reider, A.E., J.R. Mason, and L.M. Glantz
1975   "Certificate-of-need: The Massachusetts experience." American
        Journal of Law and Medicine 1 (March): 13–40.
Roth, E.
1974   "Certificate of need as a part of comprehensive health planning."
        Unpublished paper, The Johns Hopkins Medical Institutions.
Salkever, D.S., and T.W. Bice
1976a   "The impact of certificate-of-need controls on hospital invest-
        ment." Milbank Memorial Fund Quarterly/Health and Society
        54 (Spring): 185–214.
1976b   The Impact of Certificate-of-Need Controls on Hospital Invest-
        ment, Costs, and Utilization. Final report to the National Center
        for Health Services Research, U.S. Department of Health,
        Education, and Welfare, Contract No. HRA-106-74-57.
Schelling, T.
1963   The Strategy of Conflict. New York: Oxford University Press.
State of Florida, House of Representatives, Committee on Health and
Rehabilitation Services
n.d.   A Preliminary Evaluation of the Certificate of Need Program in
        Florida.
Stigler, G.J.
1971   "The theory of economic regulation." The Bell Journal of
        Economics and Management Science 2 (Spring): 3–21.
Stuehler, G.
1973   "Certification of need: A systems analysis of Maryland's experi-
        ence and plans." American Journal of Public Health 63 (Novem-
        ber): 966–972.
West, J.P.
1975   "Health planning in multifunctional regional councils: Baltimore
        and Houston experience." Inquiry 12 (September): 180–192.

The Role of PSROs
in Hospital Cost Containment

JAMES F. BLUMSTEIN

The Social Security Amendments of 1972 institutionalized peer review, through Professional Standards Review Organizations (PSROs),[1] as a means of promoting cost consciousness and assuring quality maintenance in federal medical programs. Composed exclusively of licensed physicians in an area, a PSRO is to review medical care provided to federal beneficiaries under the Medicare, Medicaid, and Maternal and Child Health programs. No funds appropriated for these federal financing programs can be disbursed for the provision of health services if those services are subject to review by a PSRO and that PSRO, applying professionally developed norms of care (§1320c-5), disapproves of the services (§1320c-7(a) (2)). This chapter will consider the contribution, if any, PSROs can make to hospital cost containment.

PSRO Responsibilities and Structure

Although the jurisdiction of PSROs is limited to reviewing the disbursement of federal health dollars under the Medicare, Medicaid, and Maternal and Child Health programs, they are seen as

[1] The PSRO law is codified at 42 United States Code §1320c et seq. For convenience, references will hereinafter omit mention of the United States Code, designating only particular sections of the statute.

prototypes for extension to private sector activities (Decker and Bonner, 1974). Where a PSRO disapproves of services, it must notify the practitioner or provider and also the individual who would have received or did actually receive the services. There is an elaborate hearing procedure (§1320c-8) by which any provider or recipient entitled to benefits can seek reconsideration by the PSRO, appeal to the State Council where one exists, appeal to the secretary of DHEW, and obtain judicial review where more than $1,000 is involved.[2]

PSROs are charged with the responsibility for review of the professional activities within their geographical area of "physicians and other health care practitioners and institutional and noninstitutional providers of health care services..." (§1320c-4(a)(1)). They must determine whether health care services and items for which payment may be made under Medicaid and Medicare (a) are or were medically necessary, (b) meet professionally recognized standards of quality, (c) or could be effectively provided on an outpatient basis or more economically in an inpatient facility of a different type (§1320c-4(a)(1)). A PSRO need only review health care services "provided by or in institutions," unless the PSRO itself, with the approval of the secretary of DHEW, seeks to expand its review capability to other health services (§1320c-4(g)). PSROs also must "utilize the services of, and accept the findings of, the review committees" of institutions in the area, provided that such institutions have demonstrated to the PSROs' satisfaction "their capacity effectively and in timely fashion" to carry out the required reviewing procedures (§1320c-4(e) (1)).

At the outset, PSRO designations are made on a conditional basis (§1320c-3(a)) for a trial period not to exceed two years (§1320c-3(b)). During this initial phase, DHEW need only require a PSRO to perform limited review functions within its capability; but by the end of the trial period, a PSRO can be considered qualified for permanent designation only if it is "substantially carrying out, in a satisfactory manner, the activities and functions" required of PSROs (§1320c-3(b)).

[2]A separate and distinct hearing procedure is involved where a sanction is sought to be imposed on a provider (§1320c-9).

The PSRO legislation alters the nature of the utilization review process. The very clear mandate is that a PSRO be composed of licensed physicians practicing in the area (§1320c-1(b)(1)(A)(ii)). Also, the law specifically addresses what former Senator Wallace Bennett, its sponsor, felt was a major irritant in the utilization review procedure under Medicare—namely, the resentment by the medical profession of having nonmedical personnel make utilization review decisions (U.S. Congress, 1972:256). The Medicare legislation required hospitals to have utilization review procedures but specified that hospital staff committees need contain only two physicians. Moreover, claims review by financial intermediaries often involved insurance company personnel in reviewing and questioning medical procedures prescribed and performed by physicians. Senator Bennett believed that "clerical personnel could not and should not make decisions as to the quality and necessity of medical services" (Congressional Record, 1972a:S16111). Accordingly, under the law no PSRO can allow anyone but a duly licensed physician to make final determinations with respect to the "professional conduct" of any licensed physician or with respect to "any act performed by any duly licensed doctor of medicine . . . in the exercise of his profession" (§1320c-4(c)).

Quite clearly, review by PSROs is intended to shift utilization control authority expressly and uniquely to physicians themselves so that "physicians can assume full responsibility for reviewing the utilization of services" (U.S. Congress, 1972:257), and is "based upon the premise that only physicians are, in general, qualified to judge whether services ordered by other physicians are necessary" (U.S. Congress, 1972:256).

Although the legislation provides for the establishment of local PSROs, the act also creates certain oversight mechanisms to advise PSROs and review their activities. In states having three or more PSROs, DHEW must establish a Statewide Professional Standards Review Council. The Statewide Council is to be composed of one representative from and designated by each PSRO in the state, two physicians chosen by the state medical society, two physicians chosen by the state hospital association, and four persons "knowledgeable in health care" who presumably are to represent consumer interests. Two of these consumer representatives must be recommended by the governor of the state before the secretary of DHEW can select them for the Statewide Council; the secretary can appoint the other two representatives from the state on his own (§1320c-11(b)).

If the appointment procedure is well defined, the duties of the Statewide Council are somewhat uncertain. The function of the Statewide Council is to "coordinate the activities of, and disseminate information and data among" the PSROs within the state, but the only specific coordinating function mentioned in the statute is the development of "uniform data gathering and operating procedures" so as "to assure efficient operation and objective evaluation of comparative performance of the several areas" (§1320c-11(c)(1)). This coordinative role is linked with a responsibility to assist DHEW in "evaluating the performance" of each PSRO in the state and to help DHEW find or organize a qualified replacement PSRO where necessary. The Statewide Council's reporting reponsibility is to the secretary of DHEW; it has "no direct authority over PSROs," but PSROs are expected to cooperate with Statewide Councils to "facilitate communication and cooperative arrangements among the PSROs in the State" (U.S. DHEW, 1974b:§530).

States that have Statewide Councils will also have advisory groups furnishing input to the council (§1320c-11(3)(1)). In states without Statewide Councils, these advisory groups will operate directly under the jurisdiction of the PSRO; the selection process is to be determined by DHEW regulation (§1320c-11(3)(2)). Since the council's provider members are all physicians, the advisory group represents an official mechanism which allows nonphysician provider viewpoints to be expressed at the statewide level. Where Statewide Councils exist, PSROs themselves have the option of establishing a formal relationship with an advisory body, subject to DHEW approval (U.S. DHEW, 1974b:§540); but in such states, PSROs are under no obligation to maintain any such formal tie.

In addition to the Statewide Councils and state or local advisory bodies, the PSRO legislation provides for the establishment of a National Professional Standards Review Council (NPSRC). This national body poses a major potential threat to the autonomy of local physicians. The regional structure of the peer review procedure was a gesture toward retention of regional control and maintenance of regional differences in medical practice. Nevertheless, as former Office of Professional Standards Review director Dr. Henry Simmons early realized, where certain procedures are by general consensus recognized to be of no use or are actually counterproductive, there is little reason to allow regional determinations of necessity or appropriateness. This tension between local or regional autonomy on the one hand and imposition of technological efficiency in disbursement of federal funds on the other is one that is left unresolved by the language of the act and predictably has generated pointed and probing questions by the medical association.

The NPSRC is charged with the responsibility of providing for the development and distribution of information and data to PSROs and Statewide Councils. These materials "will assist such review councils and organizations in carrying out their duties and functions" (§1320c-12(e)(2)). The National Council also will review the operations of PSROs and Statewide Councils to determine their effectiveness and comparative performance (§1320c-12(e)(3)), and make studies and recommendations to DHEW and to Congress about how to accomplish the objectives of the act more effectively (§1320c-12(e)(4)). Membership in the NPSRC is limited to eleven physicians, a majority of whom must be selected by DHEW only if recommended by "national organizations recognized by the Secretary as representing practicing physicians" (§1320c-12(b)). The department is also required to include as members physicians who have been recommended by consumer groups and other health care interests.

The provisions regarding composition of the NPSRC are clearly aimed at assuaging the sensitivities of physicians since all members must be doctors, and organized medical groups representing practicing physicians must recommend a majority of the members. Nevertheless, the ambiguity of the NPSRC's charge raised medical association eyebrows because of the possible usurpation (in the eyes of the AMA) of local autonomy by the national body.

The act provides for three different kinds of reviewing procedures which can be construed as sanctions. First, a PSRO can disapprove of health services and thereby deny federal payment of claims based upon provision of those services (§1320c-7). This disapproval must be based on criteria set out in the act under norms adopted by the PSRO (§1320c-4(a)(1) & (2)). Any beneficiary, recipient, provider, or practitioner dissatisfied with a claim determination (a) can seek reconsideration by the PSRO; (b) where a Statewide Council exists and $100 or more is at stake can appeal to the Statewide Council; and (c) where $100 or more is at stake can appeal to the secretary, who is obligated to provide a hearing. If $1,000 or more is at stake, an appeal to the courts is allowed (§1320c-8).

Secondly, a PSRO can report to the secretary (through the Statewide Council, where one exists) that a provider or physician has violated a duty imposed by the PSRO legislation (§1320c-6). If the secretary finds that the practitioner or provider has demonstrated an unwillingness or a lack of ability substantially to comply with his statutory obligations, then he can impose one of two penalties. He can either (a) exclude or suspend the provider from eligibility to provide health services on a federally reimbursable basis, or (b) require that the provider pay back to the government the excess charges (not to exceed $5,000). Either of these alternative penalties can be imposed only upon a finding (1) that the provider has failed in a substantial number of cases substantially to comply with the obligations imposed on him under the act, or (2) that he grossly and flagrantly violated any obligation in one or more instances (§1320c-9(b)(1)). Before imposition of any penalty, the provider is entitled to a hearing before the secretary and to judicial review of the secretary's final decision (§1320c-9(b) (4)).

Finally, the secretary can terminate a contract with a PSRO upon a finding that it is not "substantially complying with or effectively carrying out" its agreement with DHEW. In making this determination, the secretary must give notice in accordance with regulations he establishes and provide a formal hearing to the PSRO (§1320c-1(d)(2)). Statewide Councils, where they exist, will assist the secretary in evaluating the performance of the PSRO and help him locate or organize a substitute where an agreement is terminated (§1320c-11(c)(2) & (3)).

The PSRO's Reviewing Procedures

The PSRO law mandates that each PSRO "apply professionally developed norms of care, diagnosis and treatment . . . as principal points of evaluation and review" (§1320c-5). These norms are to be based on "typical patterns of practice in its regions" and are to include "typical lengths-of-stay for institutional care by age and diagnosis" (§1320c-5). The statutory provision makes it clear that PSRO educational efforts and reviewing activities are to be more than a series of ad hoc decisions, and the development and application of norms have been described as the "keystone to the PSRO program" (Gosfield, 1975:29).

The PSRO Program Manual, the primary source of authority for understanding DHEW's implementation of the law, establishes three categories for guiding PSRO operations. "Norms" are defined as reflecting typical practice; "criteria" are expertly developed guidelines against which actual practice can be measured; "standards" are professionally developed statements of an acceptable range of deviation from a norm or criterion (see also U.S. DHEW, 1973:§709). Although there is no mention of the concepts of "criteria" or "standards" in the statute itself, these constructs reflect DHEW's response to the statute's mandate that professionally developed norms accommodate actual patterns of practice.

Under the statutory provisions, the "professionally developed norms" must include "the types and extent of the health care services which . . . are considered within the range of appropriate diagnosis and treatment" for particular illnesses or health conditions (§1320c-5(b)(1)). In the formulation of these norms, "differing, but acceptable, modes of treatment and methods of organizing and delivering care" must be taken into account; and the norms adopted must be "consistent with professionally recognized and accepted patterns of care."

This language does appear to support the view that the PSRO program was aimed in part to improve techniques of practice in areas where "actual norms" diverge from "professionally developed" norms. From the legislative history, which reflects the concern for excessive utilization of unnecessary services (Havighurst and Blumstein, 1975; Blumstein, 1976), it is reasonable to conclude that the act's sponsors thought such imposition of expertise would likely cut down on unnecessary care. To the extent that physicians are prescribing care which has no benefit to patients, or which may even be counterproductive, then the "waste" control objective may be achieved through articulation and communication of professionally developed norms. Presumably, the "professionally recognized and accepted patterns of care" would effectively curtail wasteful procedures that are ordered by providers who have not been able to keep up with the latest developments.

Unfortunately, from a cost-containment perspective, this expectation would appear ill-founded. First, as a practical political matter, traditional physician concerns for professional autonomy have predictably led to erosion of national control over the development of norms. The statute nowhere grants a PSRO the authority to "develop" norms; rather the PSRO must "apply" (§1320c-5(a)) and "utilize" (§1320c-5(c)(2)) norms prepared under the supervision of the National Council (§1320c-5(c)(1)). It is the duty of the National Council to "provide for the preparation and distribution" to each PSRO of "appropriate materials indicating the regional norms to be utilized. . . ." The act contemplates NPSRC approval of regional norms "based on its analysis of appropriate and adequate data" (§1320-5(c)(1)).

Where the "actual norms of care" in a PSRO area are "significantly different from professionally developed regional norms of care," the act requires the NPSRC to inform a PSRO of the divergence. The statute then calls for a period of discussion and consultation between the National Council and the PSRO. This provision seems to be a clear expression of legislative intent to impose a professional standard of practice on regions where "typical patterns of practice" do not conform to professionally developed norms prepared at the national level. If the PSRO can show a "reasonable basis" for usage of other norms, then it can apply those norms, provided the National Council approves (§1320c-5(a)). This procedure would conform to the view that an accommodation with regional practice should be made; but the regional PSRO would have to justify its deviant practice standards, presumably as meeting special regional needs, or at least as not imposing unnecessary ("wasteful") services at increased cost. Thus, the PSRO legislation would seem to require that PSROs apply and utilize the nationally approved and professionally developed norms unless they secure approval from the NPSRC to deviate from that standard (Havighurst and Blumstein, 1975:47–51).

It appears that DHEW initially took this position. In a question-and-answer pamphlet published in December 1973—prior to release of the PSRO Program Manual—DHEW's Office of Professional Standards Review (OPSR) stated that "[e]ach PSRO will establish standards and criteria of care that reflect acceptable patterns of practice in the PSRO's area." The office went on, however, to indicate that the NPSRC "must approve norms used by a PSRO that are significantly different from professionally developed regional norms" (U.S. DHEW, 1973).

Perceiving and reacting to this apparent threat to local decision-making, the AMA raised the question, "Who would have the right to set norms and how would they be determined?" (U.S. DHEW, 1974a:2). This was obviously seen by OPSR as a very delicate issue. In response, OPSR sought to persuade the medical association that the "clear intent is to use norms, criteria, and standards developed by physicians in the PSRO area" (U.S. DHEW, 1974a) and that the PSROs would retain the "overall responsibility for the development, modification and content of norms, criteria and standards . . ." (U.S. DHEW, 1974b:§702.2). Clearly, OPSR felt under heavy pressure to come out on the side of greater local autonomy in the setting of practice norms.

The PSRO Manual reflects this decision not only in the section quoted in the OPSR Memo but also in section 709.1, which discusses development of norms. Whereas the act specifies that the National Council shall distribute materials "indicating the regional norms to be utilized" by PSROs, the manual states that the NPSRC will provide, when available, "sample sets of norms and criteria to each PSRO" (U.S. DHEW, 1974b:§709.11). The manual calls upon each conditional PSRO to review as early as "feasible" the model sets of norms "in order to adopt or adapt them for their use" (U.S. DHEW, 1974b:§709.12). Then the manual underlines the word "alternatively" and notes that the PSRO can choose "to develop its own criteria and standards and/or select its own norms." Nowhere in the section on PSRO responsibilities is there any mention of approval by the National Council, as contemplated by the act.

This position was hardly an oversight. Former DHEW Secretary Caspar Weinberger explicitly stated at PSRO Oversight Hearings in May 1974 that he believed PSROs had the authority to set norms and that if DHEW or the NPSRC in fact had that power, he would support a statutory change to remove that authority (Gosfield, 1975:55). Thus, it seems that DHEW concluded that it must rewrite the statute in order to live with the AMA. Simultaneously, the department's stance significantly waters down even the waste control authority of the NPSRC to require use of professionally developed norms by PSROs.

A second problem with the cost-containment assumptions of PSRO sponsors is that "waste control" objectives are not necessarily consistent with cost-containment goals. A program that successfully curtails unproductive or counterproductive care may not deal with broader—more fundamental—questions. Some care may be effective (that is, marginally improves the likelihood of cure or diagnosis) but uneconomic (that is, benefits do not outweigh costs). Since these procedures make a positive contribution to improved health, a purely professional standard could reasonably permit high-cost measures to be taken even if the incremental benefits are relatively small. If "waste control" is seen purely as a concept that eliminates unproductive or counterproductive care, then it is very possible that PSROs could increase rather than decrease aggregate costs.

This is a point that OPSR stressed in its early sales pitch to physicians: total cost may rise under PSRO, but this will not mean failure. The office was forced to recognize the potential conflicts between cost-containment objectives and a program limited to "waste control." But for whatever reasons, DHEW seems to have opted for "waste control," while still talking about potential cost savings (Havighurst and Blumstein, 1975:41–45).[3]

Utilization review generally incorporates an economic dimension (Stuart and Stockton, 1973), where the label "unnecessary" can

[3]For a discussion of a similar conflict in program objectives between family planning proponents and population control advocates, see Blumstein (1974).

also mean "of insufficiently high priority to warrant an expenditure." A judgment must be made in these situations whether to permit (with federal reimbursement) or require (through malpractice standards) a certain procedure in a given situation. Consider the case where a person in his twenties complains of growing near-sightedness. The symptom continues for a number of years and he ultimately goes blind. Should a physician routinely test for glaucoma in this situation when the likelihood of its occurring in persons under the age of forty is, say, 1 in 25,000? A standard based purely on technical factors might say one thing, while a consideration of cost might lead to a different conclusion (*Helling* v. *Carey*, 1974). This type of concern, however, balancing costs and benefits, cuts against the grain of the medical profession, accustomed as it has become to unchallenged underwriting by the deep pockets of third-party payers.

The PSRO statute itself calls for imposition of economic factors in the formulation of norms. Delivery of medical services can be conceived as a production process that combines a variety of inputs in order to achieve a certain outcome (Blumstein and Zubkoff, 1973). Under traditional economic theory, a production process that does not utilize inputs in a combination that brings about a given result in the least costly way is inefficient. In medical care, as in other processes, there is often a variety of treatments or combination of treatments that will bring about a desired outcome. Utilizing resources in such a way as to minimize the cost for a specified result is one way to define efficiency. One of the explicit charges to a PSRO is to determine whether health services can be provided on an outpatient rather than on an inpatient basis, or whether the services can be provided on an inpatient basis in a less costly facility (§1320c-4(a)(1)(C)). This is implicitly a responsibility to determine whether the "production process" proposed by the attending physician is an efficient one or whether, "consistent with appropriate medical care," an alternative process would utilize fewer scarce medical resources.

Improvement in the technology of producing medical outcomes is a broadly accepted goal. The controversy is who will decide what methods are effective and efficient (Blumstein, 1976). Opposition to this function of the PSRO is partly explained as professional resentment to outside supervision or control of a process that has typically been insulated from external review (Rivkin and Bush, 1974:315–324). Currently, only egregious cases, which wind up in court as malpractice cases or before disciplinary boards of medical societies, subject a physician to significant external review. A more principled objection to the exercise of this production function review by PSROs is that techniques of measurement are insufficiently refined so that a single efficient production technology is an unrealistic goal at this stage. Establishment of detailed and possibly rigid protocols for treating specific illnesses and a heavy-handed reviewing organization could lock in a specific production technology, thereby hampering experimentation or innovation.

The effectiveness and efficiency objectives, however, are not the same as faced in the glaucoma testing case posed earlier. Where unproductive, counterproductive, or inefficient care is being provided, costs can be cut without consumer sacrifice (though professional autonomy is being threatened). The glaucoma testing situation is different in that failure to test will actually result in increased health risk for some people. It is this type of problem that a cost-containment program must face if it is to keep aggregate expenditures under control. Yet a program like PSRO that emphasizes improved production function technology really does not address squarely this very basic question—whether certain expenditures are worth their cost (Fein, 1973; Fuchs, 1973, 1974; Havighurst and Blumstein, 1975; Lave and Lave, 1970).

A third problem with PSRO cost-containment assumptions is the use of and reliance on professionally developed norms of care. It is clear that formulation of norms will be a critical determinant of a PSRO's ability to pursue cost-containment goals (Gosfield, 1975:29). But the emphasis on a professionally developed standard seems likely to result in norms that impose the best available practice as the expected level of quality—with its attendant high cost. Former Assistant Secretary for Health Dr. Charles C. Edwards indicated the force of the "professional quality imperative" when he said that PSROs can be a "vehicle for change whereby the best and most effective care becomes the standard of care" (Edwards, 1973). Such an outcome could result in a mandated format of medical practice that inadequately considers forgone alternative expenditure opportunities. "Indeed, instead of serving as watch dogs on behalf of the public at large, PSROs might well become potent, and virtually unopposed, political instruments for increasing rather than containing costs" (Havighurst and Blumstein, 1975:66). This is evidently what has happened in West Germany with its counterpart to the PSRO program (Stone, 1974).

In addition to the impetus of the "professional quality imperative" in the formulation of norms, the formula for establishing norms provides an opportunity for expanding quality objectives, at the expense of cost-containment goals. Ironically, the statute implicitly contemplates development of PSRO norms which might fall below standards of customary medical practice in a PSRO area. Since this would entail a risk of malpractice susceptibility for practitioners following those more cost-conscious PSRO norms (King, 1975; Holder, 1975), the statute immunizes providers who apply PSRO norms from any form of civil liability (§1320c-16(c)). As long as providers comply with PSRO norms and standards in effect in the region where care is rendered, and apply those norms and standards with due care, they cannot be held liable for malpractice under state law (George Washington Law Review, 1974).

The malpractice immunity makes sense if PSRO norms were likely to establish more cost-conscious standards of practice for providers than currently exist under state malpractice law. But the PSRO statute, especially as implemented by DHEW, seems to set current practice patterns as the minimum upon which to build. "Criteria" are to be developed by national specialist groups under contract with DHEW, and they are likely to require more sophisticated patterns of treatment (even while weeding out some "wasteful" procedures). Thus, the manual and the statute call for establishment of a range of acceptable care, but the bottom of the range is likely to be current practice, while the "professional quality imperative" will tend to push the upper end of the range to more elaborate coverage. At the very least, the PSRO statutory references to "professionally developed norms of care" seem to dictate a higher standard than currently exists under traditional malpractice law, which relies on "customary" practice (King, 1975). The implementation formulation developed by the PSRO Program Manual would seem virtually certain to assure this result, encouraging providers who practice at the lower end of the established range to "improve" their standards by modifying their patterns of practice. If this prediction is accurate, then the malpractice immunity provision may be less significant than PSRO strategists initially thought.

While professionalism and quality goals provide an impetus for "upgrading" patterns of care at public expense, professional self-interest also cuts in the same direction. Composed of physicians who practice predominantly in a fee-for-service environment, PSROs are unlikely to look kindly on cost-containment objectives when they threaten physician incomes. This is especially true when a patient is a public beneficiary whose welfare is increased by improved quality of medical treatment and who loses a benefit if he or she does not undertake a treatment whose net health effect is positive, even if very costly. This allows the physician to have a congruence of interests with the patient, providing the "best" care unconcerned with and unconstrained by cost factors. The coincidence of the physician's pecuniary interest with the patient's welfare maximization interest is a comfortable one for the provider, alleviating the need for soul-searching about improper motivation for self-interest. Yet, this factor of self-interest has been recognized as a lurking influence in standard-setting: "Obviously there is minimal possibility of such low cost-oriented norms because the physicians establishing norms have a financial incentive to extend Medicare and Medicaid coverage to as many services as possible" (Gosfield, 1975:54, n. 37).

Impact of PSRO Authority and Structure

The problems that PSROs will have in achieving cost-containment objectives arise not only from the format and control of the standard-setting and reviewing process but also from their range of authority and their structure.

Delegation

The PSRO law stemmed in part from the Senate Finance Committee's conclusion that hospital utilization review procedures had not succeeded in curtailing excessive use of hospital services. A primary legislative concern was the apparent conflict of interest represented by internal institutional reviewing committees. Testimony showed that physicians who had a financial interest in a hospital often sat on the utilization review committee; also, because of the attendant fiscal hardship, hospitals had an institutional stake in avoiding low occupancy rates. Some evidence even supported the view that the rigor of the reviewing process decreased as the hospital's occupancy rate fell.

The Finance Committee's concern with conflicts of interest found its way into the statute. Physicians with staff privileges in a hospital may participate in reviewing services provided by that institution, but they "ordinarily should not be responsible" for that review (§1320c-4(a)(5)). Similarly, a physician is not permitted to review services provided to a patient "if he was directly or indirectly involved in providing such services" (§1320c-4(a)(6)(A)); nor can a physician review services provided by or in an institution "if he or any member of his family has, directly or indirectly, any financial interest in such institution, organization, or agency" (§1320c-4(a)(6)(B)). Nevertheless, in the final version of the act, each PSRO was required to "utilize the services of, and accept the findings of, the review committees" of provider institutions if they satisfied a PSRO that they were doing an effective job (§1320c-4(e)(1)).

While hospital review committees must apply norms established by PSROs, the manual allows PSROs to grant permission to hospitals to use their own guidelines (U.S. DHEW, 1974b:§709.42). This provision undermines much of the desired independence sought for the reviewing process. By September 1976 fewer than 30 percent of all hospitals under PSRO review held "nondelegated status"—that is, were permitting PSRO personnel directly to perform the reviewing function (U.S. DHEW, 1977:30). However, it is possible that some good can still come from the new procedure.

Presumably, if PSRO norms are applied, even by a hospital committee under delegated status, the review will be less idiosyncratic, reflecting a broader practice pattern (Havighurst and Blumstein, 1975:51). Also, PSROs have a duty to keep track of each institution's performance under delegated review status (U.S. DHEW, 1974b:§720.01); and as part of its overall responsibility for collecting and comparing data and profiles of care, a PSRO will be able to exercise some oversight.

Another plus might be the effect of delegated status on the practice in health maintenance organizations (HMOs). PSROs have jurisdiction over HMOs, and an argument can be made that the process norms being developed by PSROs are suited primarily for a fee-for-service milieu and are incompatible with the prepaid group practice mode of delivery (Havighurst and Bovbjerg, 1975; but see Gosfield, 1975:89-94). Through the delegation amendment to the act and the even more permissive provision in the manual, it is possible that some of the more onerous effects of PSRO review on HMO care might be curtailed.

Of course, it is questionable whether PSROs will have any reason to act so munificently toward HMO providers (Havighurst and Bovbjerg, 1975). And the delegation amendment certainly raises questions about the effectiveness that PSROs will have, for it seems that internal committees still continue to play the critical reviewing role as before.

Structural Aspects

The mission of PSROs, as reviewing institutions, is to determine whether a provider has furnished adequate quality care to a specific Medicare or Medicaid beneficiary and whether the government should pay for that care. It has no jurisdiction to consider trade-offs among competing allocative priorities within the health sector (for example, curative vs. preventive care) or between health and other items. PSROs' cost-containment goal has apparently become that of eliminating unproductive or counterproductive care—that is, barring payments where there is no net benefit to the patient. While PSROs have authority to enforce improvements in production technology, including requiring outpatient in lieu of inpatient treatment or inpatient care in less costly facilities (§1320c-4(a)(1)(c)), they do not have authority to reinvest these savings to spend in other ways to promote other health objectives. This is a particularly difficult structural disincentive to cost containment where PSROs are asked to curtail admittedly efficient and useful procedures on the grounds that they are of insufficiently high economic priority when balanced against competing claims on scarce resources.

It is helpful to introduce the concepts of "micro-" and macro-" quality at this point. Macro concerns emphasize the "effectiveness of the health-care sector as a whole in maintaining or improving the health status of the . . . population as a whole" (Reinhardt, 1973:177). Micro-quality, on the other hand, would place primary emphasis on the technical quality of the medical services actually provided to individual patients (Reinhardt, 1973:177). Assuming that the health industry knew how to produce either macro- or micro-quality efficiently, there would be a trade-off between achieving either goal. Given a level of resources, a health policy planner would have to face the question of determining which measure of quality is more important and which therefore should receive more weight and command additional resources.

In this context, the limited jurisdiction of PSROs poses an extremely difficult institutional problem. From a societal viewpoint, there is a very real trade-off between goals of micro- and macro-quality. There can be no objective statements about the "overall quality" of alternative allocation decisions because, for any given resource constraint, "any overall index of quality must be a weighted sum of micro- and macro-quality, and these weights can be established only through political consensus" (Reinhardt, 1973:180). Thus, one's evaluation of a health system often depends on the relative weights assigned to differing concepts of quality.

Since a PSRO does not have an option to reallocate resources, and its choice is limited to approval or disapproval of federal reimbursement for specific medical services, it is warranted in concluding that its micro-quality goal is being promoted once it determines that a medical procedure arguably will make a positive contribution to a patient's health. What such a decision ignores, unfortunately, is that society does have an option to reallocate funds to macro goals if it chooses. But reorientation to macro objectives or reallocation to important nonmedical priorities is not within the institutional competence of a PSRO, and the legislation establishes no incentive for a PSRO to be sensitive to these other societal needs.

Indeed, the PSRO legislation promotes just the opposite. Since

PSROs are organized regionally, a hard-nosed PSRO may be imposing lower standards of micro-quality on patients in its region without their receiving any tangible benefits in return. Both Medicare and Medicaid are entitlement programs whereby patients are reimbursed if they incur eligible expenses. As an organizational matter, there is no mechanism established to assure that patients in a PSRO's area will reap any reward from forgoing very expensive medical services. Savings imposed by one PSRO remain in the common pool for expenditure elsewhere or are returned to the federal treasury. These funds, therefore, are disbursed broadly, not to those who cut expenditures to reduce costs. This is an especially strong consideration and disincentive to economize where patients (and providers) in one region can accurately point to nearby PSROs which are applying more lenient standards.

In addition, the constituency to which regional PSROs are accountable includes physicians and other providers in their area. DHEW has very little maneuverability in applying sanctions to an ornery PSRO because of legislative limitations on the conditions for termination and designation as a qualified organization. On the other hand, the PSRO law gives physicians, institutional, and other providers standing to challenge PSRO judgments. Therefore, it is fair to assume that pressure on PSROs will come almost entirely from those who have a stake in maximizing micro-quality. Formal challenge procedures have been created to guarantee patients review of PSRO denial of payments, and patient interests are likely to be aroused when they are hit with medical bills that are deemed ineligible under a federal program. Providers will also press claims to reimbursement for services since many patients under Medicare or Medicaid are unable to make good on payments for already rendered care (*Mount Sinai Hospital of Greater Miami* v. *Weinberger*, 1974).

Not only is there no incentive for PSRO patients to restrain pursuit of micro-quality irrespective of cost because they will not benefit tangibly from such restraint, but also each PSRO itself has no institutional reason to face up to the difficult general allocative problems that society must confront with regard to public expenditures in the aggregate. Thus, while often promoted as a cost-containment tool that examines economic as well as medical perspectives, utilization review as carried out by PSROs may exacerbate already existent pressures for focusing on micro-quality. PSROs may therefore serve as extremely forceful political institutions influencing federal health and spending priorities generally and helping to shape definitions of quality of care. Rather than serving to contain aggregate costs, they may very well become extremely potent political lobbies that perpetuate current perspectives on medical spending and promote adoption of high standards of quality at the expense of other important social goals (Stone, 1974; Stuart and Stockton, 1973:342–343).

Regulatory Authority

The Senate supporters of PSROs identified two factors that had contributed to cost increases in the Medicare and Medicaid programs: rises in the unit prices of services, and increases in the number of services provided to beneficiaries (U.S. Congress, 1972:254). PSROs have no jurisdiction to consider pricing decisions, and therefore their effectiveness as cost-containment institutions is inherently limited. Moreover, to the extent that determinations of medical necessity include a socioeconomic judgment (Stuart and Stockton, 1973), limitations on PSRO power to concern itself with price inevitably inhibit its ability to perform a resource allocation function.

The narrow scope of PSRO authority also leaves it no role in the planning process. PSROs will generate data on utilization rates and profiles of practice and patient care; and some cooperative arrangement with the areawide Health Systems Agencies—HSAs—being set up under the National Health Planning and Resources Development Act of 1974 will be necessary (U.S. Congress, 1975). But the HSA regions have not been established to conform to PSRO regions (even though the Health Planning Act called for coordination of PSRO areas and health services areas to the "maximum extent feasible.") And there seems to be a conflict brewing between HSAs and PSROs with regard to their respective data-gathering roles (Butler et al., 1977).

In addition, the Health Planning Act requires states to establish a certificate-of-need program which applies to "new institutional health services," defined as services provided through health care facilities and health maintenance organizations. The certificate-of-need requirement vests planning and regulatory activities in another limited function organization, which will authorize expenditures on capital items. Under traditional forms of pricing arrangements, institutions will be permitted to earn a rate of return on approved capital outlays. With this approval, providers will have a much stronger claim in negotiating with PSROs that usage of the facilities should be permitted.

The Health Planning Act reflects a federal move toward more regulation in the health area, but functions typically performed by a regulatory body are now dispersed among multiple agencies. Utilization decisions for federal beneficiaries are made by PSROs; capital outlay decisions will be made by a statewide certificate-of-need body in consultation with areawide planning agencies (HSAs); and pricing decisions will be made by a third set of decision makers, typically government health officials or fiscal intermediaries.

Neither PSROs nor certificate-of-need agencies, furthermore, have any institutional incentive to curtail overinvestment or overutilization (Havighurst, 1973). This is an especially noteworthy problem for PSROs since their funding comes directly from DHEW and is unrelated to their performance in curtailing excessive utilization. Also, PSROs do not have a fixed budget to administer—either as an absolute amount or a target—so that their utilization review decisions will be made in part in a vacuum, which inevitably means the "yes-no" perception is exacerbated at the expense of the "either-or" viewpoint (Havighurst and Blumstein, 1975). Without some prior specification of a budget for a region, it becomes difficult to assess how individual decisions should be made, giving due consideration to cost factors.

Thus, the regulatory apparatus being set up in the health field will suffer even greater disadvantages than the regulatory bodies in other industries (Posner, 1971). Given the fragmentation, financing, and functional specialization, there is likely to be even less incentive and less opportunity to affect costs and to weigh different health objectives. Expansion of PSRO authority, on the other hand, has its risks, and further governmental involvement in supervising doctor-patient encounters runs the risk of invading privacy (Springer, 1975; Boyer, 1975), though not impermissibly so in the PSRO case, *Association of American Physicians and Surgeons* v. *Weinberger* (1975). This overall pattern must be part of an evaluation of the likely effectiveness of PSROs as a cost-containment instrument for hospital services and should encourage policymakers to search for additional mechanisms for pursuing cost-containment objectives.

References and Acknowledgments

Initial work on PSRO research was supported by the Commonwealth Foundation and by grant number HS 01539 from the Bureau of Health Services Research, Health Resources Administration, U.S. Department of Health, Education, and Welfare. The preparation of this study was supported by the Vanderbilt Institute for Public Policy Studies and also by the Department of Community Medicine, Dartmouth Medical School.

American Medical Association
    1972   Peer Review Manual. Chicago: American Medical Association.
Andreano, R., and B. Weisbrod
    1974   American Health Policy. Chicago: Rand McNally College Publishing Company.
Association of American Physicians and Surgeons v. Weinberger
    1975   395 F. Supp. 125 (N.D. Ill.), *affirmed* 423 U.S. 975.
Berki, S.E.
    1972   Hospital Economics. Lexington, Mass.: Lexington Books, D.C. Heath & Co.
Blumstein, J.F.
    1974   "Foundations of federal fertility policy." Milbank Memorial Fund Quarterly/Health and Society 52 (Spring): 131–168.
    1976   "Inflation and quality: The case of PSROs." Pp. 245–295, 375–380 in Michael Zubkoff, ed., Health: A Victim or Cause of Inflation? New York: Prodist for Milbank Memorial Fund.
Blumstein, J.F., and M. Zubkoff
    1973   "Perspectives on government policy in the health sector." Mil-

bank Memorial Fund Quarterly/Health and Society 51 (Summer): 395–431.

Boyer, B.B.
1975   "Computerized medical records and the right to privacy: The emerging federal response." Buffalo Law Review 25: 37–118.

Butler, L.H., et al.
1977   Cooperation between Health Systems Agencies and Professional Standards Review Organizations. San Francisco: Health Policy Program, University of California School of Medicine.

Cochrane, A.L.
1972   Effectiveness and Efficiency: Random Reflections on Health Services. London: The Nuffield Provincial Hospitals Trust.

Congressional Record
1972a   Remarks of Senator Bennett. 118, No. 152 (September 27): S16111–16112.

1972b   Remarks of Senator Long. 118, No. 168 (October 17): S18479.

Decker, B., and P. Bonner
1973   PSRO: Organization for Regional Peer Review. Cambridge: Ballinger Publishing Company.

Edwards, C.C.
1973   "Improving the nation's health care system." Address before the National Association of Blue Shield Plans. Chicago: October 25, 1973.

Fein, R.
1973   "On achieving access and equity in health care." Pp. 23–56 in John B. McKinlay, ed., Economic Aspects of Health Care. New York: Prodist for Milbank Memorial Fund.

Fuchs, V.R.
1973   "Health care and the United States economic system—an essay in abnormal physiology." Pp. 95–121 in John B. McKinlay ed., Economic Aspects of Health Care. New York: Prodist for Milbank Memorial Fund.

1974   Who Shall Live? Health, Economics and Social Choice. New York: Basic Books, Inc.

George Washington Law Review
1974   Note, "Federally-imposed self-regulation of medical practice: A critique of the Professional Standards Review Organization." George Washington Law Review 42: 822–849.

Gosfield, A.
1975   PSROs: The Law and the Health Consumer. Cambridge: Ballinger Publishing Company.

Havighurst, C.C.
1973 "Regulation of health facilities and services by 'certificate of need.'" Virginia Law Review 59 (October): 1143–1232.
Havighurst, C.C., and J.F. Blumstein
1975 "Coping with quality/cost trade-offs in medical care: The role of PSROs." Northwestern Law Review 70 (March–April): 6–68.
Havighurst, C.C., and R. Bovbjerg
1975 "Professional Standards Review Organizations and Health Maintenance Organizations: Are they compatible?" Utah Law Review (Summer): 381–421.
Helling v. Carey
1974 519 P.2d 981.
Holder, A.R.
1975 Medical Malpractice Law. New York: John Wiley & Sons, Inc.
InterStudy
1973 Assuring the Quality of Health Care. Minneapolis: InterStudy.
Jeffers, J.R., et al.
1971 "On the demand versus need for medical services and the concept on shortage." American Journal of Public Health 61 (January): 46–63.
King, J.H.
1975 "In search of a standard of care for the medical profession: The 'accepted practice' formula." Vanderbilt Law Review 28: 1213–1276.
Koos, E.L.
1954 The Health of Regionville. New York: Columbia University Press.
Lander, L.
1974 "PSROs: A little toe in the door." Health/PAC Bulletin 59 (July/August).
Lave, J.R., and L.B. Lave
1970 "Medical care and its delivery: An economic appraisal." Law and Contemporary Problems 35 (Spring): 252–266.
Mount Sinai Hospital of Greater Miami v. Weinberger
1974 376 F. Supp. 1099 (S.D. Fla.).
Posner, R.A.
1971 "Regulatory aspects of national health insurance plans." University of Chicago Law Review 39 (Fall): 1–29.
Reinhardt, U.
1973 "Proposed changes in the organization of health-care delivery:

An overview and critique." Milbank Memorial Fund Quarterly/ Health and Society 51 (Spring): 169–223.

Rivkin, M.O., and P.J. Bush
1974   "The satisfaction continuum in health care: Consumer and provider preferences." Pp. 304–332 in Selma J. Mushkin, ed., Consumer Incentives for Health Care. New York: Prodist for Milbank Memorial Fund.

Simmons, H.E.
1973   "PSRO's—An opportunity for medicine." Address before the American Public Health Association, San Francisco, November 7, 1973.
1974a   "PSRO and the quality of medical care." Address before the Indiana Medical Association, May 16, 1974.
1974b   "Federal policy on health manpower." Pp. 81–87 in Institute of Medicine, Manpower for Health Care. Washington, D.C.

Springer, E.W.
1975   "Professional standards review organization: Some problems of confidentiality." Utah Law Review (Summer): 361–380.

Stevens, R.
1971   American Medicine and the Public Interest. New Haven: Yale University Press.

Stone, D.
1974   "Professionalism and accountability: Controlling health services in the United States and West Germany." Working Paper #8742, Center for the Study of Health Policy, Institute of Policy Sciences and Public Affairs. Durham: Duke University.

Stuart, B., and R. Stockton
1973   "Control over the utilization of medical services." Milbank Memorial Fund Quarterly/Health and Society 51 (Spring): 169–223.

Tancredi, L., and J. Woods
1973   "The social control of medical practice—Licensure versus output monitoring." Pp. 327–353 in John B. McKinlay, ed., Economic Aspects of Health Care. New York: Prodist for Milbank Memorial Fund.

Theodore, C.
1974   "Towards a strategy for evaluating PSROs." Westchester Medical Bulletin (November).

U.S. Congress
1972   U.S. Senate Committee on Finance, Report 92-1230, 92d Congress. Washington, D.C.: U.S. Government Printing Office.

1975   National Health Planning and Resources Development Act of 1974. Public Law 93-641 (January 4, 1975). Statutes at Large 88: 2225.

U.S. Department of Health, Education, and Welfare

1973   Publication No. (OS) 74-5001 (December). Reprinted in 2 CCH Medicare and Medicaid Guide: ¶12,885.

1974a   OPSR Memo No. 4 (April).

1974b   P.S.R.O. Program Manual. Washington, D.C.: OPSR.

1977   PSRO Fact Book. Washington, D.C.: Office of Health Standards and Quality, Health Care Financing Administration.

Welch, C.

1973   "Professional review organizations—problems and prospects." The New England Journal of Medicine 289 (August): 291-295.

Methodological Issues in Cost-Containment Procedures

The Relationship

of Hospital Cost Measurement

to

Hospital Cost Control Programs

WILLIAM O. CLEVERLEY

Introduction

A tale that was often heard in hospital financial managers' circles during the recent Economic Stabilization Program (ESP) era best illustrates the purpose of this paper. It seems that a hospital administrator wanted to obtain some expert accounting assistance to fill out his S-52 form. To help him select the best accounting firm, he asked the partner of each firm he called what 2 plus 2 equaled. Each of the partners responded 4, until he called a partner from a certain Big 8 firm. The partner responded, after a climactic pause, "What number did you have in mind?" Obviously he got the job.

Most hospital cost regulators recognize the importance of a cost accounting system in any hospital cost-containment policy. The basic cost control measures used by hospital regulatory decision makers are in many cases the direct outputs of hospital cost accounting systems. It is necessary, therefore, to identify the relationship between hospital cost accounting systems and hospital cost control programs, and to examine those areas in the cost accounting measurement process that affect cost comparability. For unless that measurement process is reasonably standardized, effective and equitable hospital cost control programs do not appear to be feasible.

Relationship of Cost Accounting and Cost Control Programs

Cost control, whether it be exercised by an external third party or by internal management, is predicated upon the relationship between two cost measures. First, there must be some normative measure of what cost ought to be, given a specified set of circumstances. Second, there must be a measure of what costs actually were. Cost control decisions are ultimately based on the magnitude of the difference between those two measures. Consistent differences indicate either that the standard is not correct or that appropriate changes in operating behavior have not been effected. Both conclusions dictate that the controlling authority take action to ensure future compliance.

Cost accounting systems play an integral informational role in the cost control process. These systems directly provide the measures of actual cost, and in many cases provide the underlying data used to develop the normative cost measures. Given this latter role, there is a requirement that these cost accounting or measurement systems be comparable, at least within a given hospital and perhaps across hospitals.

The need for cost accounting system comparability is related to the manner in which the normative cost measure(s) are to be established. If the normative cost measures for a hospital are to be based exclusively upon prior actual cost measures of that hospital, then there is little need for cost accounting comparability across hospitals. If however, the normative cost measures of a hospital are based upon actual cost measures of other hospitals, then there is a need for comparability across hospitals.

In general, it appears that four methods for developing normative cost measures have been used to date (refer to Table 1):

1. Using a formula applied to past actual cost data of the controlled hospital.

TABLE 1   Normative Cost Measurement Schemes

Individual Hospital Formula
1. Economic Stabilization Program
2. New York Commissioner of Health

Group Hospital Formula
1. Blue Cross of Alabama
2. Blue Cross of Western Pennsylvania
3. Section 233 of P.L. 92-603

Submitted Budgets
1. Blue Cross of Southwest Ohio
2. Blue Cross of Indiana
3. Kentucky Blue Cross
4. Blue Cross of Northeast Ohio
5. Connecticut Hospital Association
6. Blue Cross of Michigan
7. Blue Cross of Rhode Island
8. Maryland (HSCRC)
9. Arizona Health Planning Authority
10. Montana Hospitals Rate Review System
11. Nebraska Hospital Reimbursement Plan
12. New Jersey Budget and Cost Review Program
13. Virginia Hospital Association
14. Washington State Hospital Commission
15. Wisconsin Blue Cross

Engineer—Cost Analyst
1. Blue Cross of Southern California
2. Blue Cross of Western Pennsylvania

2. Using a formula applied to past actual cost data for a group of similar hospitals.

3. Using submitted individual hospital budget data.

4. Using industrial engineers or cost analysts to develop hospital specific cost norms.

Of the above methods, only the first one clearly does not require cost data from other hospitals. The second method directly incorporates cost data from other hospitals, while methods three and four would appear likely to incorporate other hospital data in the development of normative cost measures. For example, Cohen (1975:129) indicates that the Maryland program, which bases its standards on submitted budgets, intends to utilize uniform financial reports from the controlled hospitals in the development of cost norms. It thus seems safe to conclude that comparability of cost data across hospitals is a highly desirable, if not essential, requirement for most cost control programs in the hospital industry.

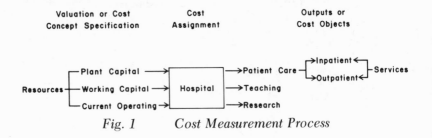

Fig. 1   *Cost Measurement Process*

Cost Accounting Process

The importance of interhospital cost comparability in hospital cost control programs has been identified. The achievement of comparability is largely affected by the nature and degree of variation in hospital cost accounting systems. Uniformity in hospital cost accounting is one approach toward the achievement of cost comparability. Uniformity of accounting implies that only one accounting treatment for a given fact situation is appropriate. Comparability would certainly be enhanced with uniformity, assuming no logical reason for accounting diversity exists.

The focus of this section is on the identification of various aspects of the cost accounting measurement system where uniform adoption of various accounting treatments may promote interhospital cost comparability. Figure 1 provides a diagrammatic representation of the cost accounting process. For discussion purposes, the costing process is categorized into three separate processes:

1. Determining the value or cost of resources acquired by the hospital.

2. Determining the relevant objects to which costs will be assigned.

3. Allocating costs or values to the designated cost objects.

Alternative Valuation Concepts

The issue of asset or resource valuation has been one of debate both among accountants and also between accountants and various user groups, most notably economists. Valuation is obviously a key concept in the entire costing process. Different measurements of value will clearly produce different measures of costs for the objects being costed and thus affect comparability.

Schwayder (1969) identified four major alternative valuation rules for assets or resources:

1. Historical cost.
2. Historical cost adjusted for changes in the general price level.
3. Historical cost adjusted for changes in the specific price level of the assets of the firm.
4. Historical cost adjusted for the inputed cost of capital.

All four of these valuation rules are based upon the initial entry value or historical cost of the assets. The last three rules may modify this value with the passage of time in a predetermined manner. For the sake of completeness, alternative valuation rules may be developed which use exit values or resale market values for costing and expense recognition (Edwards and Bell, 1964). The utility of many exit value concepts is principally for decisions in organizations that are not classified as going concerns. A relevant value of assets in those situations is their current market or liquidation value. This better represents the short-run opportunity cost of the assets.

Entry values appear more relevant for cost control decisions than do exit values for several reasons. First, many hospital cost-containment plans tie cost control to reimbursement. Equitable reimbursement from the provider's perspective must allow for the acquisition of resources required to provide needed services. Entry values of resources would appear to be more suitable than exit values for this purpose. Second, pragmatically, entry values are easier to measure and usually more objective than exit values. Thus, measurement would be easier and less costly if entry values were used as opposed to exit values.

Alternative Cost Objects

The final outcome of a cost accounting process is to attach measures of value or costs to a variety of cost objects (Vatter, 1969:25-31). Some typical cost objects would include outputs, departments, classes of customers, inventory, and many others. Specifying the cost objective determines to a large extent how initial resource values or costs are to be collected and later assigned to the relevant cost object.

The notion of relevance of the cost object relates to the type of decision for which the measure of cost is being used. Some cost objects have no informational value in certain classes of decisions (for example, costs of classes of customers are irrelevant for most management control decisions which require departmental cost measures).

To provide cost measures for a variety of cost objects, accounting systems attempt to classify the initial resource values into a very large number of elements or accounts. These elements or accounts can then be aggregated in various manners to achieve measures of costs for a variety of designated cost objectives. The chart of accounts is the mechanism used by accountants to provide the initial system of cost classification.

The chart of accounts has two basic classification dimensions: natural and departmental. The natural dimension indicates the nature of the expense, such as salaries, supplies, employee benefits, and purchased services. The departmental dimension assigns the cost to a specific department, such as administration, radiology, and housekeeping. Thus cost measures contained in the accounts can be aggregated in various ways to produce measures of costs for a variety of cost objectives. For example, the total fees paid to hospital-based physicians could be determined by adding the individual physician fee payment accounts across hospital departments.

Cost control programs in the hospital industry seek to control both the costs of services delivered and the amounts of services provided. The relevant cost objects for cost control purposes would thus appear to be the services or outputs produced by the hospital. Measures of costs for hospital services can be determined from existing charts of accounts only if there are systematic relationships between services or outputs and departments. Fortunately, these relationships do exist, because the production of identical outputs or services does not occur in different departments. Thus, a departmental classification system is, by and large, isomorphic to a service or output classification system.

Assuming this relationship between department and output structure, there are at least three possible cost objectives that may be relevant for cost control programs:

1. The hospital as a single entity.
2. The direct patient service departments.
3. The direct patient service departments and indirect or support departments.

The measure of output used in alternative one would be macro, such as patient days or admissions. This alternative was used in the recent Economic Stabilization Program (ESP) and is currently used in the New York state program. Alternative two would require allocations of costs from indirect departments to the direct departments, if total hospital costs were to be controlled. Section 233 of the Social Security Amendments of 1972 (P.L. 92-603) currently provides controls over routine inpatient nursing per diem costs. Method three would control separately the costs of both direct and indirect departments. The Social Security Administration incentive reimbursement experiment in Connecticut provided budgetary control over several indirect and direct service departments.

Alternative Cost Assignment Methods

Uniformity of valuation and cost objective specification in the cost accounting process does not ensure the comparability of costs across hospitals. Uniformity of cost assignment in the cost accounting process must also be present. In general, there are four major areas of cost assignment which provide considerable latitude in the determination of costs. To promote cost comparability, some elimination of available alternatives within these four areas should be sought. The four areas are:

1. Expense recognition patterns.
2. Departmental cost allocation methods.
3. Fiscal year end.
4. Accounting estimates.

1. The relationship of expenditures and expense recognition is crucial to accounting measurement and the discussion of accounting principles. Accountants use the term "cost" to refer to the value that is initially assigned to an asset or resource upon acquisition. This value is most often based upon an actual expenditure or the associated increase in a short-term liability, for example, accounts payable or accrued salaries. "Expense" is recognized as the asset is employed in the production of services.

In most cases, the expenditure and the expense occur in the same reporting period. For example, most labor costs are actually paid in the period in which they are used. An accrual accounting system will recognize that small amount of labor expense incurred but not yet paid at the reporting period end by charging the labor expense account and crediting an accrued wages and salary liability account.

However, there are situations where this pattern does not occur. In some cases, expenditures are made for resources which produce benefits in future reporting periods. Some common examples are plant and equipment, organization costs, bond issue costs, and in some cases supplies inventory. In other cases, benefits are realized prior to the actual expenditure. Some common examples are pension costs, vacation costs, and holiday and sick leave costs.

2. Much of the attention of hospital cost accounting experts has focused on alternative cost allocation schemes. Conceptually, there are three possible areas in which variability is created in cost accounting systems:

a. *Selection of the cost apportionment method.* At the present time four methods of cost apportionment are employed in the hospital industry: direct apportionment; step-down apportionment; double distribution apportionment; and simultaneous equation apportionment.

b. *Identification of the indirect and direct departments.* Different organizational structures will produce different listings of direct and indirect departments. Both fewer indirect and fewer direct departments may exist in smaller hospitals because of their more limited range of services. For example, small hospitals may aggregate the general administrative activities of admitting, business office, and accounting into one general administrative cost center.

Smaller hospitals may also offer a narrower range of ancillary services which would be reflected in fewer direct departments.

    c. *Identification of cost allocation bases.*

    3. The selection of reporting periods is another area that could affect the comparability of cost data. For the most part, external financial statements and cost reports are filed on a yearly basis consistent with the hospital's fiscal year. Problems of cost comparability arise when comparing costs of hospitals with different fiscal year ends. Three solutions to these problems are possible:

    a. Require all hospitals to have identical fiscal year ends.

    b. Limit comparisons to hospitals with identical fiscal year ends.

    c. Adjust cost data to create comparability.

    4. Accounting estimates constitute the final area of cost assignment that may produce cost variability to be discussed in this paper. Accounting estimates are required in a significant number of expense recognition alternatives. Some common examples are: useful lives of fixed assets, investment yields in pension expense measurement, life expectancy in pension expense measurement, and bad debt write-offs.

In general these estimates are required irrespective of the selection of accounting principles. For example, an estimate of the useful life of a depreciable asset is necessary no matter what type of depreciation measurement principle is adopted—straight-line, sum-of-the-years digits, or double declining balance. Using different estimates, given the same accounting principle, can produce different measures of periodic expense. Thus if comparability is desired, some uniformity in accounting estimates appears needed.

Evaluation of Cost Accounting Alternatives

In evaluating the various cost accounting process alternatives mentioned in the last section, the primary criterion that will be used is the promotion of interhospital cost comparability. The relevance of this criterion is based upon its central role in the determination of measures of normative cost that are essential in cost control programs. Another criterion to be considered is the promotion of intrahospital cost comparability. This criterion is of importance in those cost control programs that base their measures of normative cost exclusively upon past measures of actual cost in the controlled hospital (for example, individual hospital formula plans). Equity of provider reimbursement is also another important consideration. Since cost control programs will probably be related to reimbursement, the cost measures used in the cost control process must reflect the reasonable financial requirements necessary to provide services (American Hospital Association, 1969). Finally, some consideration should be given to the level of administrative costs associated with the selection of various cost accounting alternatives. Their adoption should not result in an excessive increase in the costs associated with maintaining the hospital's cost accounting system.

Alternative Valuation Concepts

Uniformity of valuation in cost accounting systems is presently a reality. All hospitals are required to use unadjusted historical cost valuation, if they adhere to Generally Accepted Accounting Principles (GAAP), which they must for all audited financial statements.

However, the comparability of unadjusted historical cost measures on both an interhospital basis and a temporal intrahospital basis is not good. Many difficulties are encountered in making intelligent analyses of interhospital cost data with the present-day historical cost measurement rules. Most of the major problems arise in the comparison of the cost measures for capital costs or depreciation charges. To illustrate this point, examine the data presented in Table 2. The two hospitals are assumed to be identical in every respect, except for their construction cost per bed. This difference is due to the cost at the time construction was undertaken, and is not due to any difference in the physical amounts of capital provided. With an inflation rate in construction costs of 10 percent per year, the age differential would be seven years. An individual looking only at cost per patient day might erroneously conclude that hospital A is more efficient than hospital B and argue that the $104.45 cost per

TABLE 2   Comparative Hospital Cost Data

	Hospital A	Hospital B
Bed size	250	250
Construction cost/bed	$ 50000	$ 100,000
Total construction cost	$12,500,000	$25,000,000
Depreciation (20 yr. life)	$ 625,000	$ 1,250,000
Patient days (80% occupancy)	73,000	73,000
Operating cost	$ 7,000,000	$ 7,000,000
Total cost	$ 7,625,000	$ 8,250,000
Cost/patient day	$ 104.45	$ 113.01
General price index at time of construction	100	185
Construction cost index at time of construction	100	200
Current year end general price index	200	200
Current year end construction cost index	250	250
General price adjusted cost	$ 8,250,000	$ 8,351,351
General price adjusted cost per patient day	$ 113.01	$ 114.40
Specific price adjusted cost	$ 8,562,500	$ 8,562,500
Specific price adjusted cost per patient day	$ 117.29	$ 117.29

patient day should be the norm rather than the $113.01 cost per patient day in hospital B.

Intrahospital temporal cost comparisons are also difficult for outside reviewing organizations to make. An institution that was furnishing the same set of services over time and employing the same set of resources to produce those services might show sharply increasing costs because of inflationary effects. Assuming that the cost control regulatory body wishes to control both the costs of acquired resources and the utilization of those resources, present-day cost reports would be largely inadequate for these purposes.

The equity of reimbursing hospitals for unadjusted historical costs is clearly questionable (Cleverley, 1974; Walls, 1972). In the long run, dependence upon this type of reimbursement with no allowance for an accounting profit would certainly lead to the financial ruin of the present private hospital system. Simply stated, no hospital can replace plant assets in our present inflationary economy and meet the associated debt service requirements of that replacement with reimbursement limited to unadjusted historical cost depreciation.

General price level adjusted historical cost would improve the comparability of both inter and intrahospital cost reports. For example, in Table 2 it can be seen that the increase in the general price index between the two construction points was 85 percent. Assuming that the operating costs are already stated in current terms, the general price level adjusted total costs would be much more comparable. The difference between the two now is due to the relative difference in price changes between the general price index and the construction cost index.

Intrahospital temporal comparison is more meaningful when general price level adjusted historical cost is used because of the stable monetary unit weighting built into the system. Usually cost measures expressed in dollars are indications of the value of the resources attaching to some cost objective. But dollars of one year do not have the same purchasing value as dollars of another year. Therefore, general price adjustments of prior cost measures to dollars of the current period create cost measure comparability. Changes in constant dollar costs can then be attributed to factors other than general inflation, such as increased utilization or the payment of unreasonable prices for the resources.

Reimbursement of general price level adjusted historical costs is more equitable to the hospitals than unadjusted historical cost reimbursement. As previously discussed, the major reason for this improvement in equity is the reimbursement for depreciation. However, in periods of inflation significant inequities may also result in the reimbursement of current operating costs on an unadjusted historical cost basis. Table 3 illustrates this inequity more clearly. In this case general prices are increasing 16 percent per year with the increases distributed equally among the four quarters. It is assumed that there is a one-quarter or three-month delay from the point of payment for current operating expenses and reimbursement by third-party payers. This interval may be longer for some payers, which would increase the magnitude of the shortage. Assuming that the physical quantities of resources consumed are constant but with increasing prices, the hospital would face a $480,000 shortage in unadjusted dollars at year end. If current operating expenses were price level adjusted, reimbursement in the first quarter would be

**TABLE 3   Inequity of Unadjusted Historical Cost
Reimbursement for Current Operating Costs**

Quarter	General Price Index	Unadjusted Historical Costs	Reimbursement	Shortage
4th	100	$ 3,000,000		
1st	104	$ 3,120,000	$ 3,000,000	$120,000
2nd	108	3,240,000	3,120,000	120,000
3rd	112	3,360,000	3,240,000	120,000
4th	116	3,480,000	3,360,000	120,000
Year's Total		$13,200,000	$12,720,000	$480,000

$3,120,000 ($3,000,000 × 104/100). Reimbursement in each of the following periods would match the required outlay in that period so there would be no dollar shortage during any of the periods. This assumes that the general price index used for adjustment matches the changes in prices of the conglomeration of hospital current operating cost elements.

General price level adjustments to historical cost would require more clerical effort than unadjusted historical cost, but in the days of computerized bookkeeping systems, the increased effort is not substantial, at least in the long run. In addition, it is quite probable that in the not too distant future the Financial Accounting Standards Board (FASB), the accountants' rule-making body, will change the present valuation basis from unadjusted historical cost to price level adjusted historical cost. This event becomes more probable given the continued accelerated rate of inflation in our economy.

The valuation basis that is most likely to be used, based on prior research (American Institute of Certified Public Accountants [AICPA], 1963; AICPA, 1969; Russell, 1975; FASB, 1975), is historical cost adjusted for changes in the general price level. Probably the index for historical cost adjustment would be the Gross National Product Implicit Price Deflator, largely because of its all-inclusive nature. Given this event, there would not be any increased administrative cost associated with general price level adjusted historical cost valuation, because hospitals would be required to record costs on this basis for financial reporting purposes.

Specific price level adjusted historical cost is in many respects a refinement of general price level adjusted historical cost. In this case the objective is to derive the specific replacement cost of the assets or resources used in the production of goods and services. Pragmatically, this would mean using a number of price indexes for adjustment rather than just one general price index.

Comparability and equity should be marginally better using specific indexes rather than one single index. For example, the cost per patient day in hospitals A and B in Table 2 is now identical, $117.29, using specific price adjusted cost. However, the administrative costs associated with maintaining a cost accounting system using this valuation basis could be astronomical. At one extreme, a hospital-specific index could be developed for each individual hospital resource category. Such a system would increase the cost of measurement significantly. It is doubtful that the improvement in comparability and equity would be sufficient to justify the increased cost, given a general price index alternative. Alternatively, a very limited number of externally reported specific price indexes could be used for major resource categories. This system would involve less clerical costs and the improvement in comparability and equity might be sufficient enough to justify the slight increment in cost.

The final policy adopted by the FASB is highly relevant to this decision. Maintenance of two cost measurement systems based on different valuation rules would be not only costly, but also confusing. In this vein, general price level adjusted historical cost would appear to have an advantage over specific price index adjusted historical cost.

The last valuation rule, historical cost adjusted for the imputed cost of capital, will not be discussed in great detail. Its use is more relevant for proprietary organizations where return on investment is a prime management control concern. Since most hospitals are nonprofit, the realization of a rate of return on investment is of less concern. At the same time, cost of capital is not uniform among firms but varies according to the financial structure and investment opportunities of the firm (Arditti, 1973). This valuation rule is dismissed then as a possibility for hospital cost measurement.

To summarize this analysis, it seems highly desirable to have hospitals value assets using a general price level adjusted historical cost basis. This adoption would improve cost comparability over the level that currently exists with unadjusted historical cost valuation.

Alternative Cost Objects

Controlling hospital costs using only a macro measure of total hospital costs, perhaps eliminating research and teaching costs, does not promote cost comparability. It is questionable if anyone can make appropriate cost-containment decisions by comparing the costs of a $50 million university hospital with a $4 million community hospital. Dividing by gross measures of activity such as patient days, adjusted patient days, or admissions does not help because the variations in produced services are just too large. Furthermore, grouping hospitals by size, geographical location, and metropolitan status, as is done in Section 233 of P. L. 92-603, might not eliminate a large enough percent of this service variation to be of major benefit.

Intrahospital temporal comparisons are also not valid, especially in the long run. Hospitals are constantly changing both the quantity and types of services that they deliver. Comparing total hospital cost over a five-year period is difficult, unless changes in services have been properly accounted for. The ESP, which employed a total hospital cost measure, was plagued by this problem. Had it continued for a longer period of time, the number of exception requests would have required a large army of legal, cost, and hospital specialists to account equitably for the changing nature of hospital services.

Reimbursing on the basis of total hospital costs has several equity-related disadvantages. First, given the continuance of multi-hospital payers, equity is improved when payers pay on the basis of services received and not on some proportionate basis of total cost. Second, reimbursement of total costs may hide underlying departmental efficiencies and inefficiencies. A total hospital cost measure may be viewed as satisfactory when compared to some normative total hospital cost measure, but significant departmental inefficiencies may exist. Reimbursement would not provide a strong incentive for improving performance in those inefficient departments, when determined on a total hospital cost basis.

Intuitively, the administrative costs of total hospital cost measurement might appear to be substantially less than departmental cost measurement. However, hospitals would continue to maintain departmental cost measurement systems, even if a cost control agency required only total hospital cost measurement, because departmental cost measurement is central to hospital management control. Thus, there is no rationale for selecting total hospital cost measurement over departmental cost measurement on the basis of any savings in administrative costs, at least from the hospital's perspective.

Departmental cost measures would improve comparability because the basis for comparison would be the departmental level where the degree of output homogeneity is unquestionably higher than at the total hospital level. Certainly, differences in hospital departmental outputs will be present when interhospital comparisons are made, but groupings of similar hospitals at the departmental level should eliminate some of this variability of service. Given the initial degree of service homogeneity at the departmental level, comparisons of interhospital departmental costs should be very valid. This is especially true if uniformity in valuation and other cost measurement principles is a reality.

Intrahospital temporal comparisons are also more valid at the departmental level. The establishment of new departments or the expansion of volume in an existing department is more likely to be reflected properly in departmental cost measures than in total cost measures. For example, using a cost per patient day measure over time does not properly recognize the expansion of delivered ancillary services that have been associated with a day of inpatient care. If price level adjusted departmental cost measures were used, comparability between years would be enhanced because adjustments for both changes in volume and price structure could be easily made. Better focus on controllable cost increases should result.

Equity should be improved with departmental cost measurement because reimbursement can be tied more directly to the quantity and type of services produced by the individual hospital. There is still a need, however, for some organization to assure that the delivered services are appropriate, for example, a Professional Standards Review Organization. In addition, focusing on departmental costs should spotlight departmental efficiencies and inefficiencies. Since this departmental focus parallels the hospital's own management control structure, cost control or containment decisions made by external cost-containment organizations would be made on the same basis that hospital management control decisions are made. Better focus and direction for cost-containment decisions should result.

The administrative effort involved in departmental cost measurement is influenced by the degree of departmental specification. If only direct departments are included, then allocations of indirect departmental costs are required as stated earlier. Because these allocations are likely to be arbitrary, the objectivity of cost measurement is reduced and the administrative cost is increased. Including indirect departments would remove the need for arbitrary cost allocations. Also, since approximately 40 percent of total hospital costs may be in indirect departments, separate control over those departments is likely to enhance the overall effectiveness of hospital cost-containment programs.

In summary, cost comparability would be promoted if departmental cost objectives were used in cost control programs. Furthermore, to eliminate the need for arbitrary cost allocations from indirect to direct departments, the cost objectives should not be limited to direct departments, but should include indirect departments as well.

Alternative Cost Assignment Methods

1. The availability of alternative expense recognition accounting principles can severely restrict interhospital cost comparability. By and large, the accounting profession has not taken effective steps to limit the number of acceptable accounting treatments (Briloff, 1972:24–37). For example, depreciation expense may be calculated by using any one of a number of currently acceptable methods, for instance, straight-line, sum-of-the-years digits, declining balance, and units-of-output. The amount of depreciation expenses reported in any period may be substantially different with different methods.

**TABLE 4   Comparison of Alternative Depreciation
Methods for a Group of Five Year Life Depreciable Assets**

Year Asset Acquired	Cost	Straight-Line Depreciation	Sum-of-the-Years Digits Depreciation
Current year	$1,500	$ 300	$ 500
One year ago	1,500	300	400
Two years ago	1,500	300	300
Three years ago	1,500	300	200
Four years ago	1,500	300	100
Totals	$7,500	$1,500	$1,500

Depreciation is not the only area where generally acceptable accounting principle alternatives exist; they extend to almost every area where the realization of benefits does not coincide with the incurrence of an expenditure.

While not promoting uniformity in accounting principles, the accounting profession has attempted to foster cost comparability by its consistency requirement. Consistency permits the selection of alternative accounting principles, but limits the ability of an organization to change its accounting principles over time. Adherence to consistency may foster cost comparability in the absence of uniformity in accounting principles. For example, Table 4 illustrates the effect of consistent utilization of alternative depreciation methods. Hospitals with an identical composition of assets would show identical depreciation charges for these two alternative depreciation expense recognition methods. However, the existence of inflation in asset acquisition costs would make this statement false, unless price level adjustments were made.

Given the current absence of uniformity in accounting principles, cost comparability cannot result unless some officially designated external party begins to promulgate a set of uniform accounting principles. Many public utilities already adhere to uniform accounting principles required by their regulatory agencies; most notable among these agencies is the Interstate Commerce Commission, which regulates the railroad industry (Hendriksen, 1965:32–36). A Cost Accounting Standards Board (CASB) was also recently formed by the passage of P.L. 91-379 in 1969. The primary function of this body is to develop cost accounting standards for defense contractors that will achieve uniformity and consistency. It would appear that such an organization could and should be established for the hospital industry.

2. If there is a need for departmental cost allocations, the simultaneous equation method would be the most accurate. Departmental cost allocations are necessary only when the cost objectives are limited to direct departments. We recommend using both direct and indirect departments to eliminate the necessity of these arbitrary cost allocations and also to improve the effectiveness of cost control programs.

The existence of different departmental structures in hospitals does create cost comparability problems, but the problem is not serious. To a great extent, a uniform departmental structure exists, especially among hospitals of similar size and service. Much of this uniformity can be directly attributed to the American Hospital Association (AHA) through its publication efforts (AHA, 1966; AHA, 1968). In addition, the reporting requirements of some third-party payers, Medicare in particular, have fostered departmental uniformity. Some additional minimal departmental classification might be useful and probably feasible to promote better hospital cost comparability. This is especially true if the focus of hospital cost containment is at the departmental level, as has been suggested in this paper.

The definition of allocation bases for indirect departments is another area that can potentially affect cost comparability. However, the importance of allocation bases becomes relevant only if the focus of hospital cost containment is at the direct departmental level. If both direct and indirect departments are included, no technical requirement for allocation of costs exists.

3. The comparability of cost reports between hospitals with different fiscal year ends is the third cost assignment issue. If two hospitals with fiscal year ends on December 31 and June 30 are to be compared to establish normative cost measures, are these comparisons valid? Assuming a period of inflation, the answer appears to be no. In the previous case, only one-half or six months of the two hospitals' reporting periods would be comparable. The remaining one-half would be one year apart. Cost structure can obviously change dramatically in a year's time.

Requiring all hospitals to have identical fiscal year ends is the easiest solution to this problem. However, this change might be costly to some hospitals. For example, governmental hospitals which are part of larger governmental entities with a different fiscal year end than the one which might be required would find the switch to a different fiscal year end both costly and confusing.

Limiting comparisons to hospitals with identical fiscal year ends might not be feasible. In some cases the number of hospitals in a given category, say, February 15 year ends, might be reduced significantly. If group comparisons are required for establishing normative cost measures, then this restriction could be critical because it might restrict the relevant sample below tolerable limits.

The last solution to this problem would be to adjust cost data with different fiscal year ends to create cost comparability. Using a price index to adjust cost data already stated in common dollars, as would be the case with general price level adjusted historical cost statements, would create comparability. This observation reinforces the earlier recommendation that general price level adjusted historical cost valuation be used.

4. There is often justification for different accounting estimates across institutions because not all hospitals experience the same levels of bad debts or retain fixed assets for the same periods of time. To impose uniformity in accounting estimates may in the long run produce incomparability rather than comparability across institutions.

In some cases external standards for accounting estimates exist, especially for the useful lives of fixed assets (AHA, 1966). Audits of cost reports should identify those accounting estimates that differ widely from those norms. Justification for those differences can then be documented and evaluated. Modifications could then be made on the basis of this information. Such a process should promote interhospital cost comparability.

In addition, an external agency with responsibility for developing uniformity standards in accounting estimates would be beneficial. This agency should be identical to the one recommended earlier that would be responsible for developing uniformity in accounting principles. Audits of cost reports could then ensure adherence to these uniformity standards and document any deviations.

Recommendations

The recommendations that follow relate the nature of cost information that a hospital cost-containment agency should receive. These recommendations are based largely on the need by cost-containment agencies for comparable cost data which are critical to the development of meaningful normative or standard cost measures. The recommendations follow from an analysis of the hospital cost accounting process as previously discussed and represented schematically in Fig. 1. The first recommendation relates to the valuation process, the second recommendation relates to the specification of cost objects, and the last two recommendations relate to the nature of cost assignment within the hospital.

1. *Require all hospital cost accounting systems to use general price level adjusted historical cost as the basis for valuing resources.*

The adoption of this recommendation would help achieve two basic objectives. First, cost comparability from both inter and intrahospital perspectives would be enhanced. This would be true not only for the measurement of capital cost, but also for the measurement of current operating cost. Second, to the extent that reimbursement is linked to cost control, the equity of provider reimbursement would be improved with general price level adjusted historical cost measurement. This improvement in equity will eliminate much of the current need to manipulate cost measures that presently exists in the hospital industry.

This recommendation may not constitute a radical departure from existing accounting practice. The accounting profession appears to be moving with great speed in this direction, and financial reporting may soon require price level adjusted historical cost valuation.

2. *Require hospital cost reports to present measures of direct departmental cost for both direct and indirect departments.*

Comparability of hospital cost measurement is not possible

when the cost object is the entire hospital. Costs of more homogeneous units like departments help foster both inter and intrahospital cost comparability. Groupings of similar hospitals or developing statistical cost equations will be more valid at the departmental rather than hospital level because the degree of output variability is much less.

Inclusion of both indirect and direct departments is recommended. The inclusion of indirect departments eliminates the need to make arbitrary cost allocations and will promote comparability. In addition, because of the large proportion of total costs accounted for by indirect departments, direct control in these departments is critical to effective cost containment.

3. *Establish a hospital cost accounting standards board at the federal level.*

An analogy to the defense industry can be made. The Cost Accounting Standards Board (CASB) is required to generate cost accounting standards for achievement of uniformity and consistency in the cost accounting principles followed by defense contractors (Li, 1973; Staats, 1969). The rationale for such a body is based upon the need to foster efficiency and equity in a largely cost-reimbursed industry. The hospital industry could be similarly described.

The primary purposes of the hospital cost accounting standards board should be to: (1) establish a minimum chart of accounts; (2) formulate a uniform cost report that can be used by all third-party payers and cost control agencies and (3) develop a list of generally accepted accounting principles.

4. *Require an annual audit of all hospital cost reports.*

This audit should be conducted by an independent certified public accounting firm and should not be duplicated. Currently, as many as two or three audits of hospital financial reports are performed by various third-party payers and independent certified public accountants. This unnecessary and costly duplication of audit engagements should not be continued, as it invites "gamesmanship" in the accounting process to meet the idiosyncracies of each auditor.

Certified public accountants are a logical choice for two reasons.

First, many creditors will not accept financial statements that have not been audited by certified public accountants. Thus, their involvement is a given for most institutions and their services are not capable of being assumed by any third-party payer auditor. Secondly, the major objective of the audit is to assure inter and intrahospital financial statement comparability. In the absence of uniform financial and cost-reporting standards, certified public accountants can apply their existing set of generally accepted accounting principles and requirements for consistency to promote a modest degree of comparability. If and when the public body described in recommendation three is formed and develops uniform financial and cost reports and a set of uniform accounting principles, certified public accountants can then apply those reporting requirements in their audit function.

References

American Accounting Association
    1966   A Statement of Basic Accounting Theory. Evanston, Ill.
American Hospital Association
    1966   Chart of Accounts for Hospitals. Chicago: American Hospital Association.
    1968   Cost Finding and Rate Setting for Hospitals. Chicago: American Hospital Association.
    1969   "Statement on the financial requirements of health care institutions and services." (February 12)
    1972   "Guidelines for review and approval of rates for health care institutions and services by a state commission." (February 9)
    1975a   "Analyses by state commission of rate review legislation in comparison to the principles stated in the AHA guidelines for review and approval of rates for health care institutions and services." (June 1)
    1975b   "Current status of pending rate review and prospective payment legislation." (September 4)
American Institute of Certified Public Accountants
    1963   Reporting the Financial Effects of Price-Level Changes. New York.

1969   Financial Statements Restated for General Price Level Changes. New York.

1972   Hospital Audit Guide. New York.

Arditti, F.

1973   "The weighted average cost of capital: Some questions on its definition, interpretation and use." Journal of Finance (September): 1001–1008.

Berman, H., and L. Weeks

1974   The Financial Management of Hospitals, 2d ed. Health Administration Press.

Berry, R.E., Jr.

1975   "Perspectives on rate regulation." In National Academy of Sciences, Controls on Health Care. Washington, D.C.: Institute of Medicine.

Briloff, A.

1972   Unaccountable Accounting. New York: Harper and Row.

Cleverley, W.O.

1974   "Is hospital capital being eroded under cost reimbursement?" Hospital Administration (Summer): 58–73.

Cohen, H.A.

1975   "State rate regulation." Pp. 123–135 in National Academy of Sciences, Controls on Health Care.

Cost Accounting Standards Board

1975   Standards, Rules, and Regulation as of June 30, 1975. Washington, D.C.

Dowling, W.L.

1974   "Prospective reimbursement of hospitals." Inquiry 11 (September): 163–180.

Edwards, E.O., and P.W. Bell

1964   The Theory and Measurement of Business Income. Berkeley: University of California Press.

Elnicki, R.A.

1975   "SSA—Connecticut hospital reimbursement experiment cost evaluation." Inquiry 12 (March): 47–58.

Federation of American Hospitals

1975   "State rate controls." Review (August/September): 9–34.

Financial Accounting Standards Board

1975   "Exposure draft: Financial reporting in units of general purchasing power."

Hendriksen, E.
  1965   Accounting Theory. Homewood, Ill.: Richard D. Irwin.

Lemer, R., and D. Willman
  1974   "Rate setting." Topics in Health Care Financing 1 (Winter): 1–80.

Li, D.H.
  1973   "Cost Accounting Standards Board: A progress report." Management Accounting 55 (June): 11–14.

Russell, T.A.
  1975   "An application of price level accounting." Financial Executive 43 (February): 21, 78.

Schwayder, K.
  1969   "The capital maintenance rule and the net asset valuation rule." Accounting Review (April): 304–316.

Staats, E.
  1969   "Uniform cost accounting standards in negotiated defense contracts." Management Accounting 51 (January): 21–25.

Vatter, W.
  1969   Standards for Cost Analysis. Report to the Comptroller General of the United States.

Walls, E.
  1972   "Cost reimbursement worsens capital crisis." Hospitals, Journal of the American Hospital Association (March 1): 81–86.

Wood, J.
  1975   "Medicare reimbursement." Topics in Health Care Financing 1 (Spring): 45–80.

The Use of Marginal Cost Estimates in Hospital Cost-Containment Policy

JOSEPH LIPSCOMB,
IRA E. RASKIN,
AND JOSEPH EICHENHOLZ

Although the authority of the Cost of Living Council (COLC) to regulate the health industry expired on April 30, 1974, neither hospital inflation nor the underlying cost pressures have abated. During the first twelve months after expiration of the controls became certain (congressional bills to extend controls died in committee in March), hospital service charges rose 16.5 percent compared to an increase of 10.3 percent in the overall cost of living (Bureau of Labor Statistics, 1975). At the same time, hospital expenses (both per patient day and per admission) were rising at increasing rates. Compared to the same period in the previous year, the rise in average cost per adjusted patient day accelerated steadily from 9.3 percent in the first quarter to 14.9 percent in the fourth quarter of calendar year 1974 (American Hospital Association, 1974). Inflationary pressures may very well be exacerbated in the future with the advent of any national health insurance plan. Consequently, the federal government has felt the need to maintain an active hospital cost-containment policy, both in the form of mandatory regulations related to the Medicare and Medicaid programs and through informal discussions with the hospital industry.

514

A crucial aspect of past and future regulations is the underlying cost assumptions built into the rules for hospital cost containment. We will focus on the economic concept of the marginal cost of hospital services and the role that it was meant to play in regulations established during COLC's brief existence. Specifically, some of the conceptual problems inherent in Phases II and III hospital cost regulations will be outlined in order to set the background for the changes introduced during Phase IV. A brief review of Phase IV controls, with specific reference to the underlying marginal cost assumptions, is followed by an overview of available empirical research on hospital marginal costs, primarily to illuminate the background for certain assumptions made in Phase IV. Finally, we briefly consider the derivation of marginal cost estimates as a basic problem in applied econometrics in order to highlight the methodological and empirical difficulties investigators must continue to confront if such estimates are to play a meaningful role in future cost-containment policy.

Phase II Controls: An Oversimplified Specification of Hospital Cost and Revenue Functions

The basic operational goal of the Phase II hospital regulations was to limit the increase in a hospital's aggregate revenue due to price increases to 6 percent of the previous year's revenue, subject to adjustment for changes in the volume of patients treated.[1] COLC regulations allowed hospitals to adjust their projected revenue and cost for the current fiscal year by a volume index, in lieu of actually calculating increases due to price increases versus those due to volume increases. The volume index was a weighted function of two inpatient measures of output (patient days and admissions) and one outpatient measure of output (outpatient procedures) divided by an

---

[1] There was also a profit margin limitation that prohibited institutions from either increasing "excess of revenues over expenses" or decreasing operating losses without first obtaining an exception. This provision did not, however, impact directly on most institutions because of the combined effects of the Phase II regulations themselves, changing occupancy rates, and general economic conditions.

intensity factor of 1.02. The intensity factor was designed to allow for the increasing complexity, and thus costliness, of services in hospital care; its ultimate effect was to raise the effective ceiling on increases in aggregate annual revenues to more than 6 percent. For third-party payers that reimbursed on the basis of incurred costs, Phase II provided for a maximum increase in per diem reimbursement (Federal Register, 1974:2696). The volume index was used to adjust projected revenues to what they would have been if there had been no change in the volume of services between years. If, after the volume adjustment, the projected increase in revenue exceeded 6 percent, the hospital had to file for an exception with COLC in order to maintain current charges.

However, any adjusted increase in annual revenues had to be cost justified by the hospital. Regardless of its anticipated rise in costs, the hospital could pass through no more than a 5.5 percent increase in its wage bill and 2.5 percent in nonwage expenses. A 1.7 percent factor was included to allow for outlay on new technology not directly charged to patient services. These components resulted in a 6 percent limit on increases in total costs, given the assumption that the hospital labor bill was approximately 60 percent of total costs.

It can be shown that application of this volume index to determine allowable revenue and cost changes for alternative levels of output during Phase II involved the implicit use of overly simplistic hospital cost and revenue functions, resulting in disincentives for hospital efficiency. Essentially, the volume adjustment under Phase II rules provided for an almost one-to-one correspondence between changes in volume and changes in allowable revenue and costs; that is, Phase II hospital controls implicitly assumed that all costs are variable as volume changes. Because the fixed costs component of the hospital labor bill is substantial in the short run, use of the volume index to adjust both revenues and costs had undesirable effects: it created strong incentives for volume expansion and imposed severe financial penalties for volume contraction. The perverse incentives which evolved under Phase II hospital controls are illustrated in Figs. 1 and 2.

First, let TR_r represent the (actual) total revenue function of the

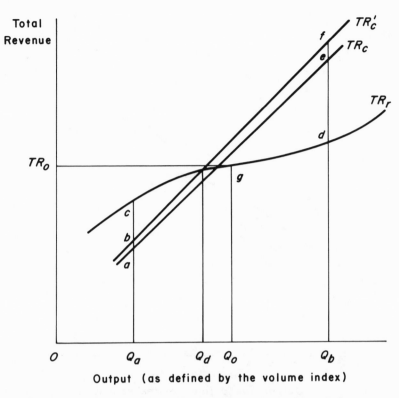

Fig. 1   *Treatment of Hospital Revenues under Phase II*

hospital in the base year prior to the imposition of cost controls. Assuming comprehensive cost reimbursement by third-party payers, TR_r approximates the hospital's (actual) base year total cost curve, TC_r of Fig. 2. However, the total revenue and cost curves implicit under Phase II rules were, in fact, linear over the typical hospital's relevant output range and not at all like the curves actually faced by the hospital. To see this, note that a hospital could receive (ignoring for now the intensity adjustment) 6 percent of the base year's revenue (or cost, under our full reimbursement assumption) as its price increase allowance for the current year. Thus, the greater the volume change from the base year (either positive or negative) the greater the difference between the 6 percent allowance and

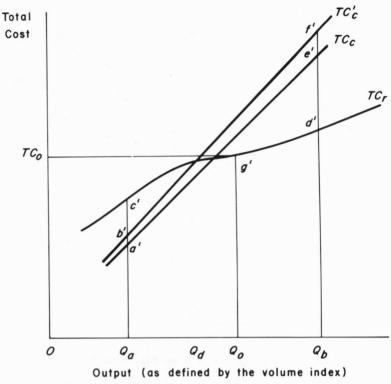

Fig. 2   *Treatment of Hospital Costs under Phase II*

6 percent of the current year's projected revenues (or costs). For example, suppose a hospital had a $1,000,000 budget in the base year and produced a Phase II-defined volume of output equal to 1,000. The hospital's price increase allowance would be $60,000. If volume were to rise 10 percent in the current year, its new allowable revenue would be $1,160,000, or $1,055 per unit of output. If the volume increase were 50 percent, allowable revenue would be $1,560,000, or $1,040 per unit of output. Similar relationships hold for volume reductions.

Generalizing, the total revenue function implicit under Phase II (ignoring momentarily the intensity factor adjustment) was $TR_c = (TR_o / Q_o) Q + (.06) TR_o$, where TR_o is base year revenue, Q is the current volume of output, and Q_o is base year output. This is shown in Fig. 1. Notice that revenue per unit of output becomes $(TR_c/Q) = (TR_o/Q_o) + [(.06) TR_o/Q]$. Thus, as Q grows large, revenue per unit approaches the base year figure (TR_o/Q_o), while as Q becomes small, TR_c increases without limit.[2]

Note that the intercept term of TR_r must invariably exceed that given for TR_c, namely $(.06) TR_o$, because of the substantial amount of hospital fixed cost in the short run. (Under comprehensive reimbursement, the hospital is granted revenue to meet this cost.) Consequently, TR_c will tend to lie below TR_r for most output levels less than Q_o and above TR_r for all output above Q_o, as indicated in Fig. 1.

Finally, we can rotate TR_c to TR'_c in Fig. 1 to reflect the additional service intensity allowance. At a given output level, a hospital's projected aggregate annual revenue had to exceed TR'_c before it was required to file for an exception. The resulting incentive to expand volume is apparent in Fig. 1. Hospitals which expanded were less likely to be required to file for exception or to report price increases than were those which experienced no change in volume. As shown in Fig. 1, an increase in output to Q_b would mean that actual total revenue would be determined at d, which is significantly below the allowed revenue (at f). Hospitals in this category were able, therefore, to increase their revenue (up to f, for

---

[2]As an administrative matter, a floor on (TR_c/Q) of \$1,030 was established for volume increases, while a ceiling on (TR_c/Q) of \$1,200 was set for hospitals expecting volume declines in the current year. These limits serve to destroy the simple linearity of TR_c (and of TC_c) at current output levels that diverge greatly from base year levels. For instance, in the numerical example presented above, a hospital's current year volume would have to be double the base year's before the \$1,030 per unit floor was reached. Correspondingly, output would have to drop to 300 units (a 70 percent decline) before the \$1,200 per unit ceiling attained. Consequently, in practice the intercept value of TR_c was not simply $(.06) TR_o$, *although a line segment consistent with such an intercept characterizes the hospital's Phase II revenue function over the relevant output range.* In fact, if a hospital's output was, for some reason, negligible in the current year, it would still have been allowed reimbursement in an amount equal to the base year's insurance, interest, and depreciation expenses.

Since most hospitals do not experience such variations in output between years, we may safely treat TR_c and TC_c as linear.

instance) by raising prices for private paying patients, increasing costs for third-party cost-reimbursed patients, or some combination of the two. On the other hand, if a hospital's output dropped below Q_d, to a level, say, of Q_a, its projected revenue would have been determined at point c, which exceeds allowed revenue (at b); therefore, the hospital would have to file for an exception.

The total cost function implicit in Phase II regulations (TC_c in Fig. 2) can be pivoted to TC'_c to reflect current year increases in input prices (recall that under Phase II the limit was 6 percent of TC_c, with separate limits on wage and nonwage components).[3] Hospitals did not have to present any cost justification unless they anticipated an increase in (output-adjusted) aggregate annual revenue. Those hospitals with declining levels of output were more likely to have to file for exceptions, and were less likely to be able to cost justify price increases. The undesirable nature of this constraint was underscored in a recent review of the Phase II hospital cost regulations:

> If the decline in volume was 5%, expenses had to be reduced by a full 5%. However, because a significant portion of hospital costs is fixed in the short run, the effect of the Phase II volume adjustment was to take away some allowable costs that had to be incurred regardless of how many patients were served. The result was that many hospitals facing declines in volume had to dip into (and perhaps exhaust) reserves in order to meet operating expenses [Federal Register, 1974:2697].

As illustrated in Fig. 2, hospitals that experienced a fall in output to Q_a would have costs of c', exceeding the allowable cost b'; the increase in costs (from b' to c') would require an exception.

In contrast, there was an incentive to spend under Phase II controls for those hospitals which experienced increased output:

> It has always been recognized that the added cost of treating more patients, particularly in a well-functioning hospital, is far

---

[3] TC_r is shown here reflecting first increasing, then approximately constant, and finally decreasing returns to scale—in classical textbook fashion. To be consistent with the empirical findings reviewed below, only minimal decreasing returns are indicated.

less than the average cost of treating all patients. As a hospital adds a few more patients, it is not necessary to add such items as more x-ray machines, nurses, or even beds. Therefore, the hospital that increased its volume of patients was permitted more allowable costs and revenues than it really needed to treat the additional patients. The requirement for cost justification meant that if these potential revenues were not actually spent, they had to be returned. Thus, there was still an incentive to spend [Federal Register, 1974:2697].

Figure 2 shows that an increase in volume to Q_b would have allowed a hospital to raise its costs beyond f' before any of the increase would be subject to exception. In fact, the hospital would have to raise costs above e' before it could even show an increase in volume-adjusted costs. In short, expansion of output under Phase II regulations gave the hospital greater cost flexibility before it ran up against the legal control limits, while output contraction had the opposite effect.[4]

Phase IV: A More Flexible Approach

The underlying rationale of Phase IV was to minimize the undesirable incentives which confronted hospitals under Phase II. A number of changes were made under Phase IV hospital regulations. These included the use of admissions as a measure of hospital volume, separation of controls in inpatient and outpatient services,

---

[4]As Mark Pauly has pointed out to us, this criticism of Phase II regulations does assume that it is short-run, and not long-run, marginal cost that is the relevant analytical consideration in cost control mechanisms. He argues that if hospitals viewed these regulations as permanent, they would have made output and input decisions on the basis of their perceived long-run cost curves.

Consequently, the above analysis should probably not be applied to hospital price and cost control mechanisms that are thought to be viewed by providers as permanent. On the other hand, because the Cost of Living Council's price control authority during Phase II had a legislated termination date (subject, of course, to extensions), it is not clear that hospitals would, in fact, view the regulations as permanent—at least with respect to important matters of federal interpretation and implementation.

and add-on allowable cost adjustments for more complex patient mix and enlarged capital outlay (the latter allowances subject to a separate review process).

Particularly important, Phase IV regulations explicitly introduced a more flexible (and realistic) assumption concerning the relative difference between the fixed and variable components of hospital costs.

In contrast with the Phase II notion of essentially a pari passu correspondence between unit change in costs and volumes, Phase IV hospital regulations directly incorporated the assumption that marginal costs, defined as costs that vary directly with output, were on average 40 percent of hospital average costs, defined as the total cost (both variable and fixed) divided by the corresponding level of output. In other words, the controls were redesigned to recognize that total cost elasticity with respect to output (the ratio of marginal to average cost) was less than unity (Allen, 1962:260–263); fixed costs were acknowledged to be a significant component of the hospital budget in the short run. This implied, on the one hand, that short-run average cost should fall as the rate of admissions increases. On the other hand, the regulations acknowledged that costs could not be expected to fall in tandem with a decrease in hospital admissions.

A marginal cost-average cost ratio of 0.4 was built into Phase IV formulas used to determine officially prescribed hospital operating allowances (Federal Register, 1974:2700). Application of this 0.4 factor, however, was qualified by a "zone of no adjustment" as well as by minimum and maximum constraints on allowable cost increases per admission. The rationale for this qualification was given as follows:

> If this volume adjustment were used from zero change in admissions, it would mean that an institution that was increasing in volume would be allowed only 40% of average cost and charge for each extra admission. The hospital that was declining in volume would be allowed to keep 60% of the average cost and charge of each lost admission, and recover the differences from the remaining patients.

There are, however, statistical indications that while the

40/60 ratio is a reasonable average, when volume of admissions increases the marginal cost may actually be somewhat higher, i.e., it costs more than 40% to service the increased admissions; and that when volume is declining the fixed costs may be higher, i.e., a hospital cannot reduce its cost per case by 40%. For this reason, and to reduce the need for hospitals to make charge adjustments for small changes in volume, a "zone of no adjustment" was created [Federal Register, 1974:2699].

A different "zone" was set up for small and large hospitals under Phase IV. The decision was made so that at least as many "small" hospitals as "large" hospitals would find themselves in the "zone" based on the historical distribution of volume changes. This was achieved in the limits that were set to define the "small" hospital under the proposed Phase IV regulations ($2.0 million in budget or 3,500 admissions, which corresponds roughly to a 100-bed hospital operating at about a 75–80 percent occupancy rate).[5]

Figures 3 and 4 below illustrate this differential "zone of no adjustment." For purposes of comparison, the effective per admission allowances for Phase II are graphed as well as those for Phase IV, even though the Phase II controls were not on a per admission basis. Instead, for comparative analysis, it is assumed in Figs. 3 and 4 that any changes in admissions under Phase II were accompanied by proportionate changes in patient days; thus the volume index, which was calculated separately for both changed days *and* admissions and then averaged, could be an explicit relationship based on units of admission.

Under Phase II, a hospital was entitled to a 6 percent price index based on the previous year's revenue, plus 2 percent on a cost basis for greater intensity. Since this 6 percent allowance was a fixed dollar amount based on the prior year's revenue, it represented a slightly falling percentage increase *on a per admission basis as volume increased*. Conversely, if the volume of admissions declined, the 6 percent price allowance represented an allowance of more than 6 percent on a per admission basis. On the other hand, the

Later revision of the regulations broadened the definition to less than $2.5 million in budget or fewer than 3,000 admissions.

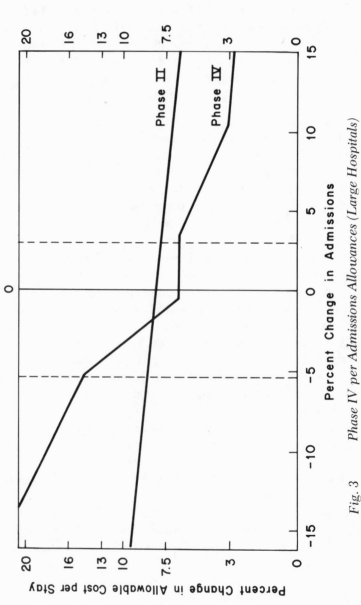

Fig. 3   *Phase IV per Admissions Allowances (Large Hospitals)*

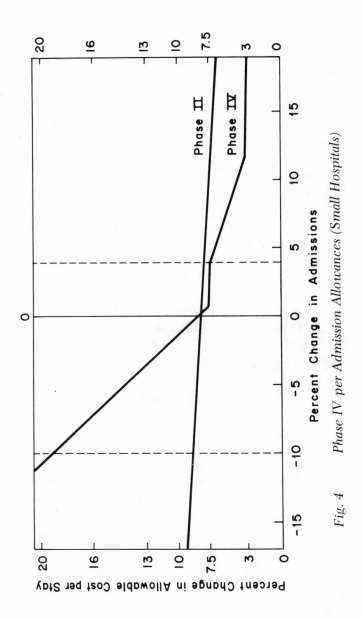

Fig. 4   *Phase IV per Admission Allowances (Small Hospitals)*

intensity allowance was a flat 2 percent of the *current* year's costs. The slightly downward slope of the Phase II allowance curve consequently reflects the *net* effect of the Phase II volume index, that is, a one-for-one increase of allowable cost (and revenue) for volume changes, a flat 2 percent per admission intensity allowance, and a fixed dollar equivalent price increase limited to 6 percent of the prior year's revenue.

Under Phase IV, for both large and small hospitals, a per admission cost increase allowance was set at 7.5 percent for a zero change in admissions. Once admissions increased, the large hospital was allowed to maintain the 7.5 percent increase as long as the actual increase in cost was less than 2 percent. In this part of the "zone," all costs were assumed to be variable. Beyond 2 percent, the marginal-costs–average-cost ratio was set at 0.4 for the incremental admissions, and the average increases allowed per admission were reduced accordingly. When the actual average cost increase reached a low of 3 percent, no further trade-offs were required and the full cost increase was allowed. The regulations for small hospitals were similar except that all costs were assumed variable for a rise in admissions up to an annual rate of 4 percent rather than 2 percent.

For institutions with declining volume the picture was different. For large hospitals, if the volume decline was 5 percent or less, the total budget was permitted to exceed that of the base year by as much as 7.5 percent. For small hospitals, this zone of no adjustment extended down to a volume decline of 10 percent. However, once a hospital's volume decline exceeded the boundary of the zone, it was required to deduct 40 percent of the prior year's average cost per admission for every admission below the zone. When the actual average cost per admission increased by as much as 20 percent, no further deductions were required.[6] Finally, note in Figs. 3 and 4 that the effect of holding the current year budget to 107.5 percent of the base year over the range of small admissions declines was to permit the percent change in allowable cost per stay to increase, as well, over these zones.

[6] The reader can refer to the *Federal Register* of January 23, 1974, for a complete review of the essential features of Phase IV regulations, including an appendix that outlines the important analytical issues.

Of primary concern here is the fact that the volume adjustment formulas actually used by COLC during Phase IV incorporated a marginal-cost–average-cost ratio of 0.4. The following section will attempt to illuminate the analytical background behind the selection of the value for this ratio.

Empirical Research on Hospital Cost Functions

Much of the frequently cited literature on hospital cost functions has already been critically reviewed and assessed elsewhere (Berki, 1972). This section will instead focus on the contribution which various studies have made to the direct estimation of hospital marginal costs.

To facilitate comparison of estimated cost relationships across the studies, we focus on the relationship between marginal and average costs. Since the definition of hospital output varies considerably among studies, it was felt that the available estimates of marginal cost were not comparable. In contrast, the marginal-cost–average-cost ratio abstracts from the particular output unit used and measures the proportional rate of increase of total cost for proportional increases in output. In addition, since average cost is more readily attainable for each individual hospital (or group of hospitals), a ratio of marginal to average cost would permit quick estimates of marginal cost. Nevertheless, as the study by Lave and Lave in this volume indicates, this ratio can be very much a function of the particular measure of output employed.

The ratio of marginal to average cost is calculated below using the authors' estimated total or average cost curves, evaluated at the mean value of the output measure used (except in those instances where the ratio or its components was explicitly reported by the author). The results are presented in Table 1, where selected studies are arrayed chronologically in terms of their date of publication or preparation. It should be noted that the marginal-cost–average-cost ratio will, in general, be a function of the *level* of output. Consequently, the ratios in the table are most reliable (in a predictive sense) for output levels in the neighborhood of the mean output levels, with which they were derived.

TABLE 1 Estimates of Marginal Cost-Average Cost Ratio (MC/AC) Derived from Selected Hospital Cost Analyses

Study (year)	Interval of Observation	Type of Hospital	Sample Size	Output Measure	MC/AC
Lave and Lave (1975)	1964–1973	Short-term, nongovernmental (AHA Annual National Survey)	507	(1) Admissions (controlling for length-of-stay)	.55–.74
Lave and Lave (1975)	1973	Short-term, nongovernmental (AHA Annual National Survey)	5,655 (partitioned into 3 bed-size groupings)	(2) Patient days (controlling for admissions)	.22–.34
				(3) Admissions (with constant occupancy rate level)	.38–.53
Berry and Carr[a] (1974)	1966	Short-term, general—all hospitals (AHA Annual National Survey)	2,700	Average daily census (ADC)	.96
Berry and Carr (1974)	1966	Short-term, general—governmental (AHA Annual National Survey)	667	Average daily census	.84
Berry and Carr (1974)	1966	Short-term, general—voluntary (AHA)	1,772	Average daily census	.94
Berry and Carr (1974)	1966	Short-term, general—proprietary (AHA)	154	Average daily census	.91
Kuenne (1972)[b]	1964–1970	General, New Jersey with 4,000–7,000 annual admissions	25	Admissions	.91
Kuenne (1972)	1964–1970	General, New Jersey with 7,000–13,000 annual admissions	24	Admissions	.65

[a] Listed sample size is estimated from author's regression analysis. Similar analysis by Berry for 1965 data (1970:67–75) could not be worked up in the same manner since mean values for average daily census were not provided in the earlier study.

[b] Premised on marginal cost functions for basic hospital costs where the overall cost function is derived from an aggregation of cost functions for a number of hospital departments.

Study	Period	Type/Location	N	Measure	Ratio
Lave, Lave, and Silverman (1972)	Second half of 1968	General, Western Pennsylvania	65	Utilization (actual bed days/available bed days)	.68
Evans and Walker (1972)	1967	General, British Columbia	90	Average occupancy rate (100 × total patient days/365 total available beds)	.80-.90
Evans (1971)	1967	General, Ontario	185	Average occupancy rate	.76-.86
Lave and Lave (1970a)[c]	14 semi-annual obs. during 1967-1971	General, Western Pennsylvania	74	Utilization (recorded patient days/available patient days)	.40-.65
Lave and Lave (1970b)[d]	7 annual obs. during 1961-1967	General, Eastern and Western Pennsylvania	109	Utilization (utiliz. as % of mean utiliz. for the hospital during 7-year interval)	.58-.68
Cohen (1970)[e]	1965	Short-term, general, members of United Hospital Federation of New York	46	Service units (a cost-weighted average of hospital services)	.67
Francisco (1970)[f]	1966	Short-term, general	4,710	Total patient days	.73-.87
M. Feldstein (1968)	Fiscal Year 1960-1961	Acute, nonteaching in England and Wales	177	Total annual cases adjusted for case-mix variation among hospitals	.21

[c] In contrast with the authors' *Inquiry* article (1970b), the methodology employs semiannual rather than annual observations (and, therefore, relatively short-run estimates of marginal costs), and a two-stage estimation procedure.

[d] As in their *American Economic Review* paper (1970a), insufficient information was provided to permit derivation of estimates of marginal costs using the model employed.

[e] This ratio was derived by using a total cost function (p. 288) and computing a mean level of service units on the basis of the author's comments concerning service units equivalents per bed (p. 290) and the average bed size of United Hospital Federation hospitals (p. 282).

[f] The range of this ratio is derived from cost equations for twenty-five groups of hospitals, classified on the basis of number of facilities and services available; estimates were secured from equations whose coefficients were statistically significant (p. 324).

Table 1—(continued)

Study (year)	Type of Hospital	Interval of Observation	Sample Size	Output Measure	MC/AC
Ingbar and Taylor (1968)[g]	Short-term, voluntary in Massachusetts	Annual obs. 1958–1959 and 1961–1963	72	Available bed days	.80–1.05
Berry (1967)[h]	Short-term, general (AHA)	1963	763	Patient days	.70–.77
Carr and P. Feldstein (1967)[i]	Short-term, general (AHA)	1963	3,147	Average daily census and patient days	.83–.97
P. Feldstein (1961)	Short-term, general (Gary Methodist Hospital in Gary, Indiana)	1956–1958	1	Patient days	.21–.27

[g] Lave and Lave (1970a) have observed, with reference to this study, that while "it is a bit difficult to come up with a single figure for percentage variable, their results suggest that marginal cost is about 80 percent of average cost" (p. 394). This is the ratio shown here. However, a review of Ingbar and Taylor indicates that the ratio of MC/AC may be greater than unity. That is, for 1959 the median number of beds for the hospitals studied by the authors was 110 (p. 18). Consequently, since (for 1958–1959) the plateau on their inverted U-shaped average cost function was at 150 beds, then marginal costs would have to exceed average costs; the latter would still be *increasing* at the size level of 110 beds. Use of the authors' mean expense per patient day (p. 21) and marginal expense per patient day (p. 43) does in fact give a ratio of 1.05 for marginal/average expense. Therefore, Table 1 shows a range of 0.80 to 1.05 for MC/AC.

[h] In order to calculate average costs for hospitals grouped according to similarity of facilities and services, it was necessary to use a later, unpublished paper by Berry which sets out the mean average daily census for each group ("Economies of Scale, Optimal Size, and Relative Savings in the Production of Hospital Services"). Of twenty-three hospital groups which exhibited a U-shaped cost curve, sixteen had statistically significant coefficients for the output variables in the published article. These groups comprised 51 percent of the sample actually used by Berry. Conversion from mean group values of ADC to mean number of patient days was also derived from the author's unpublished addendum. The range of 0.70 to 0.77 was obtained by first employing cost functions for these 16 groups and then repeating the procedure after eliminating two groups (3.3 percent of the sample) with outlier results (where MC/AC = 0.23).

[i] The range for the MC/AC ratio is derived from analysis of cost functions for five "service capability groups" of hospitals, using mean values for variables provided by the authors (pp. 59 and 61).

Most of the studies examined in Table 1 are cross-sectional or pooled cross-sectional analyses. If it is assumed that the hospitals under observation were, in fact, minimizing the cost of producing their desired output levels, one may argue that long-run cost functions have been estimated in these studies. However, short-run marginal cost (estimates of the expected near-term changes in total variable cost as hospital output increases) is probably most relevant for the development and application of cost control regulations.

Three studies listed in Table 1 have given explicit attention to obtaining short-run cost estimates: P. Feldstein (1961), Lave and Lave (1970a), and M. Feldstein (1968). Utilizing monthly cost and output data, P. Feldstein (1961) found that, on average, short-run marginal costs were 21–27 percent of short-run average costs. Lave and Lave (1970a), using semiannual data, found marginal cost to range from 40 to 65 percent of average cost. In a similar study using annual observations, Lave and Lave (1970b) found this marginal-cost–average-cost ratio to vary from 58 to 68 percent. M. Feldstein (1968) used annual data, but also included control variables for the possibility of scale adjustment *and* case-mix variations over the (relatively long) observation interval, and found that short-run marginal cost was about 21 percent of short-run average cost.

On the other hand, as shown in Table 1, the more long-run analyses indicated generally that the ratio of marginal to average cost ranged from .58 to in excess of unity. These higher results are theoretically consistent with the lower short-run estimates since, by definition, there are fewer fixed factors of production in long-term analysis.

Aside from short-run versus long-run considerations, another important factor influencing the estimated marginal cost–average cost ratio is the choice of output variables in the regression model. This is most clearly indicated in the study by Lave and Lave in this volume; with admissions as output (and controlling for length of stay), MC/AC ranged from .55 to .74. With patient days as output (controlling for admissions), MC/AC varied from .22 to .34. Lave and Lave found cost estimates to be considerably more sensitive to these specification differences than to the use of cross-sectional versus pooled cross-sectional samples from the AHA data base.

Given the range of estimates noted above, the short-run marginal-cost–average-cost ratio would appear to be less than .58; the few short-run analyses suggest, therefore, that 0.4 would not be an unreasonable estimate for hospitals. Consequently, a selected review of the literature does tend to support the use of a marginal-cost–average-cost ratio of 0.4 in Phase IV of COLC regulations.[7]

Methodological Issues in Hospital Cost Analysis

A reasonably complete analysis of the various methodological issues involved in the specification and estimation of hospital cost functions is by itself sufficient material for a separate lengthy paper. However, the main statistical problems evolve from the manner in which cost analyses deal with the multiproduct nature of hospitals, the multiple objectives of these institutions, and the impact of changes in technology on their operating decisions.

First, since the hospital is a multiproduct firm and since case-mix proportions will likely vary among hospitals in a sample, use of any single variable (such as the number of patient days or cases per time period) to represent output will imply a product homogeneity that does not exist.

This becomes an econometric problem under the reasonable assumption that the total cost of producing a certain number of patient days or cases depends on the case composition of those days or cases. If this is so, but no account of this heterogeneity is taken, one has, in effect, omitted one (or more) of the $(K + 1)$ variables that must be included. It can be easily shown that the omitted variables become part of the error term so that it is no longer randomly distributed with a mean equal to zero. If the omitted variables are not pair-wise uncorrelated with each included independent variable, all coefficient estimates for the included variables (including marginal cost) will be biased and, additionally, will not converge to the true coefficient values even in large samples.[8]

---

[7] It should also be noted that the "zone of no adjustment" described above allowed for a somewhat less restrictive imposition of the marginal cost assumption where hospital volume was in fact changing by some significant amount.

[8] Even if the pair-wise orthogonal condition should hold (which is unlikely), the

Research efforts that have attempted to account for product heterogeneity in hospitals have utilized several different approaches.[9] Of these, further refinement of the models developed by M. Feldstein (1968) and Lave, Lave, and Silverman (1972) would probably be most fruitful. That is, the hospital case would be the basic unit of output, and a vector of case-mix proportions would be included to control for relative variations in the input requirements of cases. Ideally, each case in the mix vector would be defined differentially by the input requirements for producing the case. Conversely, whenever two categories of patient stays in a hospital required significantly different input proportions, they would be recognized as two distinct cases in the mix vector.

M. Feldstein's use of hospital departments as case categories masks some of these differences (Feldstein, 1968). But the ICDA-based classification schemes of Lave, Lave, and Silverman (1972) and Lee and Wallace (1973) may permit specification of cost function models that are more sensitive to actual cost variations arising from the movement of a hospital along its production possibility surface. Among the promising alternatives to this case-mix vector approach is the development of composite output indices which would be sensitive to case-mix variations. Rafferty (1972) has reported progress along these lines. Such indices would likely have the advantage of not requiring as much detailed case-specific output and input data as the case-mix approach; in addition, multicollinearity would be reduced. But the sensitivity of these indices to variations in case cost is a matter for continuing investigation.

estimated standard errors of the coefficients of the included variables will be positively biased. Thus all *t*-tests of significance are invalidated, and one will tend to accept too often the null hypothesis that coefficients of included variables are equal to zero. The above underlies the statistical motivation for the considerable effort which has been devoted to finding appropriate case-mix measures and methods of entering them into the cost function.

[9] These approaches of which various combinations are possible include: (a) the assumption that case mix is reasonably constant within a single hospital over short time periods; (b) the stratification of hospitals into groups on the basis of facilities available; (c) the estimation of cost relationships for each of several hospital departments; (d) the development of a composite output measure; and (e) the inclusion of direct measures of case mix within the cost function.

Second, the manner in which a hospital combines inputs is a function, partially, of the underlying objectives of the hospital. For those instances in which variations in objective functions among hospitals in a sample may be expected to result in coefficient biases, there are general approaches that can be utilized. One would involve linking the observed institutional characteristics of a hospital with the nature of its objective function. That is, one may posit that profit-maximizing hospitals are characterized by a certain vector of institutional attributes, that health status–maximizing hospitals are characterized by another n-vector, and that prestige-maximizing hospitals are represented by yet another such vector. As independent variables in the cost function, the appropriate n-vector would be regarded as a proxy controlling for variations in management objectives (Lave, Lave, and Silverman, 1972). An alternative strategy would employ survey interview techniques in order to obtain the explicit objectives of hospital officials; these would be analyzed in relation to actual policy decisions of the hospital. The end result would be a categorization of these objectives from which a multichotomous management input variable could be derived.

Finally, failure to account for changes in the service intensity of hospital care can lead to biased coefficient estimates for the marginal cost parameter.[10] Inclusion in the basic regression model of variables representing the input proportions required to treat each major case category would, after further allowance for variations in input prices, tend to control for variations in the input intensity with which

---

[10]Suppose we have a time series of observations for a single hospital on total cost, the designated hospital output variable, and other relevant explanatory variables, including the case-mix vector. Now, if over this time period, service intensity (as measured by the real value of inputs used to treat a case of a particular type) increases within the hospital and no account of this is taken, a specification bias will result. This can be seen by letting X_1 be the representative hospital case produced in the first period of observation and X'_1, defined as $(X_1 + I_1)$, be the representative case in a later period, where I_1 is a "factor" representing the change in the nature of output resulting from the increase in intensity. Now if one is counting output in that later period, one still only observes X_1, but it is X'_1 which in a very real sense is produced; its I_1 component is directly influencing the value of dependent variable, TC. Consequently, failing to adjust for changes in service intensity is tantamount to omitting a relevant explanatory variable.

cases are produced. This result would be expected regardless of whether the intensity variations arise because of an uneven distribution of applied medical knowledge or variations among hospitals in how a well-known stock of technical knowledge is translated by physicians and administrators into treatment modalities.

Concluding Comments

In this paper we have argued that future federal policies governing allowable hospital price increases should be carefully designed to reflect the fact that a significant portion of hospital cost does not vary in the short term with the volume of patients served. Under Phase II it was implicitly assumed that all hospital costs were variable. We showed graphically how this policy led to perverse incentives for the hospital to maintain, and even promote, high occupancy rates regardless of patient need. Recognition of this problem by Cost of Living Council planners led to the modified cost-containment policy of Phase IV; COLC developed operational formulas which included a marginal-cost-to-average-cost ratio of 0.4 as a key input, thus taking explicit account of the fixity of some portion of hospital costs.

A survey of a number of significant empirical studies of hospital cost tended to support COLC's choice of 0.4 as the appropriate MC/AC ratio. But this finding cannot be considered conclusive. Different authors have arrived at significantly varying conclusions on the MC/AC ratio and this is itself prima facie motivation for further research into the problems of model specification, sampling, and estimation techniques involved in hospital cost analysis.

The related econometric problems that were briefly discussed are rather fundamental, even though suggestions for minimizing coefficient bias must be viewed as preliminary. As more detailed hospital data bases are developed from existing and new sources of information, there will be ample opportunity for implementing a number of alternative models. This research should be aimed pragmatically at assisting in the development of future hospital cost-containment policy. Sound estimates of hospital marginal costs are a prerequisite for cost control guidelines. Such guidelines must also be responsive *and* equitable with respect to differences in hospital size, location, and other institutional and area-specific variables.

References

Allen, R.G.D.
  1962   Mathematical Analysis for Economists. London: Macmillan and Co., Ltd.
American Hospital Association
  1974   Hospital Panel Survey.
Berki, S.E.
  1972   Hospital Economics. Lexington, Mass.: Lexington Books, D.C. Heath & Co.
Berry, R.E., Jr.
  1967   "Return to scale in the production of hospital services." Health Services Research 2 (Summer): 123–139.
  1970   "Product heterogeneity and hospital cost analysis." Inquiry 7 (March): 67–75.
Berry, R.E., Jr., and J.W. Carr, Jr.
  1974   Efficiency in the Production of Hospital Services. Final Report, SSA Research Grant No. 56002 (March).
Bureau of Labor Statistics
  1975   Consumer Price Index.
Carr, J.W., and P.J. Feldstein
  1967   "The relationship of cost to hospital size." Inquiry 4 (March): 45–65.
Cohen, H.A.
  1970   "Hospital cost curves with emphasis on measuring patient care output." Pp. 279–293 in H. Klarman, ed., Empirical Studies in Health Economics. Baltimore: Johns Hopkins Press.
Evans, R.G.
  1971   "'Behavioral' cost functions for hospitals." Canadian Journal of Economics 4 (May): 198–215.
Evans, R.G., and H.D. Walker
  1972   "Information theory and the analysis of hospital cost structure." Canadian Journal of Economics 5 (August): 398–418.
Federal Register
  1974   Cost of Living Council, Final Phase IV Regulations, Appendix to

Subpart R, Control of Hospital Costs under the Economic Stabilization Program, 39, 16 (January): 2670-2701.

Feldstein, M.S.
1968   Economic Analysis for Health Service Efficiency. Amsterdam: North-Holland Publishing Company.

Feldstein, P.
1961   An Empirical Investigation of the Marginal Cost of Hospital Service. Chicago: University of Chicago Press.

Francisco, E.
1970   "Analysis of cost variations among short-term general hospitals." Pp. 321-332 in H. Klarman, ed., Empirical Studies in Health Economics. Baltimore: Johns Hopkins Press.

Ingbar, M.L., and L.D. Taylor
1968   Hospital Costs in Massachusetts. Cambridge, Mass.: Harvard University Press.

Kuenne, R.E.
1972   Average Sectoral Cost Functions in a Group of New Jersey Hospitals. General Economic Systems Project, Research Monograph #1, Princeton University (October): supported by HEW Grant No. 5 R01 HS 00273-03.

Lave, J., and L. Lave
1970a   "Hospital cost functions." American Economic Review 60 (June): 379-395.
1970b   "Estimated cost functions for Pennsylvania hospitals." Inquiry 7 (June): 3-14.
1975   Hospital Cost Analysis: Implications for COLC Hospital Regulations. Final Report HRA 106-74-45, submitted to the National Center for Health Services Research, May. Also this volume.

Lave, J., L. Lave, and L. Silverman
1972   "Hospital cost estimation controlling for case-mix." Applied Economics 4 (September): 165-180.

Lee, M.L., and R.L. Wallace
1973   "Problems in estimating multi-product cost functions: An application to hospitals." Western Economic Journal (September): 350-363.

Rafferty, J.
1972   "Hospital output indices." Economic and Business Bulletin (Winter): 21-27.

Hospital Cost Function Analysis: Implications for Cost Controls

JUDITH R. LAVE
AND LESTER B. LAVE

Introduction

The cost of a day in a United States hospital has been increasing on the order of 13 to 15 percent per year since the passage of the Medicare and Medicaid legislation. From August 1971 to May 1974 a number of regulations designed to lower the rate of cost increase in hospitals were implemented. These regulations represent a major attempt to contain hospital costs and are the only nationwide experiment that has been executed, although a number of small reimbursement experiments have been run. The results of this experiment must be evaluated carefully to determine whether regulations of this sort can be effective.

The Phase I regulations, which froze all prices, were interpreted to freeze cost per patient day (for reimbursement purpose) for ninety days. The injustice of this regulation is apparent from the fact that hospitals which experienced occupancy rate increases had, compared with those hospitals experiencing declining occupancy rates, relatively little trouble meeting the constraint. The Cost of Living Council (COLC) attempted to handle such inequities by publishing increasingly sophisticated regulations. In particular, the problem caused by differential occupancy rate changes was met head on in the Phase IV regulations when the allowable change in

538

cost per patient day was determined by the percentage change in the number of admissions. The question faced by COLC staff was to determine the extent to which short- and intermediate-run costs vary with the bed occupancy rate; the decision on what proportion of average cost is variable was made after reviewing a not entirely relevant literature on estimated hospital cost functions.

A detailed knowledge of hospital cost functions is essential not only for the implementation of the type of regulation attempted by COLC, but also more generally for many of the current and proposed activities of the several levels of government. The reimbursement of hospitals under Medicare, required hospital planning, and the structuring of national health insurance are all activities that require a detailed knowledge of the cost structure of hospitals, if they are to be accomplished successfully.

The purpose of this paper is to estimate hospital cost functions to answer questions about: (a) the cost of an additional patient or patient day; (b) the effect of other factors on costs; (c) the similarity of cost functions in different regions and various sized hospitals; and (d) the extent of pure cost increases.

Theory of Hospital Cost Function

The hospital is a multiproduct firm. Hospitals produce not only inpatient care but also education, research, community service, and outpatient care. With respect to inpatient care, hospitals differ not only in the number and type of cases treated, but also in the complexity of cases treated as well as the quality of care (somehow defined) rendered. Thus, if one is going to estimate a hospital cost function (that is, to determine the functional relationship between costs and quantity of output produced as well as the scale of the plant), these factors must be taken into account.

Selecting the Output Measure

In estimating hospital cost functions, the first problem to be resolved is what is the unit of output. There is some debate over whether the patient day or the case (number of admissions or discharges) is the better unit of output. Since the hospital treats patients, the patient day might well be viewed as an input into the treatment process. The issue is confounded, however, because of a potential relationship between quality and length of stay. Controlling for case mix, measuring output in terms of patients presumes that nothing is lost by a stay longer or shorter than average. Using patient days presumes that the hospital's value added is proportional to length of stay.[1]

A basic formulation for a hospital cost function is shown below in equation (1) where the average cost in hospital i in period t is shown to be a function of a number of variables:

$$AC_{it} = f(Occ_{it}, B_{it}, CM_{it}, L_{it}, T_{it}, t),\qquad (1)$$

where Occ is the occupancy rate, B is the number of beds (a surrogate for the scale of plant), CM measures the hospital's case mix, L is a factor for location (to capture factor price differences), T measures the teaching programs which take place in the hospital, and t is an indication of the time period (to account for inflation).

The primary problem to be faced in estimating hospital cost functions is to find a way to control for the different outputs produced by different hospitals. A number of studies have been done in which explicit measures of hospital inpatient case mix were used (see Lipscomb, Raskin, and Eichenholz, this book; and also the

---

[1] Another problem is determining the appropriate dependent variable for an analysis of cost functions. One alternative would be to use the total cost for each hospital as the dependent variable. However, using total cost gives rise to a number of problems. Since there is such a vast difference in hospital size (from under thirty beds to more than 1,000 beds), we can expect the standard deviation of total cost to be as large as its mean. In particular, this means that the error term will be subject to heteroscedasticity, since it is inconceivable that the variance about the total cost of a thirty-bed hospital can be as large as that about the total cost of a 1,000-bed hospital. This heteroscedasticity gives rise to a number of problems in estimation. To deal with it, one must use the generalized least squares framework (developed by Aitken). This involved adjusting the variance-covariance matrix so that the error term will be homoscedastic. We have argued that the proper adjustment is to deflate by a measure of patients served. Thus, dividing by admissions or patient days should make the resulting error term homoscedastic.

work by Feldstein, 1968; Evans, 1971; Evans and Walker, 1972; Lave, Lave, and Silverman, 1972; Lee and Wallace, 1973, Rafferty, 1971). These researchers all used privileged data banks. There are little data on case mix generally available and there are no data available on a nationwide basis. Thus, if one wants to study a national sample of hospitals, some way must be found to finesse this problem.

In an earlier paper (Lave and Lave, 1970), we presented a model in which we assumed that within a particular hospital, case mix was constant over a short period of time. In subsequent work, we looked at explicit measures of hospital case mix and found this assumption was a close approximation to reality (Lave and Lave, 1971). We then compared some of the results obtained by estimating cost functions in which we had explicit measures of case mix (Lave, Lave, and Silverman, 1972) with those in which the case-mix measures were not explicitly introduced (Lave and Lave, 1970), and found them similar. With certain exceptions, we shall assume in this paper that case mix is constant over the relevant time period within our hospitals.[2]

Cost Functions Assuming Case Mix Constant over a Period of Time

Assuming case mix is constant, it need not be included in estimating the cost function for a particular hospital. For cross-section–time-series data, case mix would give each hospital a unique intercept (except in the index number and percent change formulations). Location and teaching programs are assumed to be constant over time within a hospital; however, since they are common to many hospitals, they are represented by qualitative variables in the analysis.

Before setting out the cost function explicitly, it is necessary to

[2] The period of time under observation is 1964-1973. It is unlikely that the case mix did in fact remain constant. In particular, with the introduction of Medicare and Medicaid, there was an increase in the proportion of poor and elderly. However, if the increase was uniform across all hospitals, our estimation procedure will take account of such a change in case mix.

describe how these change variables were constructed. As shown in equation (2),

$$IAC_{it} = \frac{AC_{it}}{\sum_t AC_{it}/10} \qquad (2)$$

the cost index in hospital i at time t is equal to the cost per admission in hospital i at time t divided by the average cost per admission in hospital i over the entire period (ten years). This cost index is computed for each hospital in each time period. A similar index is constructed for average cost per patient day (ACD). The index number for the other variables was constructed in the same way. The index number in hospital i for variable X at time t is equal to the original value of the variable in hospital i at time t divided by its average value over the entire period, as shown in equation (3).

$$I_{it} = \frac{X_{it}}{\sum X_{it}/10} \qquad (3)$$

[X: Occupancy rate, bed size, average length of stay, number of facilities and services].

Having defined these index numbers, we encounter the question of functional form. A wide variety of functional forms have been used by econometricians, ranging from the simple linear form to multiplicative and translog forms. In the absence of a priori knowledge of the production function or of the proper functional form, one is in the position of attempting to determine simultaneously the functional form and the proper formulation. Even with a large data set, there is little hope in answering all questions simultaneously and assuring oneself that the results are robust in the face of possible specification errors, errors of observation, and various other difficulties. In view of prior work, we decided to assume a linear function form, regarding linearity as an approximation to a more complicated functional form over the observed range. Thus, we caution the reader against making inferences outside the range of observed data, or even for the extreme observations in the sample.

Assuming linearity, the cost function can be written as in equation (4),

$$IAC_{it} = a_0 + a_1 IOcc_{it} + a_2 ILoS_{it} + a_3 IB_{it} + a_4 IFac_{it} \\ + a_5 DV_{it} + a_6 t + e_{it}, \tag{4}$$

where IAC_{it} is the cost per admission index number; $IOcc_{it}$ is the index number for the occupancy rate; B_{it} is the index number for the number of beds in the hospital; $ILoS_{it}$ is the length of stay index; $IFac_{it}$ is the index number for the number of facilities; t represents a series of dummy variables for time; DV_{it} is a set of dummy variables measuring the geographical location (both region and size of SMSA), and teaching status of the hospital; and e is a random error term.[3] In subsequent equations X_{it} will be used to represent many of these explanatory variables.

An alternative to equation (4) is a percentage change model, shown in equation (5):

$$\frac{AC_{it} - AC_{it-1}}{AC_{it-1}} = C_0 + C_1 \frac{Occ_{it} - Occ_{it-1}}{Occ_{it-1}} \\ + C_2 \frac{X_{it} - X_{it-1}}{X_{it-1}} + C_3 t + C_1 DV_{it} + e. \tag{5}$$

Rearranging terms a bit gives equation (6), a ratio model:

$$\frac{AC_{it}}{AC_{it-1}} = C_0 + 1 - C_1 - C_2 + C_1 \frac{Occ_{it}}{Occ_{it-1}} + C_2 \frac{X_{it}}{X_{it-1}} \\ + C_3 t + C_4 DV_{it} + e. \tag{6}$$

We can now write equation (4) explicitly, as in (7) (setting $\Sigma_t X_{it}/10 = \tilde{X}_i$) to show the similarity of the percentage change

---

[3] It is still possible that heteroscedasticity exists across hospitals. One could estimate a time-series equation for each hospital and test for equality of the variance of the errors across hospitals. The estimated variance could be used, within a generalized least squares framework, to increase the efficiency of the estimates (see Saxonhouse, 1976). However, with more than 5,000 observations, increasing efficiency would not seem to be a major concern.

ratio and index number formulations.

$$\frac{AC_{it}}{\tilde{AC}_i} = a_0 + a_1\frac{Occ_{it}}{\tilde{Occ}_i} + a_2\frac{X_{it}}{\tilde{X}_i} + a_3t + a_4DV_{it} + e. \qquad (7)$$

Other than a difference in the interpretation of the constant term, equations (6) and (7) differ only in whether each observation X_{it} is normalized by X_{it-1} or $\tilde{X}_i$. Indeed, the index number formulation has two advantages: (a) the first observation is not lost, and (b) the effect of an error of observation or disequilibrium is less heavily weighted; for example, if the observed value of X° is equal to $X_{it} + u$ then $(X_{it} + u)/(\tilde{X}_i + .1u)$ will be closer to $(X_{it})/(\tilde{X}_i)$ than will be $(X_{it} + u)/(X_{it-1})$. However, we will fit both functional forms.

A final cost function to be estimated is shown in equation (8):

$$\begin{aligned} AC_{it} = a_0 + a_1Occ_{it} + a_2LoS_{it} + a_3B_{it} + a_4Fac \\ + a_5DV_{it} + t + e. \end{aligned} \qquad (8)$$

This is a standard cost function for a cross-section of hospitals. We include it here for the sake of completeness, noting that it represents a retrogression since there is no control for case-mix variation among hospitals. We must assume, as did the early researchers, that hospital facilities represent a gross surrogate for case mix.

Estimating Marginal Cost

Equations (5), (7), and (8) represent the basic structure of the regressions to be estimated. Our major focus, as noted in the introduction, is to try to estimate the incremental or marginal cost of an extra admission or patient day of hospital care. The marginal costs for each formulation are shown as follows:

Marginal Cost Equations

Time-Series	*Traditional*
(Index Number)	*Cross-Section*
Formulation	*Formulation*

1. MC_1: Assuming length of stay is
   constant (while *PD and Ad* vary)

Patient day formulation: $1 + a_1$ $\dfrac{TC}{PD} + a_1 Occ$

Admission formulation: $1 + a_1$ $\dfrac{TC}{Ad} + a_1 Occ$

2. MC_2: Assuming admissions constant
(as PD and LoS vary)
Patient day formulation: $1 + a_1 + a_2$ $\dfrac{TC}{PD} + a_1 Occ + a_2 LoS$

3. MC_3: Assuming occupancy rate
constant (as Ad and LoS vary)
Admission formulation: $1 - a_2$ $\dfrac{TC}{Ad} - a_2 LoS$

The Sampling Procedure and Data

The data for this study are part of the responses of hospitals to the American Hospital Association's Annual Survey. A sample of hospitals was selected as follows. Using the 1965 Hospital Guide Issue, we began with the third hospital listed and then considered every fifth hospital thereafter. If the hospital thus selected was a short-stay, nongovernmental, nonmental hospital, and if it was in existence in 1973, it was considered a valid sample point. If the hospital was not a valid sample point, it was simply excluded and the fifth following hospital considered. This sampling procedure generated 982 hospitals, which represent a random sample of nongovernmental short-term hospitals in 1964.

We next obtained for each of these hospitals from the Annual Hospital Guide Issues (1965–1974) the following data: hospital bed size, types of affiliation, control, number of admissions, number of facilities, average daily census, average occupancy rate, number of bassinets, number of births, total expense, personal expense, and number of personnel. Complete data on each hospital were not available. Some of the hospitals in the sample reported data only on the hospital bed size, while other hospitals would occasionally fail to provide information on variables such as expenses, occupancy rates, or admissions. We had two choices: (1) We could try to estimate the

TABLE 1   Summary Characteristics of Sample Hospitals
1964

Hospital Character	Original Sample (n = 982)	Final Sample (n = 507)	Excluded Hospital (n = 475)
Mean bed size	150.66	168.12	128.37
Percent < 40 beds	24.13	15.27	24.83
Percent > 250 beds	17.92	21.60	13.48
Percent teaching	23.12	28.49	16.63
Percent of any SMSA	55.34	56.42	53.64

value for a missing observation, or (2) we could exclude entirely hospitals that failed to report critical information in any year from the data set. We chose the latter. In Table 1, we show some of the characteristics of the hospitals in the initial sample and of its two subsets: hospitals included and excluded from the final data set. The characteristics are based on 1964 data. As expected, the excluded hospitals tend to be relatively small, although there were a number of large, teaching hospitals also excluded.

While the basic data bank consisted of information from the Hospital Guide Issue, a supplementary data base was analyzed: the 1973 AHA data tape. The AHA records more detailed information than is reported in the Hospital Guide Issue and makes it available on request. An important addition is data on outpatient activity.

Before we present the results of our analysis, we summarize some of the characteristics of the data. The data substantiate the fact that the period 1964–1973 was one of rapid growth and development in the hospital sector. The average hospital size increased from 168 beds to 209 beds, with the hospitals which had relatively more beds in 1965 actually expanding their bed capacity more than the smaller hospitals. Average expense per admission increased from $286 in 1964 to $775 in 1973, and average cost per day increased from $39.53 to $102.05. The rate of increase was not at all constant, and we show the percentage change in cost between each two-year period, as well as the average length of stay (refer to Table 2). The "direct" figures are unadjusted rates of increase; the adjusted figures will be explained below.

The number of services offered is difficult to characterize. The AHA did not ask for information on the same services in each year.

TABLE 2   Changes in Cost and Length of Stay
1963-1973

	AVERAGE PERCENT CHANGE IN COST PER ADMISSION		AVERAGE PERCENT CHANGE IN COST PER DAY		AVERAGE LENGTH OF STAY (IN DAYS)
	Direct	Adjusted:	Direct	Adjusted:	
		Index % Δ		Index % Δ	
1963-1964					7.34
1964-1965	8	11.3 11.3	8	3.3 3.3	7.36
1965-1966	7	9.1 9.1	6	3.5 3.6	7.57
1966-1967	22	23.7 23.8	14	8.2 13.7	8.05
1967-1968	10	15.2 15.8	9	5.4 8.0	8.25
1968-1969	14	18.9 19.1	13	7.1 12.2	8.32
1969-1970	14	18.3 18.0	18	7.9 12.7	8.14
1970-1971	10	14.3 15.5	12	6.7 9.6	7.90
1971-1972	10	13.1 14.0	12	7.0 7.3	7.75
1972-1973	8	9.9 11.4	8	5.8 4.3	7.75

Some services (operating room) were completely excluded from the survey, other services (burn unit) were added, while still others were disaggregated (in 1964, hospitals were asked to indicate if they had a pharmacy; in 1973 they were asked if they had a full-time or part-time pharmacy). In 1964, the hospitals were asked to report on about twenty-nine services; in 1973, they were asked to report on some forty-five. Of these, only eighteen were common to both surveys. Thus, since the number of services reported each year is inconsistent, there is no simple service index; as described below, this omission leads to problems in the cross-section–time-series analyses.

Results: Cross-Section–Time-Series

In Table 3, the variables to be used in the subsequent analyses are defined and their mean and standard deviations are given. When variables are in index number form, their mean is one.

Pooling of Data Sets

The cross-section–time-series data are on hospitals representing an array of sizes, located in nine different census regions over ten

TABLE 3   Variable Definitions: Means and Standard Errors
Time-Series–Cross-Section Analysis
$n = 5070$, years = 1964–1973

Name	Definitions	Mean	Standard Deviation
Independent Variables			
Occ	Absolute mean occupancy rate	74.51	13.42
IOcc	Index number for occupancy rate	1.000	.110
POcc	Mean annual percent change of occupancy rate	.866	16.12
LoS	Average length of stay	7.84	2.16
ILoS	Index number for average length of stay	1.000	.126
PLoS	Mean annual percent change of average length of stay	2.114	40.13
Fac	Mean number of facilities	14.52	19.97
IFac	Index number for mean number of facilities	1.000	.383
PFac	Mean annual percentage change of mean number of facilities	7.177	58.66
BED	Mean number of beds	191.20	164.00
IBED	Index number for mean number of beds	1.000	.163
PBED	Mean annual percentage change of mean number of beds	3.488	21.09
AT	Advanced teaching hospital	8.1	—
T	Teaching hospital	17.3	—
S_0	Hospital not in SMSA	40.9%	
S_1	Hospital in SMSA pop less than 100,000	1.8%	—
S_2	Hospital in SMSA pop 100,000–250,000	8.1%	—
S_3	Hospital in SMSA pop 250,000–500,000	11.6%	—
S_4	Hospital in SMSA pop 500,000–1,000,000	8.9%	—
S_5	Hospital in SMSA pop 1,000,000–3,000,000	13.6%	—
S_6	Hospital in SMSA pop greater than 3,000,000	15.1%	—
	Hospitals located in census region:		
R_1	New England	9.5%	—
R_2	Mid-Atlantic	18.0%	—
R_3	South Atlantic	11.8%	—
R_4	East North Central	19.5%	—
R_5	East South Central	5.3%	—
R_6	West North Central	13.2%	—
R_7	West South Central	7.5%	—
R_8	Mountain	5.1%	—
R_9	Pacific	10.0%	—
$Y_1 - Y_{10}$	Year 1964–1973: 10% of observations in each year		
Dependent Variables			
AC	Total expense per admission	504.4	295.4
IAC	Index of expense per admission	1.00	.366
PAC	Mean annual percent change in expense per admission	13.83	49.90
ADC	Total expense per patient day	65.17	33.39
IADC	Index of expense per patient day	1.00	.371
PADC	Mean annual percent change in expense per patient day	13.29	47.66

separate years. Can these data be pooled to form a single data set? Are the cost functions in each census region and in each size hospital sufficiently different to require that a number of data sets be maintained?

In examining this issue, one question was answered unequivocally. To determine whether it was possible to aggregate across different census regions for the cross-section–time-series regression, an F-test was performed for the cost per case and cost per patient day indices. For both of these cases the F-statistic took on a value less than 1, indicating that one could not reject the null hypothesis that the cost structure was the same in each of the regions. The results were somewhat more equivocal for the aggregation by size of hospital. For the cross-section–time-series results, F took on a value of 1.25 for cost per case. The critical value for F with 28 and 4,819 degrees of freedom is 1.48, indicating that one cannot reject the null hypothesis that the cost structure is the same for each size of hospital. A contrary result appears for cost per patient day. There, F takes on a value of 1.87; since again the critical value of F is 1.48, one can reject the null hypothesis in this case. Thus, we conclude that we can pool the data across regions. We have pooled the data from hospitals of different sizes since we emphasize the cost per admission results. The results, however, should be interpreted with caution.

Analyses of Cost per Admission

The Index Formulation   In order to analyze the factors affecting the cost per admission, we first estimated the index number equations. The results are presented in Table 4. In regression 4-1, the index of total cost per admission is regressed against the index for total beds, length of stay, occupancy rate, and dummy variables for year. Over 81 percent of the variation in the index of cost per admission is explained by the regression—although, as will become obvious, the year effect is the factor which contributes most to the explanatory power of the regression. The estimated coefficients are statistically significant. The signs of length of stay and occupancy rate are as expected, while the sign of beds is negative—indicating that economies of scale exist.

TABLE 4   Factors Affecting Index of Cost per Admission

Variable Name	Regressions			
	1	2	3	4
R^2	.812	.814	.813	.813
Intercept	383.8	333.7	333.2	333.7
	(13.32)	(11.16)	(11.13)	(10.81)
$IOcc$	-.256	-.266	-.266	-.266
	(-11.42)	(-11.89)	(-11.90)	(-11.88)
$ILoS$	.519	.527	.527	.527
	(24.75)	(25.19)	(25.19)	(25.16)
$IBED$	-.045	-.070	-.070	-.071
	(-2.71)	(-4.08)	(-4.09)	(-4.08)
$IFac$		.053	.053	.053
		(6.02)	(6.01)	(6.00)
AT			5.080	5.632
			(0.62)	(0.65)
T			1.317	1.614
			(0.22)	(0.25)
S_0				Reference Group
S_1				1.149
				(0.07)
S_2				.112
				(0.01)
S_3				-.667
				(-0.09)
S_4				-1.168
				(-0.13)
S_5				-.693
				(-0.09)
S_6				-1.160
				(-0.15)
R_1				Reference Group
R_2				.037
				(0.00)
R_3				-.496
				(-0.05)
R_4				.025
				(0.00)
R_5				-.567
				(-0.05)
R_6				-.219
				(-0.02)
R_7				-1.210
R_8				.610
				(0.05)
R_9				1.076
				(0.10)
Y_1	Reference Year	Reference Year	Reference Year	Reference Year
Y_2	43.52	43.61	43.61	43.61
	(4.36)	(4.39)	(4.39)	(4.38)
Y_3	82.27	121.4	121.4	121.4
	(8.23)	(10.21)	(10.19)	(10.18)
Y_4	192.8	232.5	232.5	232.5
	(19.02)	(19.28)	(19.23)	(19.20)

TABLE 4   Factors Affecting Index of Cost per Admission (cont.)

Variable Name	Regressions			
	1	*2*	*3*	*4*
Y_5	280.5	323.5	323.4	323.4
	(27.41)	(25.99)	(25.94)	(25.89)
Y_6	406.2	429.0	428.9	429.0
	(39.26)	(39.05)	(38.96)	(38.90)
Y_7	550.7	574.5	574.4	574.4
	(53.24)	(52.06)	(51.94)	(51.86)
Y_8	684.7	704.0	703.9	703.9
	(66.27)	(65.28)	(65.07)	(64.98)
Y_9	824.7	838.7	838.5	838.5
	(79.48)	(79.14)	(78.69)	(78.57)
Y_{10}	943.9	957.2	956.9	956.9
	(90.41)	(89.99)	(89.68)	(89.54)

In regression 4-2, the number of facilities index is added. The coefficient is positive and significant. When it is added, the absolute magnitude of the coefficient of beds increases, implying that the increase in beds is usually accompanied by an expansion of facilities. (We should point out again that since a good measure of facilities, consistent across the time periods, is not available, we used the simple count of reported facilities each year as our base.) In regression 4-3, dummy variables for teaching are added, while in regression 4-4, dummy variables for the geographic location as well as for the size of the SMSA of the hospital are added. The significance of individual variables is tested by t statistics; the significance of each group of variables is tested by F statistics. Both tests indicate that the dummy variables do not make a significant contribution to regression 4-2. The failure to make a significant contribution means that neither teaching programs nor geographical location play an important role in explaining hospital cost increases, once occupancy rate, size, length of stay, and number of facilities are accounted for. Thus, these factors could be neglected in future regulations focused on containing increases in costs.

What are the implications of these estimated equations with respect to the estimation of marginal costs and time path of hospital cost inflation?

Holding bed size constant, a hospital could accommodate an increase in admissions by combinations of a change in occupancy rate and a change in average length of stay. The regressions imply that when admissions increase, holding beds and length of stay constant, the cost of an additional admission (MC_1) is about 74 percent of average total cost. When admissions increase, holding occupancy rate and bed size constant, the cost of an additional admission (MC_3) is about 48 percent of average total cost. These are very strong results. The implication is that if admissions increase, and each new patient has the same length of stay as previous patients, the additional patients will cost about 74 percent of cost per case; that is, few costs are fixed from year to year and hospitals seem to be able to forecast occupancy well and to adjust personnel and equipment accordingly. Similarly, the implication is that an increase in admissions, which is offset by declining length of stay (so that occupancy rate is constant), will increase costs by about half current cost per case.

The time coefficients characterize cost increases in each year.[4] Thus, from regression 4-1, it is estimated that the rate of inflation in cost per admission was 11.3 percent between 1964–1965, 9.1 percent between 1965–1966, 23.7 percent between 1966–1967, 15.2 percent between 1967–1968, 18.9 percent between 1968–1969, 18.3 percent between 1969–1970, 14.3 percent between 1970–1971, 13.1 percent between 1971–1972, and 9.9 percent between 1972–1973. This pattern of cost change is shown in Table 2 as the "index" column along with the unadjusted rate of cost increase. Thus, it is observed that the rate of hospital cost increase has been lower since the imposition of COLC regulations, although the rate of hospital cost inflation had begun to slow down before 1971.

The Percentage Change Formulation   We studied the factors affecting hospital costs per case by estimating the percent change model discussed in equation (5) above. The results are presented in Table 5.

---

[4] The adjusted percentage increase in cost from year $t - 1$ to year t, $(ac_t - ac_{t-1})/ac_{t-1}$ for the index formulation, is derived by dividing the difference between the coefficients of Y_t and Y_{t-1} by the coefficient for Y_t plus the intercept, using the intercept as the estimated coefficient for the first year:

$$\frac{ac_t - ac_{t-1}}{ac_{t-1}} = \frac{Y_t - Y_{t-1}}{a_o + Y_t}$$

TABLE 5   **Factors Affecting Percent Change in Costs per Admission**

Variable Name	Regressions		
	1	2	3
R^2	.290	.291	.292
Intercept	8.13	8.09	7.59
	(4.34)	(4.33)	(3.99)
POcc	−.375	−.378	−.377
	(−9.14)	(−9.22)	(−9.20)
PLoS	.666	.668	.668
	(40.71)	(40.82)	(40.83)
PBED	.109	.095	.095
	(3.53)	(3.07)	(3.08)
PFac	—	.041	.040
		(3.27)	(3.20)
AT	—	—	−.174
			(−0.08)
T	—	—	2.612
			(1.56)
$Y_1 - Y_2$	Reference Year	Reference Year	Reference Year
$Y_2 - Y_3$	−.210	1.901	1.883
	(−0.08)	(0.70)	(0.69)
$Y_3 - Y_4$	12.49	12.41	12.45
	(4.72)	(4.69)	(4.71)
$Y_4 - Y_5$	4.483	4.724	4.767
	(1.70)	(1.79)	(1.80)
$Y_5 - Y_6$	7.836	4.699	4.840
	(2.97)	(1.67)	(1.72)
$Y_6 - Y_7$	6.685	6.551	6.638
	(2.53)	(2.48)	(2.51)
$Y_7 - Y_8$	4.212	3.761	3.901
	(1.59)	(1.42)	(1.47)
$Y_8 - Y_9$	2.671	2.199	2.473
	(1.01)	(0.83)	(0.93)
$Y_9 - Y_2$	.054	.006	.065
	(0.02)	(0.00)	(0.02)

The three regressions in Table 5 are equivalent to the first three regressions presented in Table 4, except that the variables are now expressed in percentage terms (we do not show the regression in which the location variables are entered, because they are insignificant). With the exception of beds, the results are consistent with those found in Table 4. (Here the sign of *PBED* indicates that a 10 percent increase in bed size leads to about a 1 percent increase in cost per case. As in the index formulation, the coefficient of *PBED* changes when *PFac* is added; consistent with the index number results is the decrease in the size of the coefficient.)

Let us look again at the variables of particular interest. The coefficient of *POcc* is negative and highly significant, indicating that a 10 percent increase in occupancy rate will lead to a 3.7 decrease in cost per case. A 10 percent increase in length of stay is shown to lead to a 6.6 percent increase in cost per case. The coefficients of the teaching variables indicate that these are not important characteristics affecting the rate of hospital cost increase. The coefficients of the year dummy variables compare the yearly rate of cost increase with that experienced between 1964–1965. The rate of cost inflation was not significantly higher between 1965–1966 than it was in 1964–1965. However, the results indicate that it was about 12 percent higher in 1966–1967, about 5 percent higher between 1967–1968 and 1968–1969, about 6 percent higher in 1969–1970. After 1970, the rate of cost increase begins to approximate that experienced in 1964–1965. These rates of cost increase are shown in Table 2 at the "%Δ" column.

Analyses of Cost Per Patient Day

In addition to exploring factors affecting cost per case over time, we studied the factors affecting cost per day. In Tables 6 and 7, we present the results of estimating the index number and the percentage change equations, respectively. Since the location of a hospital was found not to have a significant effect on hospital cost inflation, we have excluded SMSA size and region from the regressions. We summarize the results briefly.

The coefficient estimates are consistent with those found in the cost per case regressions. As one would expect, the estimates of marginal cost are similar in the two formulations. When patient days increase and length of stay is constant (MC_1), the ratio of marginal cost to average cost is .64. When patient days increase but admissions do not change (average length of stay increases), the ratio of marginal cost to average cost is .25. Thus, when patient days increase as a result of new admissions (with length of stay constant), the occupancy rate increases and an additional patient day costs 64 percent of average cost. This is similar to the estimate of MC_1 = .74 from the cost per admission formulation. When length of stay increases, with other variables constant, each day increase in stay costs about 25 percent of average cost. Thus, cost per case can be lowered by admitting new cases and holding occupancy rate

TABLE 6   Factors Affecting Index of Cost Per Patient Day

Variable Name	Regressions		
	1	2	3
R^2	.810	.811	.811
Intercept	1425.0	1376.0	1376.0
	(48.54)	(45.15)	(45.09)
$IOcc$	-.358	-.368	-.368
	(-15.67)	(-16.12)	(-16.13)
$ILos$	-.399	-.391	-.391
	(-18.69)	(-18.31)	(-18.30)
$IBED$	-.087	-.111	-.111
	(-5.10)	(-6.35)	(-6.35)
$IFac$		.052	.052
		(5.81)	(5.80)
AT			5.096
			(0.61)
T			.973
			(0.16)
Y_1	Reference Group	Reference Group	Reference Group
Y_2	46.99	47.07	47.07
	(4.62)	(4.65)	(4.64)
Y_3	98.60	137.1	137.0
	(9.68)	(11.31)	(11.29)
Y_4	223.1	262.2	262.1
	(21.60)	(21.32)	(21.27)
Y_5	312.0	354.2	354.1
	(29.91)	(27.93)	(27.86)
Y_6	434.6	457.1	457.0
	(41.23)	(40.82)	(40.72)
Y_7	581.8	605.1	605.0
	(55.20)	(53.80)	(53.67)
Y_8	716.1	735.1	735.0
	(68.02)	(66.88)	(66.66)
Y_9	866.9	880.7	880.5
	(81.99)	(81.53)	(81.07)
Y_{10}	999.2	1012.0	1012.0
	(93.92)	(93.36)	(93.04)

constant (a new case costs 48 percent of average cost); cost per patient day can be lowered by increasing length of stay (an extra day costs 25 percent of the cost of an average day.

The percentage increases in cost per patient day are shown in Table 2. They are lower than increases in cost per admission, although the pattern over time is similar to that for cost per admission.

Time-Series–Cross-Section Analyses Continued

The primary analysis was extended for two groups of hospitals. For some of the SMSAs, a Cost of Living Index has been estimated

TABLE 7   **Factors Affecting Percent Change in Cost per Patient Day**

Variable Name	Regressions		
	1	*2*	*3*
R^2	.027	.031	.031
Intercept	8.11	8.07	7.56
	(3.88)	(3.87)	(3.56)
POcc	−.245	−.249	−.249
	(−5.34)	(−5.44)	(−5.43)
PLoS	−.100	−.098	−.097
	(−5.44)	(−5.35)	(−5.33)
PBED	.171	.150	.150
	(4.98)	(4.35)	(4.35)
PFac	—	.063	.063
		(4.52)	(4.46)
AT	—	—	−.990
			(−0.40)
T	—	—	2.841
			(1.52)
Y_1-Y_2	Reference Year	Reference Year	Reference Year
Y_2-Y_3	.316	3.578	3.568
	(0.11)	(1.18)	(1.18)
Y_3-Y_4	10.36	10.24	10.30
	(3.50)	(3.47)	(3.49)
Y_4-Y_5	4.681	5.053	5.113
	(1.58)	(1.71)	(1.73)
Y_5-Y_6	8.873	4.027	4.196
	(3.00)	(1.28)	(1.34)
Y_6-Y_7	9.426	9.220	9.335
	(3.19)	(3.13)	(3.17)
Y_7-Y_8	6.340	5.644	5.826
	(2.15)	(1.91)	(1.97)
Y_8-Y_9	4.012	3.284	3.629
	(1.36)	(1.11)	(1.23)
Y_9-Y_2	.972	.890	1.017
	(0.33)	(0.30)	(0.34)

by the Department of Labor. The first group consists of all hospitals in an SMSA for which cost of living data were available. Hospitals whose size was fixed are of particular interest because it is likely that their case mix is more constant over the time period. Thus, the second group consists of all hospitals which experienced a less than 3 percent change in bed size over the entire period.

Effect of Cost of Living on Hospital Cost   The Bureau of Labor Statistics calculates Consumer Price Indices (CPI) for selected SMSAs. It seemed reasonable to hypothesize that hospitals located in areas in which the cost of living was rising most rapidly would experience the highest rate of inflation. To test this hypothesis, we analyzed all hospitals (121) which were located in SMSAs for which there was a BLS index. We reestimated the index number regressions, including a variable for the cost of living. Would the CPI for this year or last year have the more important influence on costs? Since we were uncertain, we estimated the regressions twice, using the current and lagged CPI in turn. In equations (9) and (10) below, we present the two basic equations (the year coefficients are not reported to save space).

$$IAC = \underset{(1.78)}{.23} - \underset{(-3.07)}{.111 BED} - \underset{(-4.44)}{.24 IOcc} + \underset{(10.72)}{.46 ILoS} \tag{9}$$
$$+ \underset{(5.28)}{.121 Fac} + \underset{(.75)}{.08 CPI} + \ldots$$

$$IAC = \underset{(1.68)}{.21} - \underset{(-3.12)}{.111 BED} - \underset{(-4.44)}{.24 IOcc} + \underset{(10.72)}{.46 ILoS} \tag{10}$$
$$+ \underset{(5.29)}{.121 Fac} + \underset{(.91)}{.10 LCPI} + \ldots$$

Two results should be emphasized. First, the SMSAs with the highest inflation in the cost of living were not the SMSAs with the most rapidly rising hospital costs. While the signs of the CPI and lagged CPI are both positive, they are statistically insignificant. Second, the coefficient of $IOcc$ for these sets of hospitals is about the same as that obtained in the earlier regression, while the coefficient of $ILoS$ is smaller. MC_1 here is estimated to be about 76 percent of mean average cost while MC_3 is estimated to be about 54 percent of mean average cost. These hospitals are in the largest SMSAs and tend to be much larger than the average hospital; thus, it is heartening that these results are so similar to those for the entire set of hospitals.

Hospitals That Changed Little in Size Over ten years hospitals experienced considerable change: admissions rose, size increased, and new facilities and services were added. Hospitals which grew fastest were probably those with the most services initially, those located in cities, and those which added the most services. Yet, if the various formulations correctly reflect the cost structure of hospitals, the 190 hospitals which expanded their bed capacity by less than 3 percent should produce results similar to those of the full sample.

The results are presented in equations (11) and (12). As before, we do not report the time coefficients. Equation (12) is the standard specification; equation (11) is somewhat different from the other regressions since we have added here the admission index ($IADS$). (We chose not to do so for hospitals that expanded their bed size, since there would be considerable collinearity between $IADS$ and $IBED$.)

$$IEXA = .55 + \quad .37 \; IBED - \quad .34 \; IADS + \ldots \tag{11}$$
$$(7.01) \qquad\quad (13.49)$$

$$IEXA = .21 + \quad .04 \; IBED - \quad .17 \; IOcc + \quad .51 \; ILoS + \ldots$$
$$(.86) \qquad (4.58) \qquad (15.30)$$
$$\tag{12}$$

The coefficient of $IADS$ in equation (11) indicates that the marginal cost of an admission is about 66 percent of average cost. The coefficient of $IOcc$ in equation (12) suggests that MC_1 is about 83 percent of average cost, while MC_3 is about 49 percent of average cost. The change in the coefficient of $IBED$ underscores the relationship between an increase in admissions and increase in bed size over time. For those hospitals it is interesting to note that MC_1 is a bit higher than for the entire sample (.83 versus .74), while MC_3 is almost identical (.49 versus .48). Nevertheless, for such different sets of hospitals as the total sample of hospitals, hospitals located in SMSAs, and hospitals which minimally expanded their bed size, the results are very close.

Results: The 1973 Cross-Section

An analysis of cross-section–time-series data, such as that in the earlier section of this paper, is one way of investigating the structure of the hospital cost function; an analysis of a cross-section of hospitals is another. In this section we undertake a traditional analysis of the hospital cost function, focusing on the data on all short-term hospitals in 1973 for which complete information was reported to the AHA. The advantages and disadvantages of such an approach are well known (see Lave and Lave, in press). The 1973 data, however, are sufficiently interesting to provide some insight into the nature of hospital costs.

Description of the 1973 Data

The 1973 data set describes the 5,655 short-term hospitals that responded to all questions on the 1973 AHA annual survey of hospitals. Before we could analyze the data, we had to determine whether one could pool hospitals of different sizes and from different regions into a single equation. An F-test indicated that the structure of the hospital cost function was not the same across the different size categories (although it was the same across different regions) and that pooling of the total sample was unwarranted. We thus investigated hospital costs for three different groups of hospitals: bed size 0–99; 100–249; and over 250.

In Table 8 we present, for each of the bed size groupings, the means and standard deviation of the variables used in subsequent regressions. With the exception of "voluntary hospital," the variables are those used earlier. "Voluntary hospital" is a dummy variable that takes on a value of zero for other hospitals.

The pattern of means across the three size categories in Table 8 is as expected. For example, the mean number of facilities, the average hospital occupancy rate, the mean number of personnel per bed, and the mean number of interns and residents per bed all rise with the hospital size category. Among the three groups, the mean number of births per admission do not differ significantly while the mean number of surgical procedures per admission do. A more subtle point is that the ratio of the standard deviation to the mean falls as hospital size increases for almost all these variables (*Fac. A, Fac. B, BEDS, Occ,* and so on); thus, as might be expected, there is less variation in services offered and also perhaps in the case mix among larger hospitals than among small hospitals.

TABLE 8   Means of Variables Used in 1973 Cross-Section Analysis Classified by Hospital Bed Size

| Variable | Definition | BED SIZE | | | | | |
| | | 0–99 (n = 2939) | | 100–249 (n = 1609) | | >250 (n = 1107) | |
		Mean	Stan. Dev.	Mean	Stan. Dev.	Mean	Stan. Dev.
Fac. A	No. of facilities (1–22 on AHA 1973 list)[a]	3.36	2.54	8.53	2.96	13.44	3.24
Fac. B	No. of facilities (23–46 on AHA 1973 list)[a]	2.53	2.01	5.83	3.17	10.71	4.79
BEDS	Number of beds	52.	23.39	160.	12.78	430.	201.70
Occ	Occupancy rate	62.15	14.94	73.59	11.82	80.01	8.28
LoS	Length of stay	7.21	3.61	7.94	3.30	8.63	2.85
Op/Ad	Surgical operation per admission	.29	.17	.47	.15	.54	.13
Bir/Ad	Births per admission	.08	.06	.09	.06	.09	.06
MD/B	Full-time physician & dentist per bed	.007	.02	.01	.06	.03	.07
In/B	Interns and residents per bed	.001	.01	.01	.05	.08	.12
Em/B	Total personnel per bed	1.73	.52	2.14	.64	2.58	.62
OPV/B	Outpatient visits per bed	141.0	167.3	168.3	207.9	214.4	220.0
EMV/B	Emergency visits per bed	54.3	52.37	68.8	54.49	72.8	45.73
AT	Advanced teaching hospital	0%		2%		40%	
T	Teaching hospital	0%		9%		52%	
NT	Nonteaching hospital	100%		89%		8%	
Vol.	Voluntary hospital	41%		67%		80%	
Pro.	Proprietary hospital	18%		12%		2%	
Gov.	Government hospital	41%		21%		18%	
S_0	Hospital not in SMSA	75%		42%		10%	
S_1	Hospital in SMSA, 100,000	1%		2%		2%	
S_2	Hospital in SMSA, 100,000–250,000	4%		9%		11%	
S_3	Hospital in SMSA, 250,000–500,000	5%		8%		14%	

S_4	Hospital in SMSA, 500,000–1,000,000	3%		9%		14%	
S_5	Hospital in SMSA, 1,000,000–3,000,000			14%		23%	
S_6	Hospital in SMSA>3,000,000	7%		17%		25%	
R_1	Hospital located in New England	5%		5%		7%	
R_2	Hospital located in Mid-Atlantic	3%		16%		21%	
R_3	Hospital located in South Atlantic	11%		14%		14%	
R_4	Hospital located in East North Central	11%		18%		23%	
R_5	Hospital located in East South Central	10%		7%		5%	
R_6	Hospital located in West North Central	17%		9%		9%	
R_7	Hospital located in West South Central	20%		10%		7%	
R_8	Hospital located in Mountain	8%		4%		4%	
R_9	Hospital located in Pacific	14%		13%		10%	
AC	Cost per admission	$521.60	247.20	$779.00	427.40	$1,055.00	516.10

[a]Given in the Appendix.

TABLE 9   Factors Affecting the Cost per Admission 1973 by Hospital Size

Independent Variable	100 to 249 HOSPITAL BEDS			< 100 BEDS	>249 BEDS
	Regression Number				
	1	2	3	4	5
R^2	.39	.50	.66	.52	.81
Intercept	696.4	669.1	618.1	635.5	694.1
	(8.43)	(8.57)	(9.51)	(20.89)	(7.44)
Fac. A	4.29	6.22	7.19	8.47	2.32
	(1.17)	(1.86)	(2.59)	(4.56)	(.81)
Fac. B	32.30	22.38	14.33	12.40	13.09
	(9.94)	(7.46)	(5.69)	(5.58)	(6.21)
BEDS	-.41	-.04	.07	.02	.09
	(-1.72)	(-.18)	(.40)	(.11)	(2.13)
Occ	-4.00	-5.44	-4.86	-4.36	-6.16
	(-5.09)	(-7.29)	(-7.82)	(-17.52)	(-6.32)
LoS	43.04	45.37	43.13	32.05	71.76
	(15.91)	(17.32)	(19.77)	(32.60)	(24.71)
Bir/Ad	—	-1081.0	-844.3	-489.6	-1133.0
		(-7.93)	(-7.41)	(-8.96)	(-7.77)
Op/Ad	—	53.25	126.0	200.9	70.89
		(.96)	(2.72)	(8.78)	(1.20)
OPV/B	—	.69	.34	.21	.08
		(15.35)	(8.43)	(8.84)	(2.14)
EMV/B	—	.15	-.05	.16	-.03
		(.81)	(-.31)	(2.19)	(-.13)
MD/B	—	—	2983.0	1711.0	1902.0
			(24.22)	(13.84)	(14.63)
In/B	—	—	1187.0	1429.0	1036.0
			(7.11)	(4.24)	(12.46)
AT	275.4	210.4	168.0	—	90.32
	(3.42)	(2.88)	(2.51)		(3.72)
T	205.9	182.3	-32.37	—	-56.27
	(3.84)	(3.75)	(-.77)		(-2.32)
Vol.	-29.62	-36.33	7.97	-12.01	-34.87
	(-1.35)	(-1.78)	(.47)	(-1.61)	(-1.59)
Pro.	-12.45	-.69	11.17	-39.39	-83.29
	(-.38)	(-.02)	(.43)	(-3.65)	(-1.48)
S_0	-171.8	-148.7	-138.9	-83.52	-191.8
	(-5.31)	(-5.03)	(-5.63)	(-4.41)	(-6.46)
S_1	-116.4	-123.1	-113.7	-68.87	-103.8
	(-1.66)	(-1.93)	(-2.15)	(-1.39)	(-1.89)
S_2	-55.84	-46.65	-47.30	-25.45	-61.82
	(-13.7)	(-1.26)	(-1.53)	(-1.05)	(-2.17)
S_3	-54.20	-51.59	-79.52	-41.40	-43.96
	(-1.34)	(-1.40)	(-2.60)	(-1.81)	(-1.70)
S_4	Reference Group	Reference Group	Reference Group	Reference Group	Reference Group
S_5	33.38	26.43	16.45	14.84	48.86
	(.90)	(.79)	(.59)	(.66)	(2.06)
S_6	221.8	193.7	118.7	47.71	237.5
	(6.05)	(5.82)	(4.26)	(2.01)	(9.62)
R_1	Reference Group	Reference Group	Reference Group	Reference Group	Reference Group
R_2	-71.05	-51.12	-90.33	-44.65	-61.01
	(-1.81)	(-1.43)	(-3.02)	(-2.00)	(-2.01)

TABLE 9   Factors Affecting the Cost per Admission 1973
by Hospital Size (cont.)

Independent Variable	100 to 249 HOSPITAL BEDS			<100 BEDS	>249 BEDS
	Regression Number				
	1	2	3	4	5
R_3	−50.05	−19.46	−17.28	−86.13	−86.30
	(−1.25)	(−.53)	(−.57)	(−4.61)	(−2.63)
R_4	−104.0	−58.65	−50.94	−76.76	−57.39
	(−2.67)	(−1.64)	(−1.71)	(−4.17)	(−1.87)
R_5	−124.2	−56.21	−60.43	−84.53	−117.8
	(−2.68)	(−1.32)	(−1.71)	(−4.32)	(−2.83)
R_6	−161.5	−88.61	−95.19	−132.9	−187.2
	(−3.68)	(−2.19)	(−2.38)	(−7.44)	(−5.11)
R_7	−131.9	−56.28	−62.24	−97.66	−128.2
	(−3.03)	(−1.40)	(−1.86)	(−5.38)	(−3.21)
R_8	−59.32	−4.90	−28.91	−114.8	−62.01
	(−1.12)	(−.10)	(−.72)	(−5.88)	(−1.35)
R_9	1.65	16.73	71.67	45.86	15.56
	(.04)	(.44)	(2.26)	(2.49)	(−0.41)

The smaller hospitals tend to be located in rural areas, whereas the larger hospitals are located in metropolitan areas. For example, 74 percent of hospitals under 100 beds and 10 percent of hospitals over 250 beds are located outside SMSAs while 5 percent of the former and 25 percent of the latter are located in SMSAs with a population of over 3,000,000. The control of hospitals also differs significantly among the three groups—41 percent of the smallest hospitals and 80 percent of the largest hospitals are "voluntary" hospitals.

Factors Affecting the Cost Per Admission

in Table 9, we present a series of analyses of cost per admission. Regressions 1 through 3 are only for hospitals with 100–249 beds. In regression 9-1, cost per admission is regressed against *Fac*. A, *Fac*. B, *BEDS*, *Occ*, *LoS*, and the descriptive variables representing the hospital's location, teaching status, and control. The factors included in this regression account for about 39 percent of the variation in average cost per admission.[5] With the exception of *Fac*. A, all the variables are significant and all have the expected sign. In regression

[5] The same factors account for 40 percent of the variation in cost per case for hospitals less than 100 beds and 70 percent of the variation for hospitals greater than 250 beds.

9–2, variables representing various aspects of the hospital's case mix are added: number of births per admission, number of operations per admission, and the number of outpatient visits and emergency visits per bed. The coefficients of the earlier variables change somewhat. In regression 9–3 we include some variables which indicate special types of personnel—the number of full-time medical doctors and interns and residents per bed. The power of the regression rises to .66; but the coefficients of the other variables are again somewhat variable.

The instability of the regression coefficients reflects both the collinearity among the variables and the inadequacy of a single equation model. The coefficient of *LoS*, is however, very stable while that of *Occ* is reasonably stable, indicating that we can say something meaningful about marginal cost. (It is the inclusion of the outpatient activity that changes the coefficient of *Occ*.) Before turning to the marginal cost estimates, however, let us look at the effect of the other variables.

The average cost per case is highest in advanced teaching hospitals and lowest in nonteaching hospitals. This finding is of course consistent with the results of other work on hospital cost functions. Costs in teaching hospitals are higher for four basic reasons: (1) the cases treated are likely to be more complex; (2) for a given case, more tests and so forth may be offered; (3) the salaries of interns and residents are included in total costs; and (4) in teaching hospitals physicians are more likely to be salaried and thus physician costs are sometimes incorporated in the hospital costs. The decrease in the coefficient of the teaching variables when In/B and MD/B are entered indicates the importance of the third and fourth factors.

The inclusion of the case-mix variables increases the explanatory power of the regression. The coefficients of Bir/Ad indicate that the higher the volume of obstetrics, for a given number of admissions, the lower the average cost per admission, while those of Op/Ad indicate that as the proportion of surgery cases rise, cost per admission rises. The higher the volume of outpatient activity, the higher, as would be expected, are the costs per admission.[6]

---

[6] This same effect was observed for the small hospitals but not for the large hospitals. This result might obtain because there is less variation in the extent of outpatient

The location of the hospital has an important effect on the position of the cost function. The larger the SMSA in which a hospital is located, the higher its cost per admission. Since wage rates rise as city size increases (Hoch, 1974), one might assume that it is differential input prices that generate this result. The cost level of the hospital also varies significantly across the different census regions. In the absence of a more completely specified model it is impossible to determine whether this is attributable to differences in the level of demand (and hence case mix) or to relative differences in factor prices. In regressions 9-4 and 9-5 we present the estimated cost functions for hospitals in the other bed-size groupings. (There are no teaching variables in regression 9-4 because no hospital under 100 beds was a teaching institution.) The sign and significance of almost all the coefficients are the same as those presented in regression 9-3.

Estimates of the Marginal Cost Per Admission

Let us now turn to the estimates of the cost of an additional admission. As before we examine the two polar cases: (a) admissions increase, length of stay remains constant, and occupancy rate rises (MC_1); (b) admissions increase and the occupancy rate remains constant but average length of stay falls (MC_3).

For the hospitals with 100–249 beds we derive the estimated marginal cost per admission by assuming that admissions rose by 10 percent or by 588 admissions. Holding all other conditions constant, we determined that the occupancy rate would rise by 7.9 (from 79.75 to 87.73),[7] and hence average cost would fall to $747.05. We then determined new total expenses, the change in total expenses, and finally the "average" marginal cost of the new admissions. This calculated marginal cost (MC_1) for regression 9-1 is $427.51 or 55

activity among the hospitals with over 250 beds. We expect an increase in outpatient activity to increase costs per admission because the total costs are not net of outpatient costs.

[7] The initial occupancy rate was calculated; it was set equal to the $\left| \dfrac{\text{mean Admissions} \times \text{mean Length of Stay}}{\text{mean Bedsize} \times 365} \right|$ This is a different occupancy rate from the mean occupancy rate of 73–59.

percent of average cost, and for regression 9-3 is $354.19 or 45 percent of average cost. We then determined the marginal cost (MC_3) by determining how much length of stay would fall if the 588 new admissions had been accompanied by a decrease in overall length of stay while the occupancy rate was maintained at 79.75 percent. The calculated decrease in length of stay was .75 of a day. We then calculated the new average cost, total cost, change in costs, and "average" marginal cost. MC_3 for regression 9-1 was estimated to be $419.96 or 53 percent of average cost and for regression 9-3 it was estimated to be $416.84 or about 52 percent of average cost.

These estimates of the relationship of marginal cost to average cost should be treated cautiously. Since it seems obvious that the incremental resources needed to treat new patients are greater if, in addition to more intensive use of the ancillary services, the number of patient days (and hence laundry and food costs) also increase, MC_1 should be higher than MC_3. For hospitals with 100–249 beds MC_1 is slightly higher than MC_3. For hospitals under 100 beds, however, MC_1 is estimated to be between 45 and 49 percent of average cost, while MC_3 is consistently higher than MC_1. For the large hospitals, the results are more promising. MC_1 is estimated to be between 45 percent and 49 percent of average cost while MC_3 is estimated to be between 38 percent and 41 percent of average cost.

The 1973 estimates were obtained from a single equation model with few explicit case-mix variables. The limited case-mix measures all contribute significantly to the variation in the dependent variable. The single equation results have implications for constructing multiequation models. Chiswick (1974) has done some excellent work in modeling the interrelationship between hospital admission rates, occupancy rates, and bed rates among SMSAs. Our results suggest that outpatient activity and the expansion of facilities must also be taken explicitly into account. In addition, the factors influencing the hiring of physicians, as well as interns and residents, must be explored. The proportion of total medical expense, which is termed hospital expense, is arbitrary, since physician costs are sometimes included and many services may be treated similarly (see the arguments of Pauly and Redisch, 1973).

Conclusions

Our goal was to estimate hospital cost functions to answer questions about: (a) the cost of an additional patient or patient day; (b) the effect of other factors on costs; (c) the similarity of cost functions across regions and hospitals of various sizes; (d) the extent of pure cost inflation; and (e) the effect of the Cost of Living Council and Phases I–IV on cost increases. We analyzed a random sample of hospitals for which data were published by the American Hospital Association for the period 1964–1973. The principal problem with these data is the lack of a measure of case mix or other output measures. We attempted to finesse this problem by assuming that case mix was constant within a hospital over time.

Without a specific output measure, it became important to determine the sensitivity of results to the specifications. Thus, we estimated cost functions in many different forms. For the cross-section–time-series data, the forms were (a) average cost versus hospital characteristics, (b) an index of average cost versus indices of characteristics, and (c) the percentage change in average cost versus the percentage change in characteristics. Furthermore, both total expense per case and total expense per patient day were estimated, along with a number of minor changes in specification for each. Finally, we investigated data on almost all short-term hospitals in 1973.

Our estimates made it clear that there is a stable hospital cost structure that is relatively insensitive to these specification changes. Apparently, marginal costs can be estimated and one can isolate the effect of various hospital characteristics. The cost of an additional case whose length of stay was identical to that of previous cases (MC_1) was estimated to be between 55 percent and 74 percent of total expenses per case. The cost of an additional patient day, when admissions were constant and length of stay increased (MC_2), was estimated to be between 22 percent and 34 percent of total expense per patient day. Finally, the cost of an additional case when length of stay declined enough to hold the occupancy rate constant (MC_3) was estimated to be between 38 percent and 53 percent of total expense per case.

There was some evidence of economies of scale, although these were not of important size and did not exist for the largest hospitals. There were the usual results that teaching programs appear to add to cost, although the rate of cost inflation was no higher in teaching hospitals. The cost structure was found to be constant across regions, but not across different size (of hospital) groupings.

The time pattern of cost increases showed rapid increases in the inflation rate at the time of the introduction of Medicare and Medicaid; the rate of inflation then appeared to fall for the rest of the period. One is tempted to conclude that the acceleration in inflation was due to the expansion in demand resulting from Medicare-Medicaid; as the system adjusted to this now higher level of demand, costs increased less rapidly. While such a hypothesis is plausible, one cannot rule out other explanations.

Did Phases I–IV stop inflation in hospitals? The answer must be no; costs continued to increase faster than the CPI, and even faster than in the pre-Medicaid period. However, inflation did slow appreciably under the Cost of Living Council regulations. But, as noted above, this decline in the inflation rate started in 1970. Thus, one cannot conclude that COLC was the causal factor. Still, when one looks at inflation rates in the rest of the economy, the steady downward trend (from much higher levels) for hospitals is impressive and would seem to indicate at least a strong influence from COLC. Furthermore, hospital costs have risen to much higher levels since the expiration of controls.

While we believe that some sort of cost controls are needed for hospitals, we do not view all control schemes as equivalent. For example, freezing cost per patient day, as in Phase I, is effective but inequitable. The Phase IV regulations came close to setting out a structure that we regard as both workable and fair. However, even Phase IV fell short because of ambiguities having to do with outpatient activity and geographical location. To repair these deficiencies, better hospital cost analysis is required. These results point the way for future research. We must move from single equation models to multiequation models, and from empirical models estimated with state data to those estimated with more local data— from SMSAs, for example. The models must incorporate both the level of inpatient activity and that of outpatient activity. In addition, the staffing policies and expansion (of services and size) policies of the hospital must be modeled. To view the hospital as a producer of inpatient days is, as the 1973 results suggest, a historical anachronism.

Appendix

AHA Listing of Facilities and Services
1973

SA   (1)   Postoperative Recovery Room
      (2)   Intensive Care Unit (Cardiac only)
      (3)   Intensive Care Unit (Mixed)
      (4)   Open Heart Surgery Facilities
      (5)   Pharmacy W/FT Registered Pharmacist
      (6)   Pharmacy W/PT Registered Pharmacist
      (7)   X-Ray Therapy
      (8)   Cobalt Therapy
      (9)   Radium Therapy
   (10)   Diagnostic Radioisotope
   (11)   Therapeutic Radioisotope Facility
   (12)   Histopathology Laboratory
   (13)   Organ Bank
   (14)   Blood Bank
   (15)   Electroencephalography
   (16)   Inhalation Therapy Dept.
   (17)   Premature Nursery
   (18)   Self-Care Unit
   (19)   Extended Care Unit
   (20)   Inpatient Renal Dialysis
   (21)   Outpatient Renal Dialysis
   (22)   Burn Care Unit

SB   (23)   Physical Therapy Dept.
   (24)   Occupational Therapy Dept.
   (25)   Rehabilitation Inpatient Unit

(26) Rehabilitation Outpatient Unit
(27) Psychiatric Inpatient Unit
(28) Psychiatric Outpatient Unit
(29) Psychiatric Partial Hospitalization Program
(30) Psychiatric Emergency Services
(31) Psychiatric Foster &/or Home Care
(32) Psychiatric Consultation & Education Service
(33) Clinical Psychologist Services
(34) Organized Outpatient Dept.
(35) Emergency Dept.
(36) Social Work Dept.
(37) Family Planning Service
(38) Genetic Counseling Service
(39) Abortion Service (Inpatient)
(40) Abortion Service (Outpatient)
(41) Abortion Service (Outpatient)
(42) Dental Services
(43) Podiatrist Services
(44) Speech Therapist Services
(45) Hospital Auxiliary
(46) Volunteer Services Dept.

References

Berry, R.E.
   1967   "Return to scale in the production of hospital services." Health
           Services Research 2 (Summer): 123–139.
Chiswick, B.R.
   1974   "Hospital utilization: An analysis of SMSA differences in hospital
           admission rates, occupancy rates and bed rates." Working Paper
           No. 2, National Bureau of Economic Research.
Evans, R.G.
   1971   "'Behavioral' cost functions for hospitals." Canadian Journal of
           Economics 4 (May): 198–215.
Evans, R.G., and H.D. Walker
   1972   "Information theory and the analysis of hospital cost structure."
           Canadian Journal of Economics 5 (August): 398–418.

Feldstein, M.S.
  1968   Economic Analysis for Health Service Efficiency. Amsterdam:
          North-Holland Publishing Co.
Hoch, I.
  1974   "Inter-urban differences in the quality of life." In J. Rothenberg
          and I. Heggin, eds., Transport and the Urban Environment.
          New York: The Macmillan Publishing Company.
Lave, J.R., and L.B. Lave
  1970   "Hospital cost functions." American Economic Review 60
          (June): 379–395.
  1971   "The extent of role differentiation among hospitals." Health
          Services Research 6 (Spring): 15–38.
  in press "Hospital Cost Functions." To appear in Health Handbook,
          G. Chacko, ed. Amsterdam: North-Holland Publishing Co.
Lave, J.R., L.B. Lave, and L.P. Silverman
  1972   "Hospital cost estimation controlling for case mix." Applied
          Economics 4 (September): 165–180.
Lee, M.L., and R.L. Wallace
  1973   "Problems in estimating multi-product cost functions: An appli-
          cation to hospitals." Western Economic Journal (September):
          350–363.
Pauly, M., and M. Redisch
  1973   "The not-for-profit hospital as a physicians' cooperative." Ameri-
          can Economic Review 63 (March): 87–99.
Rafferty, J.
  1971   "Patterns of hospital use: An analysis of short-run variables."
          Journal of Political Economy 79 (January–February): 154–165.
Saxonhouse, G.
  1976   "Estimated parameters as dependent variables." American Eco-
          nomic Review 66 (March): 178–183.

Future Outlooks

Research Needs for Future Policy

RALPH E. BERRY, JR.

Introduction

As has been noted countless times, the cost of hospital care has been rising rapidly over an extended period of time. The average cost per patient day in nonfederal short-term general hospitals, for example, is approximately six times as high as it was twenty years ago. Moreover, the rate of increase of hospital costs has generally been accelerating. In fact, hospital cost inflation is not a problem of recent vintage, but represents a phenomenon with a rather long history that has displayed a marked tendency to intensify in recent years.

As hospital costs have risen, and particularly as these costs have been translated into a public burden through governmental budgets, more and more pressure has been brought to bear to control these costs. A variety of proposals designed to effect a control on hospital costs have appeared or reappeared in recent years. Incentive reimbursement mechanisms, prospective budgeting, rate regulation, areawide planning, certificates of need, and even structural reform of the medical care sector have been suggested as potential solutions to the cost problem—some have even been tried.

There has been some experience with cost containment in recent years as various mechanisms have been tried in several jurisdictions. There was even the brief period from 1971 to 1974 when price and wage controls were in effect nationally under the Economic Stabilization Program. A review of the experience to date, however, as

575

reflected in the several papers in Part III, does not inspire particular confidence in the current capacity to contain hospital costs. It seems not unreasonable to conclude that evidence from evaluation studies of specific cost-containment efforts is not overwhelming and does not indicate a significant degree of success. This book is indicative of the general concern with hospital cost inflation. Or perhaps it represents more the growing frustration with the propensity for hospital costs to rise in spite of a general awareness of the problem, specific public policy concern, and actual efforts to contain hospital costs.

What are the prospects for hospital cost containment? Do such mechanisms as rate regulation, prospective budgeting and reimbursement, planning and certificate of need, utilization review, and the like, have the potential to control or contain cost inflation in the hospital sector? As several of the earlier papers in this volume imply, the answers to these questions derive from the answers to several more fundamental questions. What is the structure of the hospital industry? What behavioral patterns are associated with varying market conditions? What are the dimensions of the problem of hospital cost inflation? What impact will various cost-containment mechanisms have on structure, behavior, costs, and productivity? In effect, several of the papers imply that the lack of success to date may be a function of a lack of knowledge and, hence, that successful cost containment may be enhanced by future research. There is also the implication that actual policies have often been designed without taking full account of even the limited available knowledge and, hence, that more successful cost containment may be enhanced by a better application of previous research.

The purpose of this paper is to outline some thoughts about the research needs for future policy. The intent is not to provide answers, but rather to ask questions. There is no presumption to offer any specific research agenda. Rather, it seems more appropriate and useful to reflect on a research strategy; to delineate the set of questions that should be asked in any research context and to consider the answers to those questions in the context of hospital cost containment.

A General Research Strategy

Whenever one sets out to research a problem, especially when the eventual objective is to define a policy solution to that problem, success usually necessitates first specifically answering several fundamental questions. In effect, in policy-related research or policy analysis, the degree of success is often related to the extent to which the approach to the research or the analysis has been systematic.

First, and perhaps foremost, it is necessary specifically to ask and to answer the question "What is the real problem of concern?" Although this may seem obvious and perhaps perfunctory, there is no shortage of unsuccessful research that can be traced essentially to a failure to formulate the right research question. Obviously, the more specifically the research questions can be formulated, the easier it is to seek answers, and the more likely it is that answers, when found, will have operational significance and provide the basis for enlightened policy. Similarly, one could cite a litany of unsuccessful policy or policy with unintended results that derives from a failure to ask the right question.

Once the question is specifically formulated, the researcher should answer a second fundamental question: "What is the ideal set of data necessary to answer the question?" Of course the ideal set of data is rarely available, but one needs to know what it is in order to specify an appropriate research design and to delineate specific data requirements. It is also useful to reflect on the ideal set of data in order to interpret and to qualify any findings generated from a less than ideal data set.

Next, the researcher must ascertain what part of the necessary data set is known or can be approximated by available surrogates. In essence, this simply requires that a systematic review of available data and relevant research literature must be undertaken.

Finally, the researcher can identify the gap between what is known and what needs to be known in order to answer the question. Closing this gap is what research is really about.

Different questions can be answered with different sets of data or information. One does, however, need a specific question to begin the process. Moreover, the appropriate degree of specificity can serve to limit the research effort and enhance the potential for success. Thus, for example, one might consider the question "What will happen if Congress enacts a national health insurance program?" But what is the real question? What will happen to what— prices? patterns of utilization? supply responses? Moreover, there is quite a difference between questions such as "Is utilization likely to increase under national health insurance?" and "Is utilization likely to increase by as much as 10 percent under national health insurance?"

The question whether utilization is likely to increase can be answered with a minimal data set. In fact, if we simply know whether there is any elasticity to the demand and supply curves we can provide an answer by reference to a simple comparative statics supply and demand analysis. Although this represents an oversimplification, and is only an approximation, it does provide an answer— and a reliable one at that. But if the question is whether utilization is likely to increase by as much as 10 percent, the data set necessary for an answer is considerably more complex. At the very least, we now need reasonably accurate estimates of specific elasticities. Questions of supply response, especially in the health sector, are exceedingly complex, and the necessary data set is more complex by an order of magnitude. It should be remembered that although we often use simple supply and demand curves to deal with questions of direction of change, with some confidence; and even use them to deal with questions of relative magnitude of change on occasion—albeit with somewhat less confidence; in fact, since we are rarely if ever concerned with competitive industries, there is really no such thing as a supply curve.

Some simple-sounding questions are often quite complex. Fortunately, some complex problems often involve relatively simple questions. But the first principle of successful research is to ask the right question. When the right research question has been formulated, there is some possibility that it can be answered. If we know the question and the ideal set of data necessary to answer it, then we can identify the gap between what is known and what we need to know. We can, in other words, identify the research needs.

Hospital Cost Containment—
What Is the Problem?

Although the phenomenon of hospital cost inflation has been around for a long time, and the problem of cost containment has received the considered attention of analysts and policy makers for much of that time, it does not seem unreasonable to argue that cost containment has rarely been defined in a clear concise way. In fact, even a casual reading of several of the papers in Part I of this volume suggests that we actually have a choice of cost-containment problems. Some view the problem in terms of the price inflation of hospital services. Others concentrate on the rate of increase of total expenditures for hospital care. A related concern would derive from the relative proportion of health expenditures, especially for hospital services, in the Gross National Product. Still others would view the problem in terms of the growing government budget for hospital services. It is not at all clear just what it is that is to be contained. Is policy to be designed to contain the rate of price inflation; the rate of increase of total expenditures; the share of GNP; or the size of the government budget?

Indeed, we might press the issue back one step to some heuristic advantage. Do price increases, total expenditure increases, shifts in GNP shares, or increases in government expenditures necessarily imply a problem at all? One could cite several hypotheses consistent with the observed increases, and not all of them would be cause for concern.

Total expenditures would be expected to increase if population increased; undoubtedly, some part of the increase in total expenditures for health services results from population growth. Moreover, changes in the mix of the population might explain part of the increase. The proportion of certain subgroups in the population, such as the aged, that tend to utilize more health services has increased over time. If policy is to be designed to contain the increase in total expenditures, what account must be taken of that part of the overall increase consistent with population growth and a changing composition of the population?

One might, as an alternative, look rather at the rate of increase of per capita expenditures. Per capita expenditures, by definition, abstract from increases induced by population growth. Are increases in per capita expenditures indicative of some problem and an unambiguous candidate for containment? Again one could postulate reasonable hypotheses that would suggest a degree of caution. Certainly some part of the increase in per capita expenditures can be traced to increased income, or put another way, hospital services are a normal good—that is, the income elasticity of demand for hospital services is positive. Now one does not usually consider constraining the consumption of normal goods when income rises, except in very special sets of circumstances. Or perhaps a relevant hypothesis would be that tastes have changed—a more difficult hypothesis to test, but a reasonable one and not necessarily indicative of a problem to be dealt with through cost containment policy.

What of relative shifts in the shares of Gross National Product for hospital services and other things? To the extent that the increasing proportion of hospital services in GNP represents an increase in the share of the nation's scarce resources used in this sector, does it not warrant containment? Perhaps, but again one could postulate certain hypotheses that would at least bear testing. The observed increases in the proportion of hospital services, given increases in income, are consistent with a hypothesis that hospital services have an income elasticity greater than one, for example. Perhaps hospital services are luxury goods. Indeed, the question whether hospital services are luxury goods or necessities is a research question that seems well worth answering. Income elasticity estimates from cross-section data imply that they are necessities—the elasticities tend to be well below one. On the other hand, time-series data imply that they may be luxuries—the income elasticity tends to be greater than one.

This particular example may be worth some elaboration in the context of our current concern. Suppose we take as given that cross-section and time-series data imply quite different income elasticities of demand for hospital services, and ask what relevance this might have to future research needs for cost-containment policy. Now the shortcomings of empirical demand estimates are well-known, and considerable care must be exercised in interpreting either cross-section or time-series estimates. One drawback to the cross-section estimate, of course, is the need to assume tastes are constant over persons and/or over space. But a similar problem arises in the time-series context—it is necessary to assume that tastes are constant over time. Our current concern is not with whether the same household at different points in time is more or less likely to have similar tastes than different households would at the same point in time, but rather with whether a given cost-containment policy would have the same effect regardless of whether the income elasticity was greater or less than one. Clearly it would not. Co-insurance rates, for example, could perhaps be applied with some success as a mechanism for constraining the quantity demanded and thus containing total cost. But if hospital services are a luxury good, then over time, as income increases, the co-insurance rate would have to be raised more than proportionately to effect the same proportionate constraint.

Perhaps more significant to future policy than the differential impact of a given policy instrument is the issue of whether different policy instruments entirely are suggested by the answers to certain research questions such as "Are hospital services a luxury or a necessity?" Suppose, for example, that we assume for present purposes that at a point in time consumers behave as though hospital services were a necessity, but that over time they behave as though they were luxury goods. Indeed, such may well be the case. It is not inconceivable that over time consumer preferences shift toward hospital services for a variety of reasons. Let me cite one plausible explanation. Suppose that consumers in general have elastic expectations relative to real or perceived technological advances and medical research. Then over time, as consumers become aware of changes in medical technology—or even anticipate that they have occurred—their preferences may shift toward medical services, and any estimate of the income elasticity over time will be greater than a corresponding cross-section estimate. Now quite apart from the issue of whether or not cost-containment policy is appropriate, given this phenomenon, if it were determined by some process that cost containment should be implemented, then an instrument that reflected this phenomenon would clearly have a greater chance of success than one that did not. Thus, a constraint on new equipment that embodied technological progress, for example, would work better than a general constraint on new equipment—particularly if the consumer were made aware of the implication of the constraint.

Of course, all that is really being argued is that we simply reflect on the demand for hospital services and recognize that the quantity demanded is a function of own price, the price of substitutes, the price of complements, income, insurance, and tastes. In this context we could cite any number of hypotheses consistent with shifts in the demand curve as well as movements along the demand curve. Moreover, to this point we have avoided those arguments in the demand function that are most likely to represent potential problems that are more obvious candidates for cost containment—prices and insurance. We might also note the obvious, that demand side considerations are only half the story.

Indeed, this line of argument was prompted by the question of just what is the problem that occasions such concern for cost containment. We have observed, in the case of hospital services, relative price inflation, increased total expenditures, a growing share of GNP, and higher government budgets. These phenomena are simply data; they represent the outcome of the interaction of such supply and demand factors as prevail in the market for hospital services. Taken alone, such data would not connote anything negative. In a market system prices are signals—rising prices signal sellers that buyers now value the good more highly and serve as an incentive for increased production. If we told someone sensitive to the issues and problems of economic development that the relative share in GNP of a particular service industry had grown consistently over the past few decades, he might think, "how fortunate." In fact, the reason that these specific data are viewed as symptomatic of a problem is because we think the market for hospital services is characterized by significant market imperfections. In effect, there is a problem precisely because we don't like the outcome—we don't think the market is working.

In a fundamental sense, the function of a market is to balance value in consumption with opportunity cost. If a market is working reasonably well, market prices tend to reflect scarcity values of both resources and consumer goods. The problem with the market for hospital services, of course, is that we can't trust prices to reflect scarcity values, especially of the consumer good in question. If we observed a particular consumer paying $100 to purchase a wool coat, we might take that price as a reasonable approximation of the value of the coat in consumption. But if we observed the same person consuming a day of hospital care that cost some third-party payer $100, we would be less inclined to accept the cost as indicative of the value in consumption. And therein lies the fundamental problem. Relative price inflation, increased expenditures, higher government budgets, and especially the increased proportion of GNP are considered indicative of the wrong rate of output.

Hospital cost containment, in any sense except that of constraining relative price increases for a given output, involves constraining the rate of output. Whether the policy instrument employed involves demand constraints or supply constraints, the implicit intended effect is the same.

It would seem that the most fundamental research question in the context of hospital cost containment is "What is the right rate of output of hospital services?" If that is the right question, is it any wonder that we are so far from an answer?

But, in fact, cost-containment efforts have been employed in the past and will undoubtedly continue to be employed. It should be clear, however, that the actual policy intent of cost containment is based on either of two implicit assumptions: (1) whatever the right rate of output is, it is less than the actual rate of output; or, (2) the actual rate of output is acceptable, but the only increases that will be tolerated are those generated by real productivity increases. Of course, given the relative success of cost-containment efforts to date, it would appear that neither constraint has been particularly binding.

Thus, we can formulate a small number of fundamental research questions in the context of hospital cost containment that involve the rate of output. First, what is the right rate of output of hospital services? Second, quite apart from the right rate of output, how can the actual rate of output, or more particularly the rate of increase of that output, be constrained? Third, given the actual output, how can we constrain relative price increases for that output?

The full implication of the first question is presumably obvious. The implications of the second and third may not be, however. In fact, if cost-containment policy is implemented and succeeds in constraining the rate of increase of actual output over time—in effect constraining increases that might have derived from income increases, population changes, or shifts in consumer preferences, for example—that will be equivalent to the normative assumption that whatever the right rate of output is, it is less than the actual rate of output. In effect, cost-containment policy would serve to reduce the gap between some unspecified desired rate of output and the actual rate of output.

If cost-containment policy is implemented and succeeds in constraining relative price increases for a given level of output, that will be equivalent to the normative assumption that the actual rate of output is acceptable, but increases in output must be limited to those generated by real productivity increases. This constraint is somewhat less binding, in principle, but increases that might have derived from income increases, population changes, or shifts in consumer preferences, for example, may well be constrained. In essence, if such increases would have exceeded real productivity increases, then this constraint is only a modification of the more binding one and implicitly involves the same normative assumption that whatever the right rate of output is, it is less than the actual rate of output.

When the implications of the second and third questions are spelled out, the relative importance of the first question is the more clear. Undoubtedly the general support for cost-containment efforts derives from the widespread acceptance of the implicit assumption that the actual rate of output exceeds the right rate of output. There is no doubt that the output of the hospital sector includes necessary services, quality, and necessary complexity, but is also includes unnecessary services, inappropriate complexity, and undoubtedly some waste. To the extent that cost-containment policy is implemented successfully, one might expect that it will serve to eliminate unnecessary services, inappropriate complexity, and waste. In effect, cost-containment mechanisms should serve to eliminate the gap between the actual rate of output and the right rate of output. But how will we know when the gap has been eliminated? The more successful any set of cost-containment instruments, the more likely we will go too far. Hence, the more research contributes to answering the second and third questions, the more critical it is to answer the first question.

Policy makers who sit in the catbird seat and must cope more immediately with the implications of accelerating hospital cost inflation and the burden of growing budgets are undoubtedly not particularly placated by such a point, no matter how correct it might be in a strict conceptual sense. They undoubtedly view the actual outcome to be sufficiently off mark as to warrant cost-containment efforts without specific knowledge or delineation of the desired outcome. Most researchers who have studied the hospital sector would probably agree. The known market imperfections are such that the relative inefficiency is considered to be of a significant order of magnitude albeit not specifically measured. Most knowledgeable persons would agree that successful cost containment would have to go quite far indeed before one had to worry much about going too far. Certainly it would have to go farther than efforts to date have succeeded in going. Thus, it would seem that research has something to offer, even research that stops short of answering the fundamental question. And on that encouraging note we might move on to the kinds of questions with operational significance that might be asked, and more specifically to a consideration of where some of the answers might be found.

Where Do the Answers Lie?

In the most fundamental sense, the relevant questions can only be answered when we have a more complete understanding of the market for hospital services, the imperfections that prevail in that market, and the implications of those imperfections. If one could will into being any set of data one wanted, the ideal set for assessing the market for hospital services would include three principal components. First, one would need consumer preferences and such data as are necessary to derive the market demand for hospital services. Second, one would need the technological and factor market data necessary to derive the production function or the relevant cost curves for hospital services. Finally, one would need the several parameters that define the relevant industry structure. Indeed, if one had such a set of data, one could even answer the question of what is the right rate of output—at least the right rate of output given the prevailing income distribution. (In fact, if one had the foresight to will into being sufficiently robust consumer preference data, one could even approximate the right rate of output for alternative income distributions.) Moreover, given the parameters that define the structure of the market for hospital services, one could assess both the causes and the extent of such allocative inefficiency as might prevail. Intervention such as cost-containment efforts to improve the performance of the hospital services industry would be rather straightforward.

Unfortunately, we can't will ideal data sets into being. Even economists are afforded such luxury only when they are either fantasizing or teaching introductory principles courses. Rather, we must make do with the less than ideal data that are available or can be generated from systematic research efforts. But a consideration of the ideal data set does serve to outline the practical data requirements and to guide the search for answers in the right general direction. In order to answer the relevant questions in the context of cost-containment policy we need at least some reasonable approximation of both the demand for hospital services and the cost of production over the relevant range of output, and some knowledge of the characteristics of the market for hospital services that might serve significantly to affect the outcome. Most especially, we need knowledge of the peculiar characteristics of supply response in the hospital services market.

Of course, the available data set is not a null set. The body of knowledge is not insignificant and research efforts over a number of years have provided useful estimates and insight. There have been several empirical studies of the demand for hospital services, for example. Thus, although not immune to specific empirical criticism, the relevant literature contains estimates of the elasticity of the demand for hospital services with respect to such as own price, price of substitutes, income, and insurance. Moreover, the influence on demand of such surrogates for taste parameters as race, sex, age, education, marital status, and the like have been estimated. Within a tolerable margin of error, available estimates of the relevant demand elasticities are probably sufficient to approximate the effect of such demand constraints as co-insurance and deductibles. This is not to say that these estimates cannot be refined and improved, or that the margin of error cannot be reduced significantly—indeed, one of the major research efforts of recent years, the Rand National Health Insurance Experiment (Newhouse, 1974), was designed for just that purpose—but rather to note the availability of specific surrogates for necessary demand data. Whether or not the available surrogates are sufficient for any specific future cost-containment policy, of course, can only be determined on an ad hoc, as-needed basis. They are probably sufficient for policy efforts that do not depend on a high degree of specificity for success. But if cost-containment policy is to become more effective and demand constraints are to have a significant role in such policy, as might be the case under certain national health insurance programs, for example, there will be a need for more refined estimates of demand elasticities. More and better demand analysis is a research need for future policy.

Much the same can be said for hospital cost analysis. Although there has been considerable research effort devoted to estimating hospital cost functions—and in fairness it should be noted that much of this research has provided useful knowledge and insight—it is still the case that much more needs to be known about hospital cost functions if they are to provide the basis for more refined or sophisticated hospital cost-containment policy. The empirical cost functions estimated to date have only limited usefulness in the context of cost containment.

The paper in this volume by Lipscomb, Raskin, and Eichenholz indicates the potential of empirical cost estimates, but it is also illustrative of the limited usefulness of currently available estimates. The authors addressed themselves particularly to the incentive under rate regulation for hospitals to adjust their volume of output because short-run marginal cost is below average cost. Their analysis of more than a dozen different hospital cost studies tended to support the modifications employed by the Cost of Living Council under Phase IV. Still, it seems fair to conclude that their analysis only supports the contention that the modification represented a move in the right direction. The range of marginal cost estimates in the several studies was rather broad and the authors were able to cite problems in model specification, sampling, and estimation techniques worthy of further research.

Of course, it could be argued that earlier cost studies were not designed to provide a basis for cost-containment policy and it is not fair to judge them by how specifically they might serve that purpose. And such is not the current purpose. Rather, the intent is only to note the nature of the available data set and indicate the extent to which it will meet the needs of future cost-containment policy. It would seem that hospital cost analysis is a prime research need.

The paper by Lave and Lave represents the potential of cost analysis designed specifically to address questions in the context of cost-containment policy. Their estimates suggest that there is a stable hospital cost structure that is relatively insensitive to certain output specifications. They were able to estimate marginal costs and isolate the effect of certain hospital characteristics. The availability of specific empirical estimates such as those generated by the Laves provide the basis for more specific rules and constraints and hence enhance the potential of cost-containment policy. In essence, they are akin to more specific demand elasticity estimates in the context of demand constraints.

The analysis completed by the Laves provides other insights with potential for future cost-containment policy. Thus, for example, they found the cost structure constant across regions, but not across hospital size. Moreover, they found that the cost effects of increasing and decreasing occupancy rates were not symmetrical. On balance, their research is exceedingly useful in its own right, and it does augur well for cost analysis designed specifically to address questions in the context of cost-containment policy. Still, the authors consider their work preliminary rather than definitive and argue for further research with more than the traditional polite caveat. In the spirit of our concern they offer several specific suggestions including the use of better estimating techniques, the use of data bases with more information, and more precise modeling of hospital supply responses.

Undoubtedly the weakest part of the available data set is that which involves the peculiar characteristics of supply response in the hospital services market. In attempting to assess the parameters that define the structure of the hospital industry one must cope with several typical problems such as differentiated products, lack of knowledge, geographical markets, and the like. But one must in addition cope with several rather unusual problems such as the dominance of nonprofit enterprises on the supply side of the market, the possibility that supply-side actors have influence on demand, and the fact that buyers and sellers are not alone in the market but are both significantly affected by the actions of third-party financiers. Some of the papers in this volume dealt with certain aspects of these problems, but perhaps not enough emphasis has been given to the fact that the real constraint on cost-containment policy may be the sheer magnitude of the gap between what is known and what needs to be known about the structure of the hospital industry and especially the behavioral patterns within the industry.

Effective public policy critically depends on the ability to predict the supply response to varying market conditions and specific public policy instruments. One can only expect cost containment to be as effective as the policy makers' ability to take specific account of the impact of varying mechanisms and instruments on hospital behavior and hence to predict supply response. The traditional theory of the firm that postulates a producer attempting to maximize profits (or a specific utility function with profit as a dominant argument) subject to technological and market constraints is useful because it allows prediction of supply response. But as noted before, the conceptual framework alone is sufficient only for predicting the direction of supply response. Specific empirical testing of the model in actual markets is a necessary condition for predicting the relative magnitudes of supply response because actual behavior depends not only on the utility function being maximized, but on the nature of the constraints imposed as well. Thus, for example, if one is willing to assume behavior consistent with profit maximization, one can predict the likely impact of an oil embargo or general energy shortage. In the short run prices can be expected to rise, profits will increase, and efforts to increase supply will be made as prevailing market conditions allow for the processing and refining of a supply characterized by higher marginal cost. Moreover, if the relative shortage persists, one would predict an increase in investment in a variety of contexts in the long run. But without specific empirical data concerning the structure of the oil industry and behavioral patterns among firms in the industry, there would be no way to predict precisely how much prices would rise, how much profits would increase, or how much investment would take place. In essence, neither the short-run nor long-run supply response could be approximated with any degree of precision without some specific empirical knowledge.

The economic behavior of nonprofit enterprises has drawn considerably attention in the past decade, especially from economists interested in the market for hospital services. But studies to date have been essentially conceptual and somewhat speculative in nature. Those who have attempted to model hospital behavior have concentrated on specifying utility functions for nonprofit hospitals. Hospital utility functions have been postulated in terms of such arguments as quantity, quality, prestige, net income, and the income of the medical staff. These conceptual efforts are important, but little has been done to test these models empirically. Without specific empirical testing of hospital behavior models in actual markets, they cannot provide the basis for predicting the relative magnitudes of supply response either to varying market conditions or to specific cost-containment mechanisms.

The problem, of course, is analogous to the simple supply and demand analysis of any market. One need only know that supply and demand have some elasticity in order to predict the direction of change likely with any given change in market conditions. But, in order to predict the relative magnitude of the change, one needs specific empirical estimates of the elasticities. Similarly, knowing that quality and the complexity of services are in the objective function of hospital decision makers is sufficient to predict that any demand increase induced by increased income, increased insurance, or new government programs will result in a supply response that includes a higher quality, more complex service. But one would need specific empirical data in order to predict the precise nature of the supply response. Therein lies the dilemma for cost-containment policy. Containment implies constraining the extent and the nature of the supply response. Just as the policy maker would need specific elasticity estimates in order to determine how much of a deductible or co-insurance to apply to generate a given demand constraint, he would need specific empirical estimates in order to constrain the supply response to effect a given supply constraint.

It would seem that the general lack of success of prior cost-containment efforts can be viewed in the context of the lack of specific knowledge concerning the characteristics of supply response in the market for hospital services. Certainly several of the papers in Part III of this volume would tend to support this contention either directly or indirectly. Hellinger, for example, has summarized the findings of evaluation studies of several prospective reimbursement schemes. In general, the studies did not find hospital costs to have been lowered significantly. Although one might suggest several viable explanations for the specific findings, including the confounding effect of national wage and price controls in certain instances, the voluntary nature of several of the reimbursement experiments, and even the methodological shortcomings of certain evaluations, there is reason to suspect that significant cost containment might not have been expected. A systematic review of the several mechanisms employed, for example, suggests that the instruments implemented to contain costs were formulated in the absence of sufficient empirical knowledge of their likely impact on hospital behavior, and more especially of hospital reaction to that impact. Rate regulation by formula in New York is among the strictest forms of cost containment implemented to date, for example. Still, the net effect of cost containment even in that context is modified considerably by induced adjustments in hospital behavior. It may be, as Bauer concluded, that "rate setting . . . is just a highly complicated tinkering operation, plugging up leaks in one small section. . . ." In any event, it seems not unreasonable to conclude that the failure to contain costs is related to the failure to understand or more fully account for likely hospital reaction to specific market constraints.

Salkever and Bice have provided more direct evidence of the influence of unintended supply response in frustrating actual cost-containment efforts. They have analyzed the effect of certificate-of-need regulation by examining its effect on investment patterns and costs while controlling statistically for other factors that influence investment. In essence, they found that certificate-of-need constraints have no significant impact on total investment but rather serve to encourage a redirection of investment from bed expansion to the addition of new services and facilities. They conclude that the net effect of certificate of need not only was not cost containment, but might actually have exacerbated hospital cost inflation.

Effective cost containment will depend critically on the ability to predict the supply response to varying market conditions and specific cost-containment instruments. Undoubtedly the weakest part of the available data set is that which involves the characteristics of supply response in the market for hospital services. Conceptual models of hospital behavior have been formulated and help us understand the cause of past failures. But since specific empirical testing of such behavioral models in actual markets is a necessary condition for predicting the relative magnitudes of supply response, it would seem that such efforts are a prime research need for future cost-containment policy.

What Are Some of the Gaps?

In assessing future research needs, whatever the aspect of the problem, it is probably safe to conclude that efforts could be productively directed at generating better data, applying improved estimating techniques, and empirically testing conceptual models.

Although the emphasis on each might and probably should vary, the same general conclusion is valid for demand analysis, cost analysis, and analysis of supply response in the market for hospital services. Moreover, there are undoubtedly external economies that will derive from even incremental advances in any case, since there is a clear interdependence among data, estimation, and theory as well as across demand, cost, and supply response.

There is, of course, a considerable body of existing research that can be reviewed to some advantage both to serve policy in the near term and to guide future research for policy in the long term. The state of knowledge has expanded rather dramatically in the past fifteen years as researchers have responded to the significant public policy relevance and the intellectual challenge of this rapidly growing sector of the economy dominated by nonprofit enterprises and often characterized by atypical economic behavior.

Since most of this research has been systematically reviewed and summarized periodically, the task of assessing what is known and identifying specific gaps in knowledge is considerably eased. Most of the research published before 1965 has been summarized by Klarman (1965), and his extensive survey represents a basic reference for earlier research not only on hospitals, but on health economics in general. Research relevant to hospitals has been reviewed rather extensively by Berki (1972). The essay in this volume by Lipscomb, Raskin, and Eichenholz sets out many of the findings of hospital cost analysis as they relate to the concept of marginal cost. Finally, most of the econometric studies of health economics have been reviewed recently in a particularly systematic and useful way by M. Feldstein (1974).

The purpose of this section is not to undertake a systematic and extensive review of existing research, but rather to reflect on some of the gaps that remain and represent research needs for future policy. Although it will often prove useful to refer to representative previous research in order to facilitate the flow of the discussion, there will be no attempt to be either complete or critical in what follows.

Albeit the demand side of the problem has received little attention in this volume, it has been well researched in general. As noted above, there have been a considerable number of empirical studies of the demand for hospital services. Moreover, it seems fair to conclude that in relative terms demand analysis has progressed somewhat further than either cost analysis or analysis of supply response in the market for hospital services—such is certainly the case in an empirical sense.

In general, demand studies have employed econometric techniques to estimate a traditional demand equation with the quantity of hospital services dependent on own price, prices of substitutes and complements, income, insurance, and such surrogates for taste parameters as race, sex, age, education, marital status, and the like. While most researchers have specified rather complete demand equations, the state of knowledge has been advanced by varying the emphasis on the several factors likely to influence demand as well as the preciseness with which the several independent variables were approximated.

Thus, for example, earlier demand studies, such as that by Rosenthal (1970), tended to concentrate on own price elasticity. Given the widespread contention that hospital utilization was not responsive to price, but was determined exclusively by technical medical considerations, the early demand studies that demonstrated a negative price elasticity were of some significance. Of course, given the importance of insurance, considerable care must be taken in interpreting price elasticity estimates. Later demand studies that specifically accounted for the fact that the net price paid by the patient depends on both the gross price of hospital services and the extent of insurance coverage, such as that by M. Feldstein (1971), facilitated the interpretation of price elasticity estimates. Additional demand studies that have concentrated on the role of insurance in the demand for hospital services, such as those by Phelps and Newhouse (1972) and Rosett and Huang (1973), have served to clarify still further the interrelated influences of price and insurance. Finally, several recent studies, including those by Acton (1972) and Grossman (1972), have introduced the patient's time as an integral part of the total price.

Although most demand studies have tended to emphasize own

price elasticity, some research has begun to analyze cross-elasticities and the influence of substitutes and complements on the demand for hospital services. Davis and Russell (1972), for example, estimated the cross-elasticity of inpatient care with respect to the price of outpatient services and found the expected direct relationship. Martin Feldstein (1971) included the numbers of general practitioners and medical and surgical specialists per capita in his demand equation. His findings suggest that general practitioners represent substitutes for inpatient care and that specialists represent complements.

As noted above, most demand studies have found the income elasticity to be rather low. The work of Anderson and Benham (1970) and P. Feldstein and Carr (1964) are representative and their results, as those of most cross-section studies, imply that hospital care is a necessity.

Even this somewhat brief and incomplete review of demand studies is indicative of the volume of research that has been completed. What is perhaps not indicated is the extent to which future policy and research can benefit from the economies of scale implicit in that volume. Thus, for example, the sheer number of estimates provides a useful range and a basis for approximating relevant elasticities. Moreover, a systematic analysis of comparable and related elasticity estimates can provide a basis for assessing the relative magnitudes of bias that derive from several sources, most notably general data problems, specification and estimation problems, and the interaction of insurance and price elasticity. Last, but not least, they serve collectively to point the way for future research.

Any future research that serves to refine the several elasticity estimates or to reduce the bias in such estimates will enhance future policy. In a general sense better data and better estimation would serve to close a research gap. One gap that exists in this context is especially significant—the inability to date adequately to capture product heterogeneity in the dependent variable. Very little has been done to account for product differences—quality and complexity of hospital services—in the demand function.

One gap on the demand side, however, would seem to be of

primary significance—not enough is known about the role of the physician in determining the demand for hospital services. Are hospital services final goods, or intermediate goods? Estimating a demand equation that has the quantity of hospital services dependent on own price, other prices, and such consumer characteristics as income, insurance coverage, race, age, sex, education, and the like, is equivalent to assuming that hospital services are a final good. Virtually all empirical demand studies have followed this route. An alternative perspective would view the consumer's demand to be for "medical care." Physicians would be viewed as entrepreneurs who combine several inputs, including their own time and hospital services, to produce medical care. The demand for hospital services, in effect, would be a derived demand. Such a perspective was outlined in some detail by P. Feldstein (1966), and has been alluded to by others rather often, but little if any empirical demand research has been based on such a conceptual model.

Suppose in fact that consumers do enter the market to demand medical care from physician entrepreneurs who in turn demand hospital services to combine with other inputs to produce that product. The demand for hospital services, as any factor of production, would depend on the marginal revenue product and the marginal cost of hospital services.

As an aside, it is interesting to notice how this formulation of the problem provides a simple and logical explanation of Roemer's Law that the supply of hospital beds creates a demand for their use. If hospital services are an input to the physician's production of medical care, one would expect the physician to demand more or less as the price was lowered or raised—that is, a movement along the relevant demand curve. But what is the "price" that physicians pay for hospital services? It is certainly not a money price (except in the sense that out of the total price of medical care the physician receives less as the patient pays more on a separate bill to the hospital—in which case the money aspect of price is likely to be reflected in the marginal revenue product). Rather, the price is expressed in terms of such as peer pressure and pressure from hospital administrators and perhaps trustees as the individual physician's demand for beds varies. Thus, for example, for a given number of beds it is likely that any physician who seems to be using more than his fair share would feel the pressure, however subtle. What effect does the supply of beds have? Clearly as the supply of beds varies the relevant price of beds varies to the individual physician. An increase in the supply of beds will lower the pressure (there may even be a different form of pressure to use the beds), and at the lower "price" the physician will demand more beds.

Is the demand for hospital services to be considered in the context of consumers maximizing their utility as would be the case if they are treated as a pure final good? Or is it to be considered in the context of physician entrepreneurs maximizing their utility as would be the case if they are treated as a pure intermediate good? It seems likely that neither extreme represents the state of the real world. An alternative that is intermediate and has considerable intuitive appeal would treat the physician as an agent for the patient in the market for hospital services. This is a relatively new idea and holds much promise for learning more about the role of the physician in determining the demand for hospital services.

Ross (1973) has done some preliminary theoretical modeling of agency in a general equilibrium context; and M. Feldstein (1974) has speculated in a general way on the potential of the agency relationship for understanding behavior in the health sector; but no specific conceptual models of the physician as agent have been formulated; and of course no empirical testing of the agency model in actual markets has been done. It would seem that future research directed at analyzing the extent to which the physician is an agent might be fruitful.

A crucial question, of course, is the extent to which the agency relationship holds. At one extreme, if the physician is a perfect agent, then the existing demand estimates are quite appropriate—in principle there is no difference between a consumer maximizing his own utility and an agent maximizing it for him. At the other extreme if the physician is not an agent (a perfect nonagent?), then the existing demand estimates are quite inappropriate—the correct model would involve the physician as an entrepreneur maximizing utility, and the demand for hospital services should be treated strictly as a derived demand. More likely, the agency relationship is relevant but it holds in a more or less imperfect form. Several alternative forms could be postulated and tested. Closer to the perfect agent form, for example, one might treat the physician as a utility maximizer, but include the patient's utility as an argument in the relevant maximand. Closer to the nonagent form, one might consider the case where the physician seeks to maximize utility subject to the constraint that the patient's utility (health care) is maintained at some minimum level (standard).

Indeed, this formulation of the problem serves to put the role of the physician and its potential impact on the cost of hospital care into proper perspective. Few would argue with the contention that a physician, entrusted with the care of the patient, should seek to maximize the patient's well-being. In fact, even those who are most concerned with cost containment in their public roles would at least secretly hope that if the need arose in their own cases, their physicians would seek to maximize their well-being, and perhaps even "spare no cost" in so doing. But the present structure of the market for hospital services puts the physician in an untenable position. If he is to act as an agent for the individual patient, he cannot simultaneously act as an agent for society. Future cost-containment policy would be well served by any research that contributes to the development of mechanisms that keep the physician on one side or the other.

There has also been considerable research effort devoted to hospital cost analysis. Most of the earlier cost studies tended to concentrate on the question of whether or not hospital services were produced subject to economies of scale. On balance, the weight of evidence is that economies of scale, however significant statistically, are not of a significant order of magnitude in real terms. Whatever hospitals may be, they do not have the long-run cost curves of a natural monopoly. Approximately constant returns to scale can be inferred from the long-run data analyzed in this book by Lipscomb, Raskin, and Eichenholz. This is consistent with the findings of M. Feldstein (1968) for British hospitals and Evans (1971) for Canadian hospitals. These latter two studies are significant in this regard since the availability of case-mix data in England and Canada allows product-mix differences to be taken into account and hence avoids a source of bias that prevails in most cross-section studies of U.S. hospitals.

In the short run, marginal costs tend to be significantly below average costs. This result is rather consistent among all cost studies and has some relevance for cost-containment policy as outlined in Lipscomb, Raskin, and Eichenholz's paper.

Hospital cost analysis has been hindered by the lack of available data to account adequately for the known heterogeneity of hospital output. Most researchers have tried to cope with the problem with varying degrees of success, but none has succeeded in overcoming it. Hospitals are multiproduct firms both in terms of their products— patient care–teaching–research—and the quality and complexity of these products. Even abstracting from the problems of isolating the influence of teaching and research—which is feasible for a large subset of hospitals—the problems inherent in patient care output measures remain and represent a research need of primary significance.

Recent cost studies and related efforts have approached the problem of product heterogeneity from several directions. Extensions of certain of these approaches would seem to have sufficient promise to warrant further research. One such approach is to use explicit measures of hospital case mix in estimating cost functions as was done for a subset of U.S. hospitals by Lave, Lave, and Silverman (1972) and Lee and Wallace (1973). A related approach would involve the development of an index of output based on case-mix variations building on the work of Rafferty (1972). Unfortunately, such efforts are currently constrained by a lack of data. There is very little case-mix data generally available for U.S. hospitals—there is no case-mix data available on a national basis. The gap in this context is a data gap.

An alternative approach would be to attempt to group hospitals to minimize the degree of heterogeneity in the output measure. Berry (1973) has grouped hospitals according to facilities and services. In fact his groupings are based on inputs rather than outputs, but the technique has some merit, and the implications for certain cost-containment mechanisms seem obvious.

However limited the knowledge of hospital cost functions, even less is known about the production function for hospital services. There are no engineering production functions, and a lack of relevant data constrains attempts to generate empirical estimates. Moreover, the restrictive assumptions required to apply available estimating techniques are hardly met by the conditions that prevail in the market for hospital services.

Production function information is not generally available for most products, but it is of special concern in the case of hospital services and in the context of cost containment. In general, it is expected that market incentives will suffice to stimulate firms to select reasonably efficient factor combinations and output levels. But in a sector dominated by nonprofit enterprises, with supply-side actors influencing demand, and reimbursement by third parties serving to scramble the signal of scarcity values to both sides, it is quite unlikely that the market serves this function reasonably well, if at all. If cost-containment policy is to be brought to bear to improve the performance of the hospital sector, then policy instruments have to be designed to stimulate the selection of more appropriate factor combinations and/or output levels. The irony of intervention is exposed in its classic form in this context. How can you fine-tune what you cannot see? This is a gap of considerable magnitude, but even partial closing of it would enhance future cost-containment policy by a comparable order of magnitude.

The production function is obviously related directly to supply response. In the previous section it was noted that the weakest part of the available data set is that which includes the characteristics of supply response in the market for hospital services. Although that is the case, even that set is not empty. Some important conceptual work has been done and several models of hospital behavior based on the maximization of specific utility functions have been developed.

Newhouse (1970), for example, has postulated that hospitals seek to maximize prestige, which is a function of quantity and quality. Lee (1971) suggested prestige maximization as well, but defined it more in terms of the conspicuous production of complex quality services. Evans (1970) postulated that hospitals seek to maximize surplus. Pauly and Redisch (1973) have modeled the hospital as a physicians' cooperative that seeks to maximize the income of the medical staff.

These conceptual efforts are important, and can be used to predict hospital behavior. The gap in this context is that the theories have not been tested empirically in any rigorous way in actual markets. Hence, they cannot provide the basis for predicting with any degree of certainty or confidence the relative magnitudes of supply response to varying market conditions or to specific cost-containment mechanisms.

On balance, it would seem that there is a major gap in the context of supply response. The real constraint on cost-containment policy may well be the sheer magnitude of the gap between what is known and what needs to be known about hospital behavior and supply response.

On the other hand, however limited, there is a minimal data set. It can be used to some advantage in predicting input and output behavior of hospitals in response to certain cost-containment policy instruments, albeit in a gross directional sense. In fact, several of the papers in Part III of this volume imply that in part the lack of success of cost-containment efforts to date reflect an apparent gap between what is known and what is applied.

A Final Note on Cost Containment

As hospital costs have risen, and particularly as these costs have been translated into a public burden through governmental budgets, pressure has increasingly been brought to bear to control these costs. The exuberance for cost containment reflects the growing dissatisfaction with the performance of the hospital sector. The widespread support for some form of cost-containment policy is indicative of the general acceptance of the notion that the hospital sector is not producing the right rate of output in some sense. Policy makers and most others have come to the conclusion that the extreme market imperfections preclude an acceptable performance in this sector without some form of external intervention.

But what form should the intervention take? There is a range of choice. Given the failings of the existing sector, should it be replaced, regulated, or repaired?

There are those who believe the choice is clear-cut. Interestingly enough, those would include supporters of each of the three alternatives. Perhaps the choice is not so clear-cut.

The basic presumption of this volume is that the general level of performance in the hospital sector is unacceptable and some policy effort is in order to affect the outcome. On balance, whether intended or unintended, taken as a whole this volume would seem to come out closer to the regulation alternative. Perhaps this derives from the selection of papers. Perhaps it reflects the nature of prior cost-containment efforts. Perhaps it is simply indicative of the likelihood that regulation will prevail over the foreseeable future. Many would hold that such emphasis is appropriate. They would argue that the relevant question is not should the hospital sector be regulated, but rather how should it be regulated. But others would undoubtedly hold that such emphasis is not appropriate. Some would argue that the failings of the existing sector are not such as to be amenable to regulation. They would cite the failures of regulation efforts as well as the failures of the sector and conclude that only a new planned health system was capable of performance consonant with social objectives. Still others would argue that the system could and should be repaired. They would also cite the failures of regulation—not only in health—and conclude that the baby ought not to be thrown out with the bath water. They would note with some concern that it is not that improving the market has been tried and found wanting—rather, it has not been tried.

In the last analysis, whether the policy choice is to replace, regulate, or repair the existing market for hospital services, such efforts will depend critically on what is known and what needs to be known in order to effect the desired outcome. Ironically, if one could will the ideal data set into being, there would be little to choose among the three alternatives. But since the policy maker will have to make do with something less than an ideal data set, in making his choice, he would do well to consider the practical implications and limitations of what is known and what might be generated by feasible research. As policy moves from certain interventions to improve the market to more sophisticated changes, through regulation designed to affect supply constraints by modifying supply response, or eventually to replacing the market for hospital services, the necessary data and knowledge base becomes increasingly more complex. The gap between what is known and what needs to be known in order to affect the outcome in the desired way increases by a significant order of magnitude.

The available data set would seem to be most likely to serve the needs of policy designed to unscramble the signals of scarcity values in the market for hospital services. One possibility in this context would provide incentives for the consumer to become more cost-conscious through reform of the current insurance system. The use of co-insurance and deductibles could effect a demand constraint by limiting moral hazard. In fact, by the straightforward mechanism of eliminating all but catastrophic health insurance, the consumer would be in a position to reflect directly on scarcity values in all but extreme cases. The available data set does lend some credence to this argument, and in any event, the research needs to effect policy along such lines seem quite tractable.

The available data set is somewhat less likely to serve immediately the needs of policy designed to modify the influence on demand of supply-side actors. An interesting possibility in this context would involve the encouragement of a system of competitive HMOs. Now variations of this policy instrument have in fact been implemented with rather less success than might have been expected by some. One way to view the HMO is as an agent for the patient. If HMOs are competitive, presumably the ones that perform the agency role better will be more successful. An alternative way to view the HMO is as a producer of medical care that must face the real cost of the hospital services input. Presumably the introduction of cost consciousness will mean that those that use the input more efficiently will be more successful. Perhaps the lack of success in previous HMO policy might be in part due to asking the wrong question, or at least clouding the right question by mixing it up with several other questions. In fact, it would seem that the critical question is whether or not it is possible to devise a mechanism for putting the physician on the demand side of the market for hospital services. The potential improvements in performance likely in this context would seem to warrant research efforts, and the research needs would seem to be feasible.

The available data set would seem least likely to serve the immediate needs of policy designed to effect specific containment objectives through modifying the supply response in a sector dominated by nonprofit enterprises. Such regulatory efforts as rate regulation and certificate of need are hampered by a lack of knowledge specific to behavior patterns and have been frustrated by unintended or perhaps unanticipated supply responses. The research needs in this context are significant, but certain of them seem feasible.

It was not my intention to develop a treatise on policy choices, or to present a balanced assessment of the arguments pro and con for any alternative. Nor did I intend to analyze any of them in terms of political feasibility, or even to predict the likely choice. Rather, I intended only to reflect on each briefly from the perspective of the research needs that must be met if success is to be expected from the pursuit of any particular policy choice.

The fundamental question in the context of cost containment is "What is the right rate of output of hospital services?" The answer to this question must be phrased in several dimensions. First, what is the appropriate level of output in the aggregate; how much of the nation's scarce pool of resources is to be devoted to the production of hospital services? Second, given the level of aggregate output, what particular mix of services is to be produced? Third, what is the appropriate way to produce any desired output; what combination of inputs represents a reasonably efficient production choice? Fourth, what is the appropriate pattern of distribution of hospital services among the population; who gets what part of the total output? The first three questions refer to the relative efficiency of the allocation of resources. The fourth question refers to the equity of the distribution of the produce of those resources.[1]

[1] Some would argue that the equity question is more properly treated in the context of income distribution, and that the issue of the right rate of output should be resolved

In assessing the potential for any policy choice it is necessary to reflect on how it will serve to answer these questions. In determining the research needs for any policy choice it is necessary to reflect on the gap between what is known and what needs to be known in order to answer these questions.

A planned system and a regulated system would answer the question of the aggregate level of output by means of setting a specific supply constraint. But even abstracting from the ultimate supply constraint, several critical questions remain to be answered, and the available data set does not augur well for answering them in the near term.

What particular mix of hospital services is to be produced, for example? How much coronary care, cancer therapy, renal dialysis, and so forth, will be included among hospital output? What will be the proportions of inpatient care and outpatient services? However one views the mechanisms that serve to answer those questions in the current system, or the answers that obtain, one should not lose sight of the fact that the questions will have to be answered in any event and under any alternative system. More important, one should be aware of the kinds of data needed to answer them and the likelihood that they will be sufficient to render the answers less rather than more arbitrary.

Given the level of aggregate output and mix of services, what factor combinations are to be employed in producing them? In the absence of production function information, it is not clear how questions concerning input mix are to be answered.

What will be the pattern of distribution among the population of the given output? Now some might think that removing health care from the market would negate such a question. Not so. It is not quite clear what making health care a right would imply in this context, but it is not likely that any aggregate supply constraint chosen would ever allow for consumption by all to the point where the marginal utility in consumption was zero, for example. Rather more reason-

for the given income distribution. Others hold the view that health care is a right and that the distribution of health care among the population should not depend on the prevailing distribution of income. Since our current purpose is limited and would not be particularly served by resolving this issue one way or the other, it seems reasonable to leave the question.

able conceptual alternatives would be consumption to the point where the value in consumption was equal to marginal cost, or consumption up to some point necessary to provide a given minimal health standard for all. There would seem to have to be a more practical alternative, given any likely total supply constraint for the system, but what data would provide for even an approximation to such a solution? Clearly no such data set currently exists. Still some answer must be found to the distribution question. If the system does not provide enough renal dialysis for all who might benefit from it, for example, who will get it and who will be left out?

There is no question about the relatively poor performance of the hospital sector. Similarly there is no doubt but that some form of cost-containment policy will be in place in the years to come. In a world of perfect information and perfect policy instruments, rational cost-containment policy could be implemented to bring about the right rate of output in the hospital sector—to eliminate unnecessary complexity and waste while retaining necessary complexity and quality. Unfortunately, this is a world of poor information and less than perfect policy instruments. At present, there are no data sufficiently robust to discriminate among quality, necessary complexity, unnecessary complexity, and waste. We do not have sufficient production function information. Not enough is known about the role of physicians and how to modify their influence on the demand for hospital services. And too little is known about the peculiar characteristics of supply response in this sector. Research is needed to close the several gaps. But judicious selection of policy alternatives is needed as well to take advantage of what is known and to move in those directions that can be aided by feasible research.

References

Acton, J.P.
    1972   "Demand for health care among the urban poor, with special emphasis on the role of time." Santa Monica, Calif.: RAND Publication R-1151-OEO/NYC. October.

Anderson, R., and L. Benham
  1970   "Factors affecting the relationship between family income and
          medical care consumption." Pp. 73-95 in H. Klarman, ed.,
          Empirical Studies in Health Economics. Baltimore: The Johns
          Hopkins Press.
Berki, S.E.
  1972   Hospital Economics. Lexington, Mass.: Lexington Books, D.C.
          Heath & Co.
Berry, R.E., Jr.
  1973   "On grouping hospitals for economic analysis." Inquiry 10
          (December): 5-12.
Davis, K., and L. Russell
  1972   "The substitution of hospital outpatient care for inpatient care."
          Review of Economics and Statistics 54 (May): 109-120.
Evans, R.G.
  1970   "Efficiency incentives in hospital reimbursement." Unpublished
          doctoral dissertation, Harvard University.
  1971   "'Behavioral' cost functions for hospitals." Canadian Journal of
          Economics 4 (May): 198-215.
Feldstein, M.S.
  1968   Economic Analysis for Health Service Efficiency. Amsterdam:
          North-Holland Publishing Co.
  1971   "Hospital cost inflation: A study of nonprofit price dynamics."
          American Economic Review 61 (December): 853-872.
  1974   "Econometric studies of health economics." In M. Intriligator
          and D. Kendrick, eds. Frontiers of Quantitative Economics II.
          Amsterdam: North-Holland Publishing Co.
Feldstein, P.J.
  1966   "Research on the demand for health services." Milbank Memo-
          rial Fund Quarterly 44 (July): 128-165.
Feldstein, P.J., and W.J. Carr
  1964   "The effect of income on medical care spending." Proceedings
          of the Social Statistics Section, American Statistical Association:
          93-105.
Grossman, M.
  1972   "On the concept of health capital and the demand for health."
          Journal of Political Economy 80 (March-April): 223-256.
Klarman, H.E.
  1965   The Economics of Health. New York: Columbia University
          Press.

Lave, J.R., L.B. Lave, and L.P. Silverman
  1972   "Hospital cost estimation controlling for case mix." Applied
           Economics 4 (September): 165-180.
Lee, M.L.
  1971   "A conspicuous production theory of hospital behavior." South-
           ern Economic Journal 28 (July): 48-58.
Lee, M.L., and R.L. Wallace
  1973   "Problems in estimating multi-product cost functions: An appli-
           cation to hospitals." Western Economic Journal (September):
           350-363.
Newhouse, J.P.
  1970   "Toward a theory of nonprofit institutions: An economic model
           of a hospital." American Economic Review 60 (March): 64-74.
  1974   "A design for a health insurance experiment." Inquiry 11
           (March): 5-27.
Pauly, M., and M. Redisch
  1973   "The not-for-profit hospital as a physicians' cooperative." Ameri-
           can Economic Review 63 (March): 87-99.
Phelps, C., and J. Newhouse
  1972   "Coinsurance and the demand for medical services." Santa
           Monica, Calif.: RAND Publications R-964-OEO. May.
Rafferty, J.A.
  1972   "Hospital output indices." Economic and Business Bulletin
           (Winter): 21-27.
Rosenthal, G.
  1970   "Price elasticity of demand for short-term general hospital
           services." Pp. 101-117 in H. Klarman, ed. Empirical Studies in
           Health Economics. Baltimore: The Johns Hopkins Press.
Rosett, R., and L. Huang
  1973   "The effect of health insurance on the demand for medical care."
           Journal of Political Economy 81 (March-April): 281-305.
Ross, S.
  1973   "The economic theory of agency: The principal's problem."
           American Economic Review 63 (May): 134-139.

Policy Coordination and the Choice of Policy Mix

IRVING LEVESON

Introduction

The devotion of vast resources to hospital care has led to increased concern about the unit costs of services, the way in which those services are combined into treatments, and the efficacy of treatments in improving health outcomes. While many services are of immeasurable benefit and advances are constantly being made, it is no longer acceptable to allow budgets to increase automatically without questioning the benefits which are derived. Today the issue is no longer whether hospitals will be regulated but rather how.

The challenge to open-ended financing of hospitals has come at a time of heightening interest in societal opportunities for improving health. There is an increasing recognition that the current level of inpatient service is arbitrarily high because of the effect of availability on use. It has also become clear that, under present financing methods, when substitutes for inpatient care are developed, concerted action rather than market forces is necessary to shrink the capacity to deliver inpatient care.

When the primary focus of public policy is on improving the efficiency of medical care, attention is drawn to details of delivery systems. Under the conditions that exist today society is more willing to accept serious dislocations in the hospital sector in order to achieve economies in total spending and encourage other ap-

609

proaches to improving health outcomes. These shifts in thinking are tempered by nagging uncertainties about whether the huge investment in clinical medicine and halfway technologies is finally beginning to pay off. But they are also fostered by a desire to introduce restraints before further expansion of health care financing creates new inefficiencies or makes existing ones more difficult to overcome.

Efforts to contain hospital costs have been of two types: (1) those that provide a basic resource constraint and allow the hospital to decide the details of production, and (2) those that exert control over aspects of hospital operations such as mix of services and length of stay. Evolving techniques would increase both kinds of regulation. On closer examination the details necessary to implement even the broadest methods of control introduce important constraints on the nature as well as the scale of production. As a result of the dependence of regulatory effectiveness on complex details, numerous questions arise about the effectiveness of specific techniques or combinations. At the same time there are serious questions as to the total amount of regulation that can be introduced without excessively compromising the ability of hospital managers to manage and having counterproductive effects on innovation and health status improvement.

Approaches to Cost Containment

Insurance Coverage

The most widely used method of dealing with hospital costs has been to spread out their impact over time and across individuals through the use of insurance. But the insurance itself, by lowering the out-of-pocket cost to the consumer, raises demand, adding to cost. Furthermore, by making all patients responsible for the additional costs incurred by each patient, insurance provides a further incentive for utilization to expand as new technologies are introduced. Even if some technologies avoid hospitalization and lower the cost of care, hospital beds are filled as long as they are available and the intensity of medical care performed inside the hospital continues to increase.

One approach for overcoming these effects is to make patients responsible for a larger part of the cost of care through methods such as co-insurance. But strong public preferences for avoiding the risk of large medical bills prevent any extensive retrenchment in insurance. There has been heightened interest in forms of catastrophic insurance that would cover the most costly treatments but would reduce the degree to which lower cost treatments would be reimbursed; for example, a system that would reimburse all costs above 10 percent of income. Such catastrophic plans will do little to curb the demand for hospital care since so much of the cost would be covered anyway. Their main value would be in avoiding similar problems in other parts of the health care delivery system. But any such system serves to make the most costly forms of care least costly to the consumer, providing built-in incentives for cost-increasing innovation. There have been growing attempts by consumer representatives and others to express their views at the stages where health insurance premiums are determined but premiums are destined to reflect cost increases that have been approved earlier in the process.

Supply of Capital

Until recently the principal method of attempting to limit the cost of hospital care has been to control the supply of capital. Certificate of need, which began with New York's program in 1964, is now almost universal. The study by Salkever and Bice in this volume found that certificate of need has not succeeded in controlling capital expenditures (see also Hellinger, 1976).

Salkever and Bice also found that certificate of need, while it does slow the growth of hospital beds, is thwarted by an offsetting increase in capital expenditures per bed. The authors do not make clear why certificate of need should result in an increase in expenditures on equipment. They suggest a number of interesting possibilities but do not test which are important. One explanation that they have not considered appears to require particular attention.

The lower the bed supply in an area the greater are the pressures to admit more patients to the beds that are available. Under these conditions admissions tend to rise and lengths of stay to fall. But the treatment of patients with shorter lengths of stay often involves more intensive services—more tests, more physician hours, and so forth, per day of care than would be provided on the same day of a longer stay. Greater use of equipment may be an appropriate response to this greater intensity of care. Faster patient turnover typically reduces cost per admission by significantly more than the greater intensity per day of care raises it. Consequently, a shift from beds to equipment under certificate of need that did not produce a saving in capital cost might reduce operating cost. If this explanation is correct the findings on capital cost will be misleading.

The book is still wide open on the effectiveness of certificate of need. We do not know whether in the past states were more likely to institute certificate of need where the pressures for capital expansion were greatest. In that case there would be a strong tendency to underestimate the effects of the program. My experience with the New York state system and with variations in impacts among localities leads me to speculate that in its first decade certificate of need may have been effective in areas with many small hospitals requiring consolidation, but that in areas with more highly developed medical systems the effects may have been nil or even perverse. There is no presently available test that compares effects on delivery systems at different stages of evolution. Furthermore, existing studies predate the current fiscal climate and attitude toward health costs and the new conditions may produce greater impacts than in the past, at least as long as pressures are generated by general economic conditions.

There is current interest in developing more effective methods of delicensing existing beds considered excessive and/or below quality. This is especially important in areas that authorized large expansions in bed supply in the late 1960s in anticipation of demand from national health insurance and without taking adequate account of the growth of nursing homes and other sources of out-of-hospital care. In many central cities the problem is further compounded by unanticipated declines in population. Many of the approved beds were delayed in construction by a combination of inflation, recession, and ESP. Since that time thinking has shifted toward reducing reliance on hospitalization. That hospitalization is closely related to bed supply implies a policy of reducing the number of beds. There is widespread agreement that when this is done it is generally better to close whole hospitals than parts of many hospitals. In part this is because hospitals that have excess capacity will tend to be a continuing source of pressure for expansion of utilization.

Certificate of need, the principal method of determining bed supply, is almost paralyzed for the purpose of closing hospitals for three reasons. First, the availability effect makes it all but impossible to develop "scientific" standards of need. Second, there are strong legal limitations on denial of license. Third, it is generally impossible to determine that a particular hospital is the unnecessary hospital. Rather, there is a general oversupply and those institutions that face adjustment need not differ greatly from those that do not. In subsequent discussion we shall maintain that under these conditions reimbursement approaches may be far more effective than licensing.

The one area where control over bed supply has clearly worked is in the reversal of policy to promote bed expansion. The Hill-Burton program, which had as its initial objective the encouragement of equalization of bed supply between rural and urban areas, has been curtailed and its vestiges reoriented toward renovation of existing facilities, including those in urban areas and those providing ambulatory care (Lave and Lave, 1974). It should be noted that this shift in policy is a reimbursement approach.

There have been a variety of proposals to use a capital budgeting approach in which capital spending is explicitly allocated among institutions. The present system incorporates amortization and depreciation as well as interest payments in an all-inclusive rate per patient day of care. In the past the accumulated reserves allowed hospitals to replace themselves without regard to public need. Today these reserves are small compared with costs of replacement. Reimbursement at a rate which was designed to cover amortization continues after a mortgage is paid off, adding to operating costs. A comprehensive program for allocation of capital funds was set forth in President Carter's health care cost-containment proposal of April 1977.

Manpower

If a supply control strategy is necessary because supply creates demand, then it is important to limit the supply of manpower as well as facilities. Various studies have shown relationships between physician supply and medical care use and particularly a tendency for patients to be hospitalized more frequently when there is a large supply of specialists (Feldstein, 1971). An important part of the way physician supply affects hospital utilization is through the pressures which are generated to build more beds.

The supply of physicians in the United States has continued to increase, both to allow for growing demand and to offset the effects of rapidly declining hours of work that have occurred with increasing physician incomes.[1] But there has been a major redirection of efforts away from the almost universal training of sub-specialists of only a few years ago to put emphasis on family practice and primary care specialties. There have also been rapid changes in the functions of nurses, representing a movement away from reliance on even more specialized physicians. Growth of paraprofessional occupations not tied to nursing has been much more limited. There are indications that the rapid growth of nursing and other specialties is also producing occupations whose supply creates its own demand, often in a way that increases the intensity of care rather than the number of admissions or length of stay.

Rate Reimbursement

The most direct means of controlling hospital costs is to limit the amount of money available for operating expenditures. The principal method of containing operating budgets is the setting of reimbursement rates per patient day of care. In most cases such rates are determined after the fact on the basis of a hospital's actual cost. This

---

[1] Federal policy has sought to accelerate the training of physicians in order to increase the supply. However, the emphasis on this strategy has subsided. The recent removal of rules which made it easier for foreign medical graduates to enter the country is a move toward a tighter supply, relative to what otherwise would have occurred, but the supply of physician hours per capita is likely to continue to increase.

leaves it to the hospital to determine its basic mission and the mix and intensity of services to accomplish that mission.

The criterion of "reasonable cost" has not prevented the rapid escalation of hospital costs. As a result several states have established prospective reimbursement systems under which each hospital is given a per diem reimbursement rate in advance of the coming year, instead of a blank check to be filled in after the fact. Many states have shown interest in this approach and the President has proposed its use at the national level for all third-party payers. A prospective rate-setting system can be viewed as consisting of two elements: determination of the reimbursement rate in advance and setting the rate lower than it otherwise would have been. If the rate were set so as to cover the same expenditures as before no effect on costs would be expected.

The Social Security Administration's "experiments" to assess the effectiveness of prospective reimbursement show mixed results. Some programs do not produce effects that are statistically significant. Others, while significant, may be attributable to the effects of the national Economic Stabilization Program rather than to state prospective reimbursement efforts. A test of the effectiveness of prospective reimbursement when the rates are set lower than they otherwise would be can be obtained by looking at the experience in New York City and surrounding areas. Prospective reimbursement in downstate New York is believed to be the toughest in the nation.[2] There, Dowling (1975) has found that prospective reimbursement did have a significant effect on the growth of hospital costs in comparison with similar areas.

The interpretation of the findings for downstate New York is clouded by differences in the behavior of cost per admission and cost per patient day. Cost per patient day clearly rose less rapidly than in the areas used for statistical controls. But length of stay in New York did not fall as rapidly, so that there was little difference in the comparison of cost per admission. If hospitals facing a ceiling on reimbursement per patient day resisted national tendencies toward

[2] New York is the only state using prospective reimbursement whose formula is based on "efficient production of services" rather than "reasonable cost."

declining length of stay in order to maintain revenue (that is, if prospective reimbursement caused length of stay to increase relative to what it would have done) then the net effect of prospective reimbursement on cost was at best very small. Dowling endorses this interpretation. The authors of the Abt Associates study of prospective reimbursement in upstate New York arrived at the same conclusion (Abt Associates, Inc., 1976; see also Berry, 1976, and Cromwell, 1977). The gains that might have occurred from prospective reimbursement were negated by an associated rise in length of stay.

Even in New York's "relatively tight" system there have been numerous methods by which hospital costs could increase in excess of the cost of living. Initial trending formulas used a moving average that relied on base periods that included the rapid cost increases after Medicare and Medicaid. A special increase was granted in 1975 to cover the costs of a post-ESP catch-up collective bargaining agreement. Costs rise where new or expanded services accompany facilities changes that were approved under certificate of need. The trending of costs is applied to a hospital's previous costs rather than to its reimbursement rate. This means that if a hospital's costs exceed its rate the difference is automatically folded into its rate two years later (subject to limitations in relation to group averages). Increases of about $30 million dollars per year are approved on appeal (including accounting differences as well as service changes). However, these rules are undergoing rapid change.

It is not at all clear that the federal government should move rapidly into a national prospective reimbursement system. State and local programs provide a testing ground from which a more universal program might evolve. But we still do not know enough about the value of local diversity or the impacts of various provisions. The possibility of perverse effects on length of stay offer a warning as to what can happen without appropriate changes in the incentive structure. A strong federal move at this time could lock us into the wrong system or have adverse effects that are hard to reverse. However, it is clear that whether we evolve local or national systems and whether federal efforts are immediate or deferred, we must move away from the piecemeal setting of rates with different levels, rules, and procedures for different classes of payers.

There are crude indications that since 1975 state prospective reimbursement systems may have become more effective. This appears to be a response to several factors, including the recession, the generally more conservative fiscal climate, changing attitudes toward social programs, increasing concern about hospital costs over the long run, and immediate reactions to the explosion of costs after the lifting of wage and price controls.

Economic Stabilization Program

The Economic Stabilization Program was the first national attempt to set hospital reimbursement rates prospectively. The program lasted in its various phases from August 1970 to April 1974. Paul Ginsburg's study of the ESP experience in this book indicates that wage controls significantly slowed the growth of costs. However, there is serious doubt about whether other costs were contained by the program. Furthermore, Ginsburg's findings are in sharp contrast with the analyses of cost behavior during the ESP period in the evaluations of prospective reimbursement experiments. Because of varying methodologies and the limited period of observation, differences in interpretation are likely to persist.

The experience of ESP does not indicate what would happen with price controls alone. One possibility is that wages would continue to rise more rapidly than in other industries and staff would grow more slowly or decline. The effects of this would have on the nature of care and inpatient turnover are unclear and can be better learned from evaluation of existing prospective reimbursement efforts.

As a temporary measure ESP must be looked at very differently. There was a surge in per diem reimbursement rates after the controls were lifted so that many of the gains were very short-lived. Because of this surge there is no reason to believe that costs were lower at the end of 1975 than if there had been no controls.

The program also may have acted as a catalyst, encouraging interest in strong prospective reimbursement in subsequent years. As we have noted, this demonstration effect may account for part of any increase in effectiveness of prospective reimbursement in 1975 or 1976.

Budget Systems

A variety of suggestions have appeared for the use of budgeting systems, either for the nation, the region, or the individual hospital. These possibilities are important because they would impose a known limit on the costs of care in the coming period. However, they raise a number of complex questions that have received little attention. How would resources be distributed among institutions? Would the method of distribution change the base budgets of institutions? How would we prevent hospitals from reducing the quantities of services provided if the budget is predetermined? If the budget is contingent on levels of output, in what ways does it differ from prospective reimbursement?

There has been a growing interest in budgeting approaches that would relate a number of dollars to a specific population rather than to institutions. Unfortunately, the most frequently discussed methods run a high risk of either creating geographic monopolies or placing control in a coordinating body whose effectiveness there would be good reason to question. The most promising approach for relating resources to people continues to be the development of Health Maintenance Organizations.

Health Maintenance Organizations

Encouraging the development of Health Maintenance Organizations has been a major objective of national policy for at least a decade. The use of a prepaid annual premium per enrollee serves to fix the budget of the HMO. At the same time HMOs may own their own hospitals, exerting direct control over the bed supply. The organization is generally managed by a group of physicians and/or administrators who are independent of those who directly provide care. Salaried practice may minimize incentives to overuse hospital resources for enhancing private fees. Group practice may offer additional advantages in economy and continuity of care. For whatever combinations of reasons HMOs have shown significant savings compared with other current structures.

HMOs are the one mechanism that has been effective in reducing the number of hospital admissions. HMOs may also have had some success in preventing a rate of cost increase over time prior to Medicare and Medicaid. However, they appear to have been unable to resist pressures for rapid cost increases once these broad-based financing systems came into effect (Leveson and Rogers, 1976).

With increasing tendencies for physicians to enter into group, hospital-based, and salaried practice, the transition to HMOs or at least medical foundations (which retain fee-for-service and typically are controlled by those delivering service) should be much easier than before. But in spite of the lowering of these barriers HMO development has been a difficult and slow process, mainly because as a newly introduced organizational form HMOs are particularly vulnerable to retardation from the effects of regulation.

The "landmark" HMO bill can be viewed largely as an attempt to allow prepayment to be offered to the elderly after Medicare precluded it by establishing separate fee-for-service payments under Part A and Part B. "Medicaid waivers" are an attempt to overcome the program's restrictions to fee-for-service, to permit enrollment of a broader than Medicaid population, and to allow requirement of cost separation and other features. The HMO legislation specifies a broad range of services that makes HMOs more costly than conventional health insurance coverage even if they are less costly for an identical package of services. Exemption of employer health insurance premiums from the personal income tax reduces the employee's cost of conventional insurance, but the additional costs of broader HMO services are paid out-of-pocket without such an exemption. Rules requiring HMOs to absorb all of the financial risk in contracting for hospital services preclude payment on a basis that encourages the hospital to reduce length of stay. Many states limit the formation of proprietary HMOs. In view of the extent of the restrictions it is not surprising that the development of HMOs has been extremely sluggish.

Utilization Review

Utilization review occurs at a variety of levels, including surgical second-opinion programs, tissue review committees within hospitals, and outside organizations such as Professional Standards Review Organizations. It may occur before admission, during hospitalization, or after discharge. Many programs are also part of the patient management process or of efforts to improve quality of care.

The effectiveness of utilization review has been very spotty. Many programs, particularly PSROs, are too new to judge or have not yet been followed for a long enough time. Where successes have been reported, the principal gains have been in reducing length of stay rather than in lowering the admission rate (see, for example, Flashner et al., 1973).

Efforts to impose utilization review from the outside have tended to require physicians to certify that a patient must continue to stay in a hospital if they wish to keep the patient there longer. This approach imposes administrative burdens on the hospital and the doctor and often is little more than a paper process with little or no effect on the decision to hospitalize.

An alternative approach is available whereby hospitals are reimbursed at a rate that varies with length of stay in order to provide an incentive to keep patients for a shorter time. The hospital is then free to set up its own procedures to determine how, when, and for which patients shorter stays are most appropriate. The hospital also receives a higher rate to cover the costs of the greater intensity per day when it does reduce length of stay. The incentive approach appears to be a clear improvement over the case-by-case method. This option will be discussed in detail shortly.

Further Possibilities

The certificate-of-need process used for controlling the supply of hospital beds and equipment is a licensing process. As such it faces serious limitations as a tool for determining medical care resources. Historically the emphasis has been on meeting hospital codes. In concordance with this emphasis on architectural standards the primary focus of cost review has been on construction costs. Often there is little control over the intensity of services and their financial impact. The financial feasibility tests, in which the ability to finance services is considered, critically depend on the willingness of the state to meet the costs. Yet the state commits itself to cover the operating costs associated with capital projects through rate increases at the time the services are introduced or expanded.

As we have noted, the ability to control the capacity of the system is limited because the "availability effect," which makes restriction necessary, also precludes the development of scientific standards of need and typically makes it impossible to say that a particular hospital is the unnecessary one. At the same time it is constrained by strong legal limits on denial of license. Furthermore, applications are generally accepted on a first-come-first-served basis with little opportunity to consider the ability of competing institutions to provide care at lower cost, of higher quality, or with greater responsiveness to community needs.

The certificate-of-need process can be used as a building block in a more complete system of health care regulation rather than overloading it with mandates that it has limited ability to fulfill. Much of the basic machinery can be expected to continue because it is necessary for the legal establishment of organizations. Additional attention can be paid to operating costs in the review of financial feasibility if the certificate-of-need system remains. There are a variety of ways in which decisions can be coordinated with the planning activities of the Health Systems Agencies and the state. But there are also fundamental questions about how far we should go with certificate of need. There is strong reason to believe that far more can be accomplished with a reimbursement than with a licensing approach.

At present we tend to control high-cost services largely by keeping rates tight under prospective reimbursement. This method may prevent the initiation of expansion of high-cost services. However, it requires hospitals to forgo services simply on the basis of cost rather than on cost effectiveness. Prospective reimbursement, by itself, implicitly determines which hospitals carry on an activity not on the basis of the hospital's capabilities in that area but rather on the basis of total hospital finances.

One approach to limiting the expansion of costly services is to have the state issue a special increase in reimbursement for specific institutions, contingent on provision of a particular volume of specialized services with an estimated differential cost. This offers an opportunity to limit supply to designated providers since denial of reimbursement often precludes provision of high-cost services. Furthermore the choice of provider could be based on a range of criteria including relationship to regionalization objectives, cost, and expected quality and could be based on a review period whose length is far more flexible than certificate of need.

The approach of separating out rate differentials for specialized services and authorizing them for specific institutions need not be limited to cases in which the hospital requests a change. The same approach could be used to take services out of some institutions and place them in others when that is appropriate. This might mean moving specialized services to tertiary care institutions in some cases. But in other cases, such as treatment of childhood leukemia, where less costly services may be needed after the therapy is decided, it may mean taking services out of tertiary care institutions.

The rate differential approach is applicable only for services whose cost significantly exceeds the hospital's current rate. Many services of a specialized nature will not exceed the rate, either because they are inherently not of relatively high cost or because they are located in institutions whose reimbursement rates are high because of a concentration of costly services. It is possible to exercise the same degree of choice in paying for specialized services whether or not they are of high cost through a grant-type system that provides funding to designated providers. An example of this approach, limited to capital costs, is the current method of federally financed centers for the treatment of spinal injury.

The present method of reimbursement assumes that all duly licensed hospitals will be reimbursed for services regardless of the direction in which public policy seeks to move. Broad financing systems pass along the costs to all consumers and make it very difficult to limit the use of services. One approach to overcoming this limitation is to substitute a "purchase of services" model in place of cost pass-through. Under this approach the state purchases services in a given volume from (or up to the capacity of) a given set of institutions. Only the services in designated institutions are reimbursed under general health insurance programs. Private patients may continue to use other providers and private insurers to cover the cost but their activities would be greatly reduced. This method can be used to close existing hospital beds as well as to concentrate existing or proposed specialized services in a more limited number of providers. The purchase of services approach avoids extended legal battles and allows flexibility in criteria and method of determination.

Toward a Public Choice Model

The principal thrust of efforts in hospital cost containment has been facilities control plus a model of rate regulation patterned after utilities with standardized products. The primary function of utility rate regulation is to prevent excessive increases in the price of a given set of services. Criteria such as "efficient production of services" clearly have the same connotation of doing whatever is being done at lower cost.

The utility rate regulation model was never designed to deal with the question of choosing the appropriate mix of services, choosing among qualities of care, or limiting production to those combinations of services that are considered most effiacious or most proven in improving health outcomes. The real primary function of hospital rate regulation is to prevent unwarranted increases in the levels and rates of services. It is used as a mechanism for choosing something less than the most intensive method of care or most expensive treatment as a norm. It provides an incentive for hospitals not only to limit the rate of increase of intensity but also to question the efficacy of treatments, especially when they involve high cost.

When seen in these terms, the use of hospital rate regulation must be considered along with a variety of other methods by which the consumer can make a choice among types and levels of care. The possibility of applying a "purchase of services model" to choosing the level of hospital inpatient services to be reimbursed under third-party payment systems has already been noted. There is considerable interest in the introduction of a "prudent buyer" concept in the establishment of reimbursement rates for specific services within the hospital in a way that would achieve greater uniformity across hospitals in the reimbursement for the same service.

It should be noted that the prudent buyer concept is not identical to that of purchase of services (although the term has been used by some to cover both situations) since prudent buyer suggests one price for a given service while purchase of services implies a choice among possible levels of care. The two concepts can be brought together in what might be termed a "public choice" model.

If hospital rate regulation systems are an attempt to choose levels of care, then it will be necessary to broaden the criteria of reimbursement. We will have to move not only from reasonable cost to efficient production of services but also to a principle that implies deliberate choice of service levels as well. Hospital rates might be set in accordance with a principle of "public choice and efficient production of services." It is important that such criteria be made explicit so that rates which are set in order to accomplish choices of levels of care can stand up to legal challenges.

Policy Coordination and Policy Effectiveness

Policy Effectiveness

A number of elements enter into the effectiveness of a cost-containment policy. (1) Effectiveness is critically dependent on the establishment of a definite resource constraint—whether in the form of budget, capitation rate, unit cost, beds, or manpower. The more potent the leakages through deficiencies in formula, appeal, political override, and so on, the less is cost controlled. (2) The more broadly the resource constraint is imposed the smaller is the chance for evasion and distortion of the delivery systems. Thus, a capital budget would not be expected to create substitution of spending on equipment for beds, as the uneven pressures in certificate of need appear to have done. A budget system would not encourage greater utilization to maintain revenues as can occur with unit cost (although it could permit redirection of efforts to a few services with high unit cost). (3) Highly specific resource constraints such as the staffing patterns dictated by nursing home codes do not allow management discretion to choose optional ways of producing an output as conditions change (of course they often are intended to serve other purposes such as setting standards for quality of care). (4) Once the basic resource parameters are defined the specifics of the way they are applied can be of utmost importance. Prospective reimbursement will have no impact unless the rate is set lower than it would have been. It will be far less effective if the method of trending incorporates earlier costs in excess of the rate. (5) Significant gains can be achieved by building incentives into the process. A system that financially penalizes hospitals for low occupancy rates can lead to voluntary requests for decertification of beds. (6) Policies interact with one other and that interaction may create important opportunities to design more effective cost-containment systems.

Policy Interaction

There are numerous examples of areas where policy coordination may have a potentially significant impact. The effects of rate setting clearly differed in the presence of wage controls. Certificate of need, by creating pressures on existing beds, may create an incentive to establish or make greater use of a utilization review program. Prior approval of special rate increases for costly specialized services may be made a condition of financial feasibility in certificate of need. State facilities loan funds, where they exist, may be reserved for capital projects found to be of high priority in certificate-of-need review.

The importance of the details of regulation, the nature of opportunities to introduce incentives, and the way in which the use of policies in conjunction with one another can make or break a cost-containment program are illustrated in discussions of (1) techniques and policy issues involved in introducing financial incentives to reduce length of stay, and (2) possibilities for coordination between planning and reimbursement.

Length of Stay Reimbursement

There are several possible ways to modify the reimbursement system to foster reductions in length of stay. The simplest is to adjust reimbursement to pay incremental costs rather than average costs. Consider as an example a hospital with an average length of stay of ten days and a reimbursement rate of $200 per day for a total reimbursement per admission of $2,000. Suppose that a day more or less cost 60 percent of an average day, or $120. If the average length of stay rises to eleven days, the hospital would receive $2,120 rather than $2,200 with the public saving the remaining. The new rate is equal to $192.73 per day.[3]

If the average length of stay were reduced from ten to nine days, reimbursement per admission would fall to $1,920. The new rate expressed per patient day would be $213.33. If it fell to eight days, the hospital would receive $1,840, or $230 per day.

Such an incremental cost reimbursement system accepts the hospital's present length of stay whatever its level. That is, the existing length of stay is the financial break-even length of stay. If a hospital remains at that length of stay its reimbursement remains unchanged. In principle, it is possible to set the break-even length of stay at a lower level. This can give the hospital a strong financial incentive to reduce its length of stay to the break-even level.

Suppose in the preceding example the break-even length of stay were set at eight days. If the hospital reduced its length of stay from ten days to eight days, it would receive $1,840 per admission, sufficient to cover costs, just as if it had done so without the threat of penalty. However, the days above eight would be reimbursed at less than incremental cost. For example, if the added days were reimbursed at half of incremental cost and the hospital reduced its length of stay to only nine days, it would receive $1,900 or $211.11 per day, rather than $213.33 per day. If the additional days added nothing to reimbursement and the length of stay fell to nine days, the hospital would receive $1,840, or $204.44 per day. Because this requires budget cuts when a hospital does not make a sufficient adjustment it is a kind of base budget system.

Another approach is to reimburse hospitals on the basis of cost per admission rather than cost per case. Under this method, the hospital receives no additional reimbursement if length of stay

---

[3]It does not matter whether the rate is expressed per day or per admission. As long as the same principles are used the amount of reimbursement would be the same. For example, the same rate could be obtained by saying that the per diem reimbursement rate is reduced by $7.27 when the length of stay rises by one day.

increases. The hospital is given a powerful incentive to reduce length of stay because it continues to receive the same reimbursement per case when length of stay falls. A per admission system also contains an implicit break-even length of stay since if the rate is lower than at present, the hospital must reduce length of stay to bring costs into balance with revenue.

There are two very serious disadvantages with reimbursement per case. The days that are eliminated do not cost as much as an average day and the saving from the difference is retained entirely by the hospital. Secondly, a hospital expanding admissions of very short-stay cases can receive additional reimbursement in an amount totally inconsistent with the costs. An incremental cost system provides a natural middle ground between the extremes of per day and per case reimbursement.

In part to avoid the problem of expansion of short-stay admissions under per stay reimbursement, there have been some efforts to develop systems for reimbursement on the basis of cost per admission with allowance for case mix. These systems use an assumed average cost per admission for each case type and compute the hospital's reimbursement per admission by taking a weighted average across cases, where the weights are the numbers of admissions in each category. If the cases in each category had a uniform or random length of stay so that all systematic variation in length of stay occurred between categories, the hospital would not be able to profit from changing its case mix. To the extent length of stay variation exists between categories the opportunity for manipulating case mix to increase reimbursement continues. However, there is no reason why an incremental cost formula could not be applied to variations in length of stay within case mix categories.

A major problem arises with respect to admissions when length of stay is reduced. The number of admissions tends to rise substantially when the availability of beds is increased. The emptying of beds with a decline in length of stay can be expected to have the same result. Cost savings from a lower length of stay may be dissipated in higher admissions. In fact, since the added admissions involve shorter stays, cost may actually increase.

The problem can be overcome by applying incentive reimburse-

ment methods to admissions as well as length of stay. Changes in
admissions beyond a base period would be reimbursed at significantly less than full cost. The penalty could be waived where
necessary to encourage hospitals to consolidate or where it is
appropriate to use empty facilities in lieu of new construction.

As length of stay falls occupancy rates will then decrease. A
system of penalties for low occupancy can be used along with
incremental cost reimbursement to encourage hospitals to apply for
delicensing of the beds that become empty when length of stay falls.

Coordination of Planning and Regulation

The enormous efforts that have gone into local health planning in
this country have not produced the hoped-for benefits. While areas
and times differ, a number of generalizations appear to be warranted. The need to balance diverse interests has involved large and
often cumbersome boards, often performing what could be staff
cuntions in a less political atmosphere. Planning agencies have been
swamped by "review and comment" on proposals, leaving insufficient capacity to analyze basic issues in depth. They have been
asked to develop "end state" rather than "incremental" plans which
place undue emphasis on "filling in all the boxes" rather than
focusing on major issues and policies, and which tend to commit for
years to courses of action when new alternatives are constantly
developing. At the same time they have been pressed into spending
inordinate amounts of time on a small number of hot issues that
involve the most thankless problems of choosing among providers.
And they have had insufficient resources to significantly strengthen
underdeveloped functions.

Perhaps the single most important deficiency is the limited
relationship of the activities of the Health Systems Agencies to the
processes of reimbursement. HSAs have little incentive to impose
resource constraints at the community level or to provide state and
federal officials with the guidance they need to develop a delivery
structure consistent with the resource levels chosen. As a result, local
agencies feel left out, the main decisions too often are made at
higher levels of government, and across-the-board resource deci-

sions do not take sufficient account of local conditions. Local agencies may always be likely to act as advocates, but with an important measure of input into fiscal decisions they may also better contribute to the development of plans that are responsive to existing fiscal conditions.

There are many possible ways to tie HSAs and other planning bodies into the reimbursement process. Reviews could be conducted (1) to advise on which hospitals should receive a special rate increase or grant to cover the cost of specialized services; (2) to advise on which hospitals should receive waivers of the volume adjustment intended to prevent increases in admissions when length of stay falls, if there are opportunities to consolidate institutions or use existing facilities more intensively in lieu of building new ones; or (3) to advise on priorities for access to state construction loan funds. Or (4) to suggest which providers should be designated where a purchase of services model is used. The content of reviews could be broadened to consider both capital and operating costs, regional impacts, and quality of care.

Present HSA procedures may not be appropriate for the kinds of review that would be required if the linkages to reimbursement were more fully developed. Smaller groups could be formed by choosing the most capable individuals willing to consider the interests of the community rather than by using exact formulas for balancing representation. Specialized committees might conduct the review where quality issues are involved. More of the recommendations could be promulgated by review committees rather than by the entire HSA board or executive committee to allow rapid response and reduce politicalization.

Some Distribution Issues

Efforts to limit spending or improve the efficiency of the health care delivery systems may alter the distribution of services among population groups. A dramatic example occurred in the recent efforts of some states to limit Medicaid reimbursement while Medicare rates were unchanged. The concentration of cutbacks came in the program most under control of the states and in which they shared the cost. Hospitals faced an incentive to shift from treatment of Medicaid patients to other population groups and possibly to increase Medicare length of stay to fill the beds.

There is little remaining racial discrimination in inpatient care and there is substantial financing for services for the poorest and most disabled. Hospital utilization is determined largely on the basis of availability of beds, and much use is discretionary. In this environment such shifts in the distribution of inpatient services do not spell the difference between life and death. The issue is rather one of equity in the distribution of services.

Equity issues related to the effects of regulation on inpatient services have been a source of concern when they involved the distribution of patients among systems of care. Public hospitals have typically served a disproportionate share of medically indigent patients and so acted as residual suppliers of medical care for the poor. Thus, any reimbursement changes that are concentrated in the Medicaid program can cause voluntary hospitals to steer Medicaid patients to municipal hospitals at the same time that municipal hospital finances are most severely affected.

There are important questions about the appropriate role of public hospitals in a health care system financed by broad-based insurance programs (see Lieberman, 1977). But these issues should be resolved as a matter of deliberate policy choice rather than as a side effect of piecemeal efforts to control costs.

Some patients do not require inpatient care for medical reasons but remain hospitalized because of slow placement processes for nursing homes, limited availability and financing for alternative sources of care, problems with the home environment, and insufficient incentives for the hospital to avoid retaining them. Cost-containment efforts, if not carefully carried out, can lead to dumping of these persons on the community without available alternative services.

Questions of equity become particularly apparent when we focus on activities in the outpatient sector. There is some indication that mortality of young black children fell more than would have been expected after the introduction of Medicaid (Leveson, 1976).

Since much of the care they receive is ambulatory this suggests that the distribution of outpatient care may have implications for health status as well as equity in the distribution of services.

Nominal costs per visit to outpatient departments and emergency rooms are far greater than per visit costs in private doctors' offices. This reflects the inclusion of the costs of laboratory, pharmacy, and x-ray. Emergency patients are more expensive to treat. Patient mix may also differ if physicians refer more difficult cases, especially in the Medicaid population for which office visit rates may be set at low levels. The longer length of outpatient department visits may also reflect the effects of salaried practice compared with fee-for-service on physicians' work efforts.

The reported costs of outpatient care include not only the effects of the above factors but also a tendency to shift some of the costs of inpatient care to the outpatient department. This is the result of practices such as allocating overhead costs on the basis of floor space when outpatient departments are not operated twenty-four hours a day or staffed as intensively as inpatient units. In some cases revenue associated with outpatient care is also reported on the inpatient side. The effect of these practices is to produce a deficit in outpatient budgets that is often quite large. To this are added the legitimate deficits resulting from fees that are below cost and difficulties in collecting fees from low-income patients.

Whether the deficits are real or not, efforts to control inpatient reimbursement can have serious consequences for outpatient care. If the hospital spends more on inpatient care than it is reimbursed, it will have to cover the costs from unrestricted grants or other income. If these were previously being used (actually or nominally) to cover ambulatory care deficits, there will be pressures to reduce ambulatory services as well as to raise fees. The impact of this can be seen in the decline in the number of hospitals with organized outpatient departments under the Economic Stabilization Program.

To the extent that outpatient deficits are artificial, the tendency for programs to suffer under rate regulation can be overcome by introducing truer accounting practices. This would induce the hospitals to make adjustments on the inpatient side when that is where the real losses are occurring.

Some Possible Next Steps

A number of actions can be immediately carried out that would help to lay the groundwork for better systems to contain hospital costs.

1. A change in reimbursement criteria under Medicare from "reasonable cost" to "efficient production of services" would facilitate prospective limits in the rate of Medicare hospital per diem increases as well as other measures. There is a tendency among policy makers to try quietly to redefine reasonable costs to include efficiency considerations. However, it may be necessary to obtain legislation that clearly states the principle so that a wide range of cost-containment policies can hold up in court.

2. Certificate-of-need programs attempt to define bed need in terms of "scientific" standards of need while the availability effect implies that for most services no such standards exist. A more appropriate approach is to define need at a target level consistent with public policy. The policy may be defined as reduced reliance on inpatient care.

3. The National Health Planning and Resources Development Act prescribed that new accounting principles should be implemented within one year of the law. At the time of this writing regulations for these changes had not been issued. Efforts of this kind can reduce cost and revenue spillovers among components of the health system that distort pricing and permit inefficiencies to be subsidized.

4. Introduction of incremental cost reimbursement for changes in length of stay, together with penalties for increases in admissions; and possible break-even lengths of stay below current levels in areas where stay is long could significantly reduce hospital utilization.

5. Coupling of Medicare and Medicaid hospital reimbursement rates could prevent perverse changes in utilization in one program when rates vary in the other.

6. Experimentation with case-mix reimbursement systems (with built-in incentive reimbursement elements if necessary) could facilitate the evolution of base budgeting methods.

7. The growth of technology has had a major impact on medical care costs. Under the cost pass-throughs of broad-based reimbursement systems technologies may be used that are ineffective, premature, or unproven. The next step clearly is a greater investment in efficacy testing. However the issue of what should be done once the results of the tests are available or until they arrive raises all of the issues of the effectiveness of cost-containment techniques in health care delivery.

Conclusion

The discussion has focused more on the question of what might be done to contain hospital costs than what is being done. A close look at activities actually being carried out raises serious concerns that efforts to contain costs will involve excessive regulation and costly bureaucracy. Detailed rules and complex approval processes can stifle the very innovations to which we look for improvement. The experience with Health Maintenance Organizations provides a disturbing example of how this can happen.

Those who have been concerned about excessive regulation have tended to focus on broad systems such as hospital-wide budgets. But as we look closely at the service aggregate resource constraints, numerous questions arise as to what services would be specified as a condition for payment. As we have seen, the way details such as this are resolved can have a critical impact on the outcome of regulation. There has been insufficient recognition of the possibilities for introducing incentives to improve performance and of what can be achieved by coordination of policy tools that have often been looked at in isolation in the past.

There has also been a tendency on the one hand to introduce all of the regulatory methods at once and on the other hand to seek to determine what can be eliminated. Our thinking about policy coordination suggests that the issue is not the number of tools so much as the way they will be used. In general we expect reimbursement approaches to be more effective than licensing. Society will wish to retain basic mechanisms for legal establishment, for quality assurance, for planning and reimbursement. Some elements can be expected to work especially well in combination with one another. The challenge is one of design—to evolve a cost-containment system that is in harmony with other goals and makes effective use of basic principles and policy interactions.

References and Acknowledgments

This paper has benefited greatly from discussion in the New York State Health Advisory Council, and particularly from discussion with Herbert Klarman and Mildred Shapiro. The views expressed are those of the author.

Abt Associates, Inc.
1976   "Analysis of prospective payment systems for upstate New York." Report to the United States Social Security Administration, April.
Berry, R.E., Jr.
1976   "Prospective rate reimbursement and cost containment: Formula reimbursement in New York." Inquiry 13 (September): 288–301.
Cromwell, J.
1977   "What we have (and haven't) learned from prospective payment programs." Paper presented at the Eastern Economic Association meetings, April 14–16.
Dowling, W.L.
1975   "Analysis of the effect of prospective reimbursement on costs and utilization in downstate New York hospitals." Report to the United States Social Security Administration, June.
Feldstein, M.S.
1971   "Hospital cost inflation: A study of nonprofit price dynamics." American Economic Review 61 (December): 853–872.
Flashner, B., et al.
1973   "Professional Standards Review Organizations, analysis of their development and implementation based on a preliminary review of the hospital admission and surveillance program in Illinois." Journal of the American Medical Association 223 (March 26): 1473–1484.

Hellinger, F.J.
  1976   "The effect of certificate of need legislation on hospital invest-
          ment." Inquiry 13 (June): 187–193.
Lave, J.R., and L.B. Lave
  1974   The Hospital Construction Act. Washington, D.C.: American
          Enterprise Institute.
Leveson, I.
  1976   "Some policy implications of the relationship between health
          services and health." Paper presented at the annual meeting of
          the American Public Health Association, October 20, 1976; HI-
          2501-P, Hudson Institute, September 15.
Leveson, I., and E. Rogers
  1976   "Hospital cost inflation and physician payment." American
          Journal of Economics and Sociology 35 (April): 161–174.
Lieberman, M., ed.
  1977   The Impact of National Health Insurance on New York. New
          York: Prodist.

Index

Abrams, Rosalie, 404
Abt Associates, Inc., 452, 616
Access to care, 11, 33, 43, 44, 72, 81–83, 92, 94–95, 98, 112, 113–121, 130, 251, 255
Accreditation, 15, 258
Actual cost data: and cost accounting, 21, 490–491, 498; and New Jersey prospective rate setting, 44
Acute care stays, 39
Acute conditions, 105, 106, 107
Administrators, hospital: decision-making problems, 3, 5; present cost control methods, 14, 320; extent of control, 14–15, 219–220; definition of cost containment, 14, 244–245; concerns of, 167–168; in Hospital Cost Containment Act, 169; and Talmadge proposal, 186; and medical staff, 231–232, 247, 320, 362, 373, 375; incentives for cost containment, 246, 259–260; cost-containment tools, 246–249; and government, 254–255; expectations from cost containment, 260–261; view of quality, 270; and rate reviews, 329, 361; and CON, 436; and HMOs, 618
Admissions, hospital: and Hospital Cost Containment Act revenue limit, 1, 17, 26, 171–179 *passim*, 196, 204–205; as physicians' decision, 3, 13, 227–229; and ESP, 22, 295, 514, 515, 521–526, 539; certification of, 57, 259; rate in Europe, 65–66; in utilization review, 67, 113, 620; urgency of need and, 110, 111; emergency, 257; as output measure, 303–304, 495, 503, 531, 538, 539; in ESP model study, 308, 309, 310, 313, 314; and unit cost, 331; costs per, 378, 379, 386, 387, 390, 391,

393, 394, 542–545, 546–547, 549–554, 555, 558, 563–567, 615; Maryland charge, 421; and CON, 429, 450, 612; and HMOs, 618; and length of stay reimbursement, 625–629, 632
"Advocacy" theory, 274–275
Age, 114–119, 131, 309, 311, 347
Albany, N.Y., Blue Cross–Blue Shield, 143
Amalgamated Clothing Workers of America, 146
Ambulatory care, 331, 453; supply of, 9, 37–38, 90, 613, 631; insurance and, 39, 46–47, 63, 90, 127–128, 133, 224; in other countries, 65, 66; and urgency of need, 106–110, 111, 112–113; surgery, 113; use by age, 115; and price elasticity of demand, 126, 127; and national health insurance, 126; technology in, 273; treatment costs compared with hospitalization, 277. *See also* Outpatient services
American Hospital Association, 8; national health insurance plan, 10–11, 94–97; management improvement program, 76–77; on cost increases and unit input costs, 221–222; and ESP, 306; rate-setting policy, 330; data from, 307, 390, 391, 545, 546, 559, 567; uniform departmental structure, 507; listing of facilities and services, 569–570
American Medical Association: and PSROs, 8, 465, 469, 470; on trustees, 220–221; position on salaried physicians, 237
Ancillaries, 7, 13, 14, 41–42, 127, 220, 223, 226–227, 373
Anesthesiologists, 239
Appeal, in Hospital Cost Containment